Atlas of
Sectional Anatomy

The Musculoskeletal System

Torsten B. Moeller, MD
Department of Radiology
Caritas Hospital
Dillingen, Germany

Emil Reif, MD
Department of Radiology
Caritas Hospital
Dillingen, Germany

796 illustrations

Thieme
Stuttgart · New York

Preface

Magnetic resonance imaging (MRI) of the musculoskeletal system has become an integral part of routine investigations for the diagnosis of diseases of the joints, soft tissues, bones, and bone marrow. Continual improvements in image quality have been accompanied by increased demands on knowledge of anatomic details. Those who are unable to identify normal findings on imaging can find it difficult to recognize pathologic findings.

This book was written to fulfill three demands: to provide high-resolution images with detailed and precise labeling of all relevant structures while, at the same time, providing a clear overview of the area being imaged. High-quality imaging can be obtained with most modern MRI technology, and many images in this book have been produced with 3 Tesla equipment. A 32-channel magnetic resonance tomograph with overlapping surface coils was used for the whole-body scans.

Although a highly complicated and time-consuming procedure, we produced all of the ink drawings ourselves to ensure the precise reproduction of the detailed images. No currently available computer program is able to produce images that can emphasize important structures and omit less important ones as well as a human being. The illustrator must also have sufficient knowledge about the structure she or he is dealing with before beginning to draw because the width of a line and its course often depend on this knowledge.

The complex colored illustrations and strict adherence to a consistent concept have ensured both clarity and a high degree of detail in this book. All images are accompanied by corresponding colored illustrations. Particular structures are always illustrated in the same color, e.g., muscles are always shown in different shades of red and brown, so that each group of muscles is represented by a distinct shade. This makes it possible to differentiate even large, connected groups of muscles quickly. The illustrations are also presented in an order that makes it easier to locate the desired slices.

The Atlas starts with an overview in the form of a whole-body image and the temporomandibular joint, and the rest of it is divided into three large chapters: the spine, upper extremity, and lower extremity. In the last two chapters the cross-sectional images of the arms and legs are displayed from proximal to distal to produce an uninterrupted illustration of the transverse anatomy. This layout especially facilitates recognition of structures extending beyond the joints. These images are then followed by images of coronal and sagittal slices, with the exception of the shoulder and the jaw. Reproductions of these structures are presented parallel (paracoronal) and perpendicular (parasagittal) to the supraspinatus muscle or the head of the temporomandibular joint in accordance with international conventions.

To further facilitate rapid orientation, the illustrations are accompanied by corresponding MRI slices, and the orientation diagrams at the bottom of each page provide relational information about the sides of the body part being illustrated, for example which side is the radial or ulnar, or dorsal or ventral, side. We have consistently used official terminology when labeling the illustrations. If a structure may be referred to by several different terms, we have used the most common ones.

This book could not have been produced without the active support of many committed assistants, to whom we are most grateful. We would like to offer special thanks to our radiographic assistants, Silke Köhl, Sabine Mattil, Stefanie Müller, Heike Philippi, Brigitte Schild, and Petra Weber. We also wish to thank our medical colleagues Sigrid Roth and Simone Zenner for intense discussions and encouragement.

This Atlas is based on almost 25 years of personal experience in the field of practical MRI and has profited from the knowledge accumulated during the publication of more than 15 textbooks during the past years. We ourselves benefited enormously from over a year and a half of intensive deliberations on the anatomy of the musculoskeletal system. We have also thoroughly enjoyed the "artistic" aspect of producing this book and—also thanks to the luxurious layout—are proud to present a work that is not only informative but a collector's item. It is, therefore, not surprising that we can say that the entire project provided us with a great deal of pleasure, which more than compensates for the time and effort spent on preparing this book.

We hope that our readers will also benefit from our experience and wish them little effort, great success, and lots of fun while using this book.

Torsten B. Moeller
Emil Reif

Table of Contents

Anatomic Structures Color Code: Whole Body

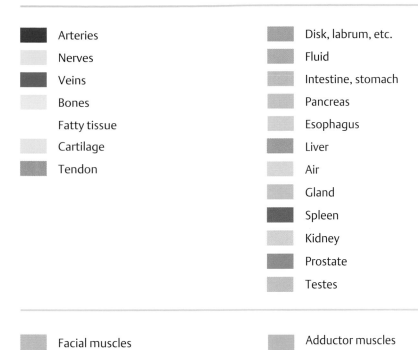

Arteries

Nerves

Veins

Bones

Fatty tissue

Cartilage

Tendon

Disk, labrum, etc.

Fluid

Intestine, stomach

Pancreas

Esophagus

Liver

Air

Gland

Spleen

Kidney

Prostate

Testes

Facial muscles

Quadriceps, short muscles
of head and neck

Shoulder, hip, and thigh
(except adductors muscles

Trunk, shoulder girdle,
and dorsal muscles of upper arm

Erector spinae (medial tract)
and triceps surae muscles

Erector spinae (lateral tract)
and ventral muscles of upper arm

Muscles of the thoracic wall

Prevertebral cervical muscles
and radial muscles of lower arm

Volar muscles of lower arm

Dorsal muscles of lower arm

Adductor muscles
(of thigh)

Peroneus muscles

Popliteus muscle

Muscles of lower leg
(extensors)

Muscles of lower leg
(flexors)

Small finger muscles

1 Temporal muscle
2 Lateral pterygoid muscle
3 Longus colli muscle
4 Cervical spine
5 Sternocleidomastoid muscle
6 Anterior scalene muscle
7 Acromioclavicular joint
8 Trachea
9 Coracoid process
10 Deltoid muscle
11 Supraspinatus muscle
12 Humerus (head)
13 Internal jugular vein
14 Common carotid artery
15 Serratus anterior muscle (middle and lower parts)
16 Biceps brachii muscle (long head)
17 Right lung
18 Pectoralis major muscle
19 Right ventricle
20 Ascending aorta
21 Intercostal muscles and ribs
22 Pectoralis minor muscle
23 Liver
24 Left ventricle
25 Ileum
26 Stomach
27 Cecum
28 Jejunum
29 Anterior superior iliac spine
30 Transversus abdominis muscle
31 Urinary bladder
32 Internal oblique muscle
33 Iliacus muscle
34 External oblique muscle
35 External iliac artery and vein
36 Gluteus medius muscle
37 Tensor fasciae latae muscle
38 Gluteus minimus muscle
39 Pectineus muscle
40 Rectus femoris muscle

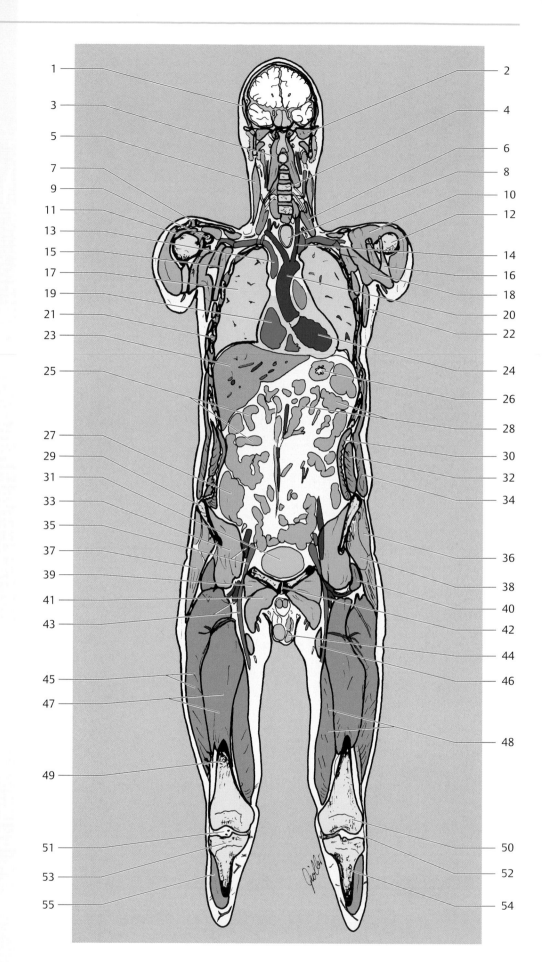

41 Adductor longus muscle
42 Symphysis
43 Superficial femoral artery and vein
44 Scrotum
45 Vastus lateralis muscle
46 Sartorius muscle
47 Vastus intermedius muscle
48 Vastus medialis muscle
49 Femur (shaft)
50 Femoral condyle
51 Knee joint
52 Lateral collateral ligament
53 Tibia (head)
54 Tibia (shaft)
55 Tibialis anterior muscle

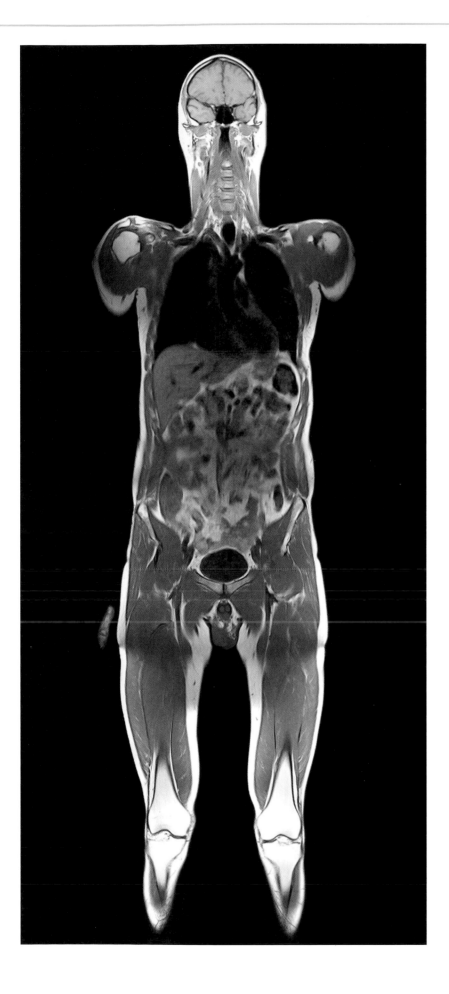

Cranial

Right
Lateral

Left
Lateral

Caudal

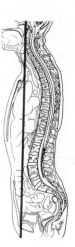

 1 Parotid gland
 2 Temporomandibular (jaw) joint
 3 Sternocleidomastoid muscle
 4 Atlanto-axial joint (median)
 5 Anterior scalene muscle
 6 Clavicle
 7 Acromioclavicular joint
 8 Acromion
 9 Supraspinatus muscle (and tendon)
10 Humerus (head)
11 Coracoid process
12 Pectoralis minor muscle
13 Deltoid muscle
14 Biceps brachii muscle (long head)
15 Coracobrachialis muscle
16 Aortic arch
17 Biceps brachii muscle (short head)
18 Pulmonary artery
19 Superior vena cava
20 Left lung
21 Cephalic vein
22 Left ventricle
23 Serratus anterior muscle (middle and lower parts)
24 Diaphragm
25 Right atrium
26 Stomach
27 Intercostal muscles and ribs
28 Jejunum
29 Liver
30 External oblique muscle
31 Abdominal aorta
32 Internal oblique muscle
33 Ilium (superior margin of the iliac crest)
34 Transversus abdominis muscle
35 Psoas major muscle
36 Ilium (acetabular roof)
37 Iliacus muscle
38 Femur (head)
39 Gluteus medius muscle
40 Deep artery of the thigh

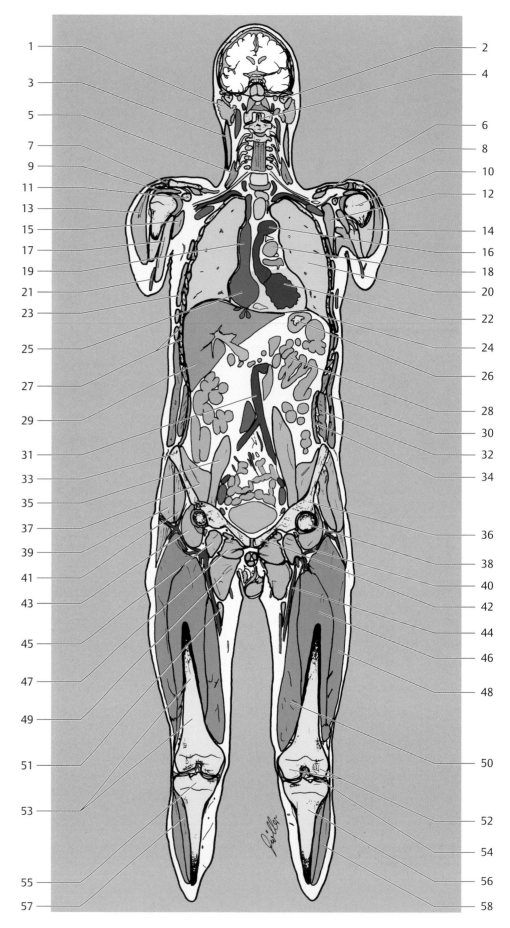

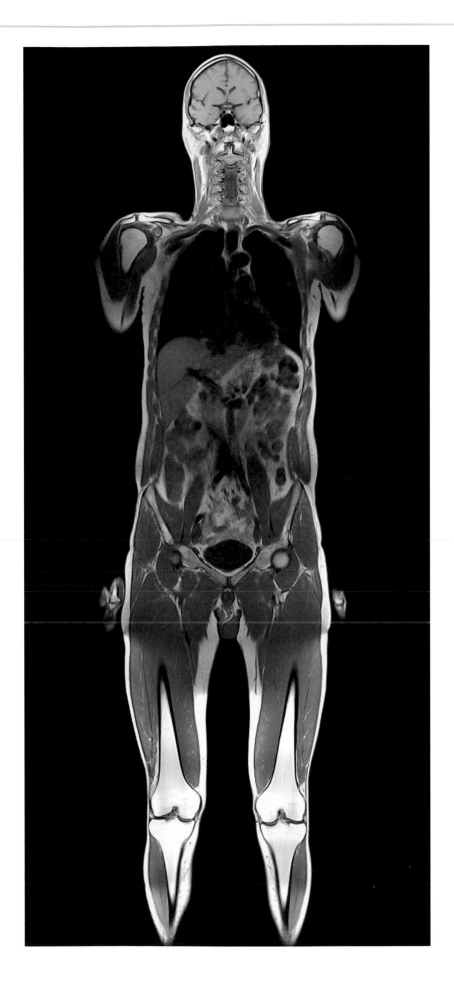

41 Gluteus minimus muscle
42 Pubis
43 Iliopsoas muscle
44 Superficial femoral artery and vein
45 Pectineus muscle
46 Vastus intermedius muscle
47 Adductor brevis muscle
48 Vastus lateralis muscle
49 Adductor longus muscle
50 Vastus medialis muscle
51 Sartorius muscle
52 Medial and lateral femoral condyles
53 Femur (shaft)
54 Knee joint
55 Tibia (head)
56 Tibia (shaft)
57 Tibialis anterior muscle
58 Extensor digitorum longus muscle

Cranial

Right
Lateral

Left
Lateral

Caudal

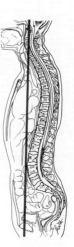

1 Sternocleidomastoid muscle
2 Levator scapulae muscle
3 Middle scalene muscle
4 Spinalis cervicis muscle
5 Trapezius muscle (transverse part)
6 Posterior scalene muscle
7 Acromioclavicular joint
8 Clavicle
9 Supraspinatus muscle
10 Acromion
11 Infraspinatus muscle (tendon)
12 Coracoid process
13 Humerus (head)
14 Axillary artery and vein
15 Teres minor muscle
16 Deltoid muscle
17 Subscapularis muscle
18 Coracobrachialis muscle
19 Biceps brachii muscle (short head)
20 Biceps brachii muscle (long head)
21 Right lung
22 Aortic arch
23 Pulmonary vein
24 Pulmonary artery
25 Serratus anterior muscle (middle and lower parts)
26 Left ventricle
27 Right atrium
28 Stomach
29 Liver
30 Abdominal aorta
31 Internal and external oblique muscles
32 Psoas (major) muscle
33 Transversus abdominis muscle
34 Iliacus muscle
35 Ilium (iliac crest, superior margin)
36 Ilium (acetabular roof)
37 Common iliac artery
38 Hip joint
39 Gluteus medius muscle
40 Femur (head)

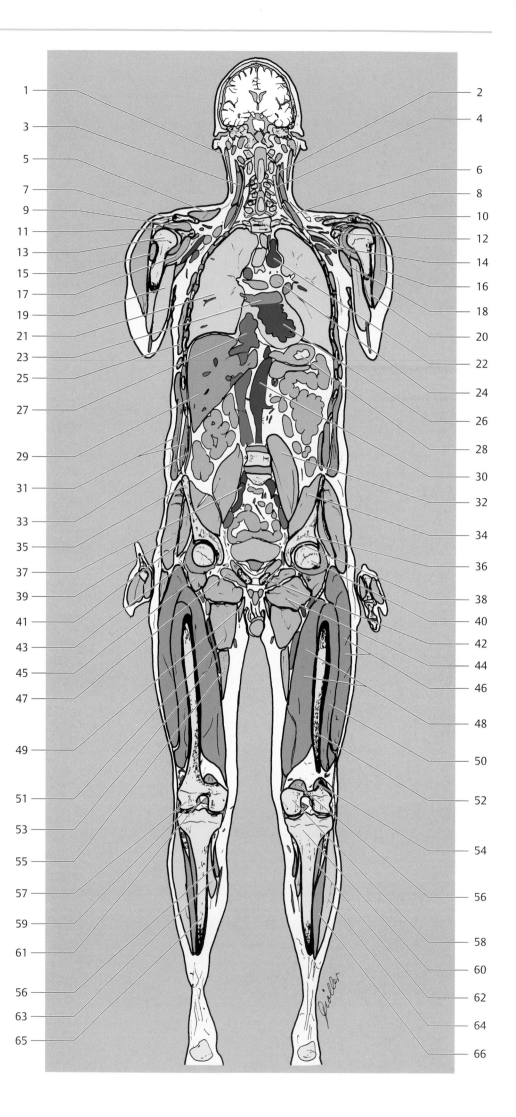

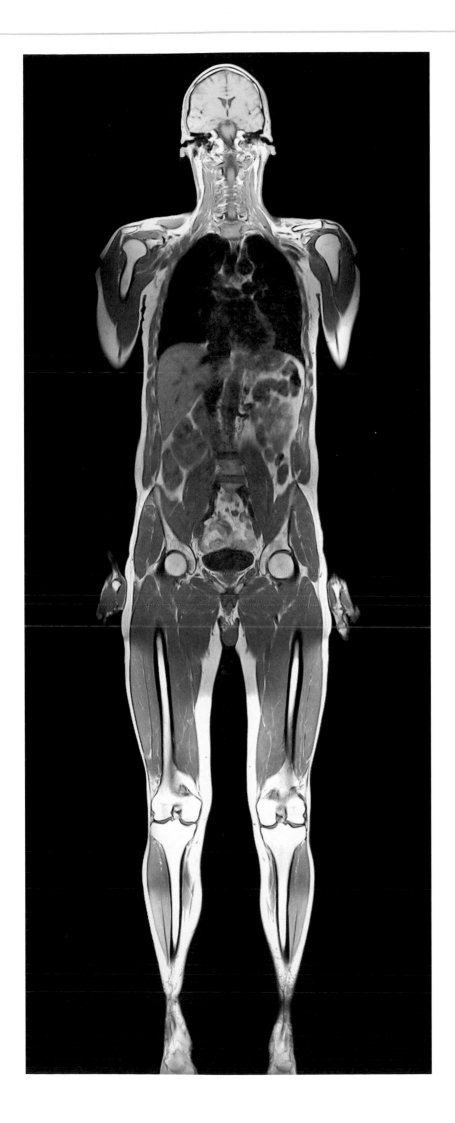

41 Gluteus minimus muscle
42 Pubis
43 Iliofemoral ligament and capsule of hip joint
44 Adductor brevis muscle
45 Iliopsoas muscle
46 Vastus lateralis muscle
47 Obturator externus muscle
48 Vastus medialis muscle
49 Gracilis muscle
50 Vastus intermedius muscle
51 Adductor longus muscle
52 Femur (shaft)
53 Superficial femoral artery and vein
54 Gastrocnemius muscle (lateral head)
55 Sartorius muscle
56 Gastrocnemius muscle (medial head)
57 Lateral femoral condyle
58 Medial femoral condyle
59 Knee joint
60 Tibia (head)
61 Anterior cruciate ligament
62 Tibialis anterior muscle
63 Flexor digitorum longus muscle
64 Peroneus longus muscle
65 Tibia (shaft)
66 Extensor digitorum longus muscle

Cranial

Right
Lateral

Left
Lateral

Caudal

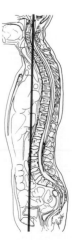

1 Obliquus capitis inferior muscle
2 Splenius capitis muscle
3 Splenius cervicis muscle
4 Sternocleidomastoid muscle
5 Multifidus cervicis muscle
6 Levator scapulae muscle
7 Trapezius muscle (transverse part)
8 Clavicle
9 Joint socket
10 Acromion
11 Infraspinatus muscle
12 Supraspinatus muscle
13 Subscapularis muscle
14 Humerus (head)
15 Teres minor muscle
16 Serratus anterior muscle (upper part)
17 Deltoid muscle
18 Axillary artery and vein
19 Trachea (bifurcation)
20 Aortic arch
21 Biceps brachii muscle and
   coracobrachialis muscle
22 Pulmonary artery
23 Brachioradialis muscle and humerus
   (shaft)
24 Left lung
25 Serratus anterior muscle (middle and
   lower parts)
26 Left atrium
27 Liver
28 Stomach
29 Internal and external oblique muscles
30 Intercostal muscles and ribs
31 Transversus abdominis muscle
32 Abdominal aorta
33 Iliacus muscle
34 Extensor carpi radialis muscle
35 Gluteus minimus muscle
36 Ilium (superior margin, iliac crest)
37 Ilium (roof of acetabulum)
38 Psoas major muscle
39 Femur (head)
40 Gluteus medius muscle

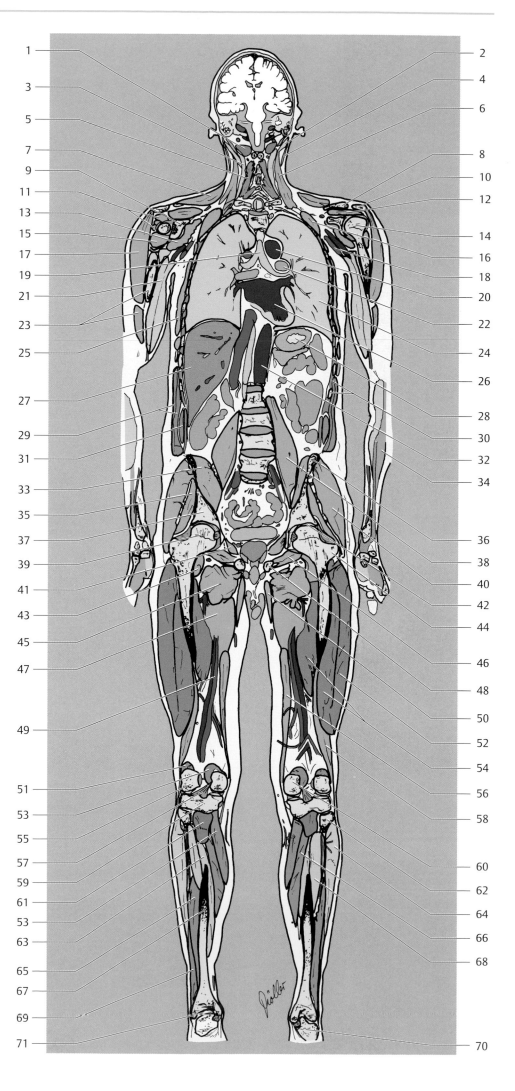

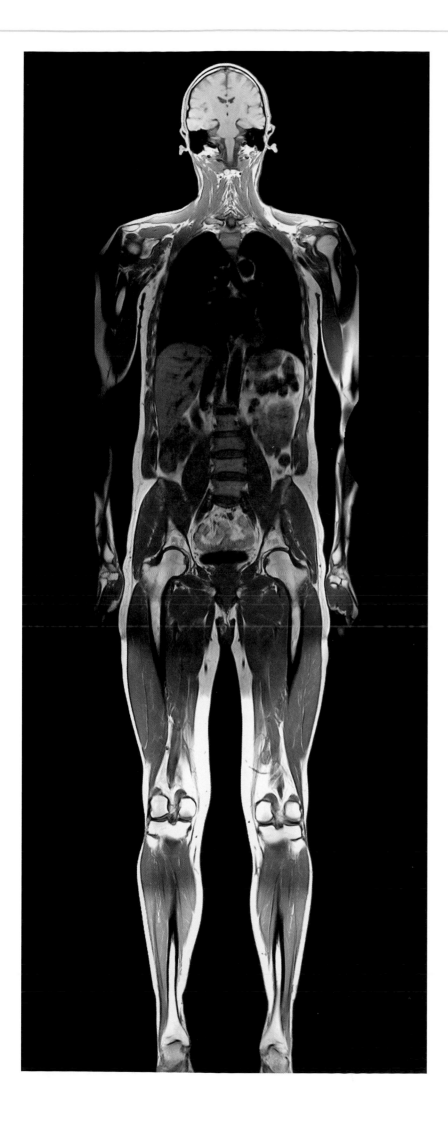

41 Obturator internus muscle
42 Hip joint
43 Iliopsoas muscle
44 Greater trochanter
45 Adductor brevis muscle
46 Obturator externus muscle
47 Adductor longus muscle
48 Ischium
49 Superficial femoral artery and vein
50 Gracilis muscle
51 Gastrocnemius muscle (lateral head)
52 Vastus lateralis muscle
53 Gastrocnemius muscle (medial head)
54 Vastus intermedius and medialis muscles
55 Lateral femoral condyle
56 Sartorius muscle
57 Posterior cruciate ligament
58 Biceps femoris muscle
59 Tibia (head)
60 Medial femoral condyle
61 Popliteus muscle
62 Fibula (head)
63 Flexor digitorum longus muscle
64 Peroneus longus muscle
65 Extensor hallucis longus muscle
66 Soleus muscle
67 Tibia (shaft)
68 Tibialis posterior muscle
69 Extensor digitorum longus muscle
70 Talus
71 Tibiotalar joint

Cranial
Right Lateral   Left Lateral
Caudal

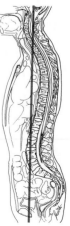

1 Obliquus capitis inferior muscle
2 Obliquus capitis superior muscle
3 Splenius capitis muscle
4 Semispinalis capitis muscle
5 Semispinalis cervicis muscle
6 Longissimus capitis muscle
7 Levator scapulae muscle
8 Trapezius muscle (transverse part)
9 Serratus anterior muscle (upper part)
10 Supraspinatus muscle
11 Acromion
12 Infraspinatus muscle and head of humerus
13 Suprascapularis muscle
14 Joint socket
15 Teres minor muscle
16 Deltoid muscle
17 Triceps brachii muscle (medial head)
18 Aortic arch
19 Posterior circumflex humeral artery
20 Serratus anterior muscle (middle and lower parts)
21 Humerus (shaft)
22 Biceps brachii muscle and coracobrachialis muscle
23 Right lung
24 Triceps brachii muscle (lateral head)
25 Liver
26 Brachialis muscle
27 Internal and external oblique muscles
28 Descending aorta
29 Transversus abdominis muscle
30 Brachioradialis muscle
31 Iliacus muscle
32 Psoas major muscle
33 Gluteus maximus muscle
34 Flexor pollicis longus muscle
35 Gluteus minimus muscle
36 Extensor digitorum muscle
37 Radius
38 Gluteus medius muscle
39 Femur (head)
40 Ilium

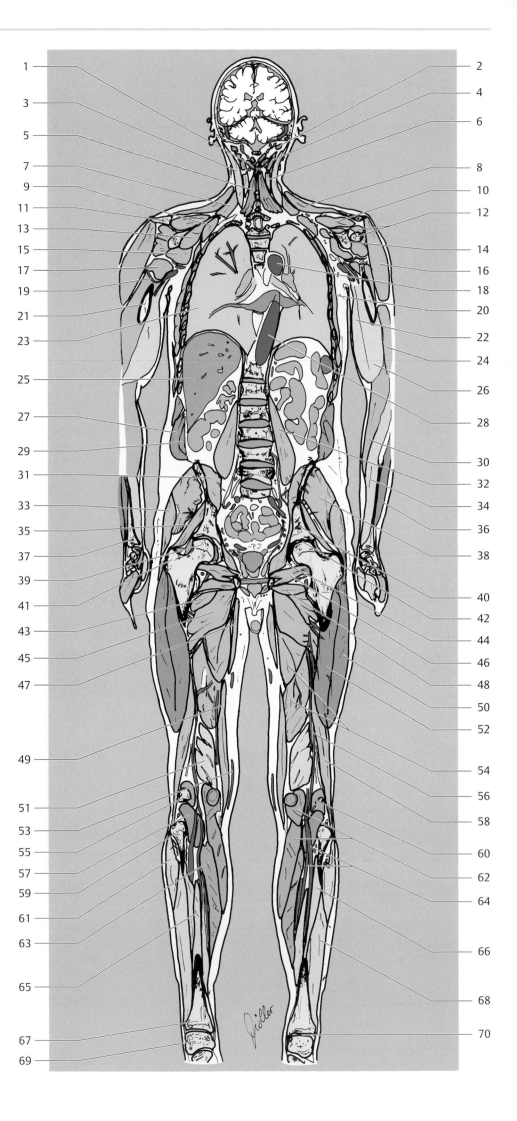

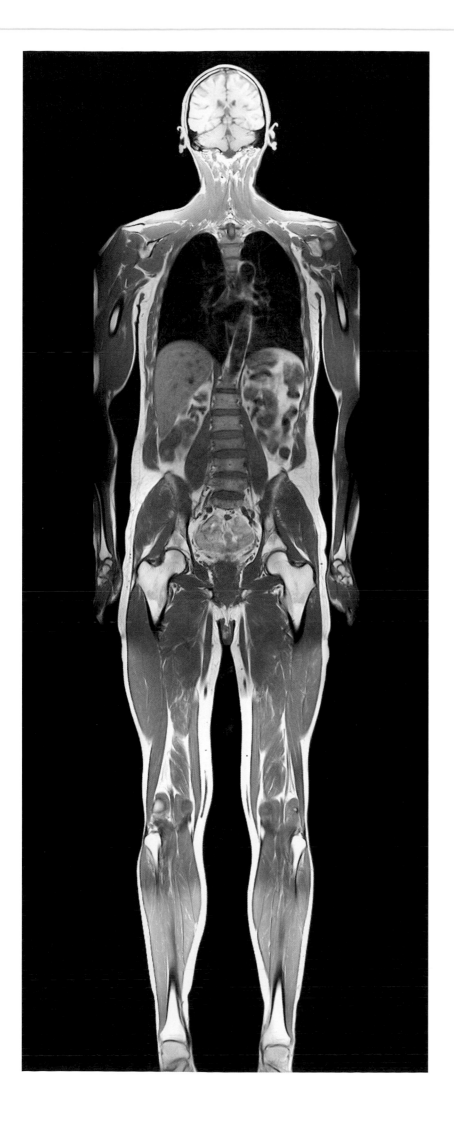

41 Greater trochanter
42 Hip joint
43 Pectineus muscle
44 Obturator internus muscle
45 Adductor brevis muscle
46 Obturator externus muscle
47 Gracilis muscle
48 Adductor minimus muscle
49 Sartorius muscle
50 Vastus lateralis muscle
51 Semimembranosus muscle
52 Vastus intermedius muscle
53 Great saphenous vein
54 Adductor magnus muscle
55 Lateral femoral condyle
56 Superficial femoral artery and vein
57 Popliteus muscle
58 Biceps femoris muscle
59 Fibula (head)
60 Gastrocnemius muscle (lateral head)
61 Peroneus (fibularis) longus muscle
62 Gastrocnemius muscle (medial head)
63 Soleus muscle
64 Popliteal artery and vein
65 Tibialis posterior muscle
66 Flexor hallucis longus muscle
67 Tibia
68 Peroneus brevis muscle
69 Talus
70 Talocrural joint of the ankle

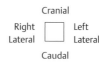

Cranial
Right Lateral — Left Lateral
Caudal

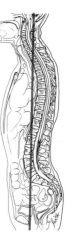

1 Semispinalis capitis muscle
2 Splenius capitis muscle
3 Rectus capitis posterior major muscle
4 Semispinalis cervicis muscle
5 Trapezius muscle (descending part)
6 Splenius cervicis muscle
7 Trapezius muscle (transverse part)
8 Levator scapulae muscle
9 Supraspinatus muscle
10 Serratus anterior muscle (upper part)
11 Infraspinatus muscle
12 Scapula (spine)
13 Teres minor muscle
14 Subscapularis muscle
15 Teres major muscle
16 Deltoid muscle
17 Right lung
18 Triceps brachii muscle (lateral head)
19 Serratus anterior muscle (middle and lower parts)
20 Latissimus dorsi muscle
21 Triceps brachii muscle (medial head)
22 Cephalic vein
23 Humerus (shaft)
24 Diaphragm
25 Coracobrachialis and biceps brachii muscles
26 Spleen
27 Liver
28 Intercostal muscles and ribs
29 Right kidney
30 Psoas major muscle
31 Iliocostalis lumborum muscle
32 Internal and external oblique muscles and transversus abdominis muscle
33 Quadratus lumborum muscle
34 Interspinous ligament
35 Gluteus medius muscle
36 Sacro-iliac joint
37 Ulna
38 Gluteus maximus muscle
39 Sacrum (lateral mass)
40 Piriformis muscle

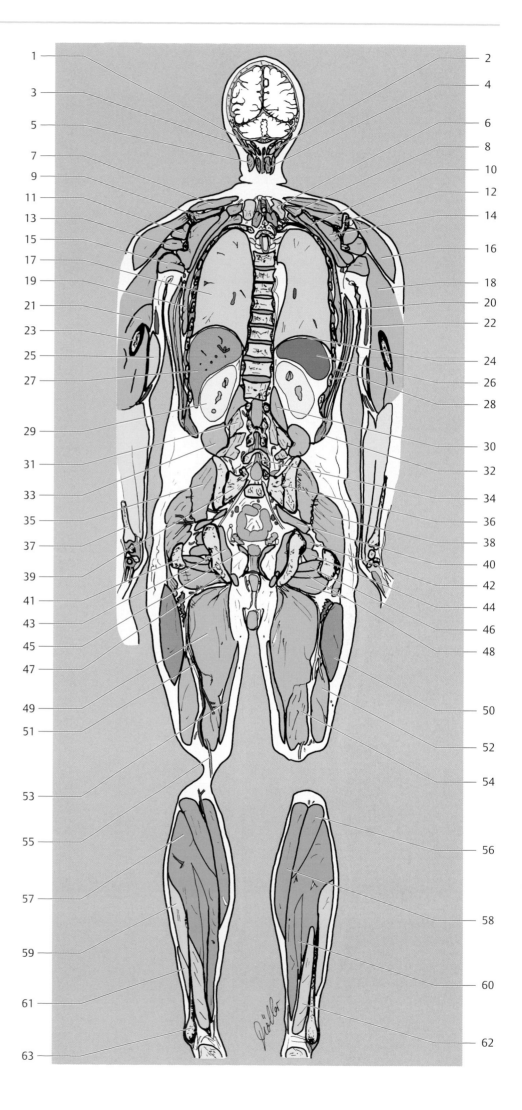

41 Intertrochanteric crest
42 Gemellus superior muscle
43 Obturator internus muscle
44 Obturator externus muscle
45 Levator ani muscle
46 Gemellus inferior muscle
47 Ischium
48 Quadratus femoris muscle
49 Adductor magnus muscle
50 Vastus lateralis muscle
51 Sciatic nerve
52 Biceps femoris muscle (long head)
53 Gracilis muscle
54 Semimembranosus muscle
55 Semitendinosus muscle (tendon)
56 Gastrocnemius muscle (lateral head)
57 Soleus muscle
58 Gastrocnemius muscle (medial head)
59 Peroneus longus muscle
60 Tibialis posterior muscle
61 Peroneus brevis muscle
62 Flexor hallucis longus muscle
63 Fibula (lateral malleolus)

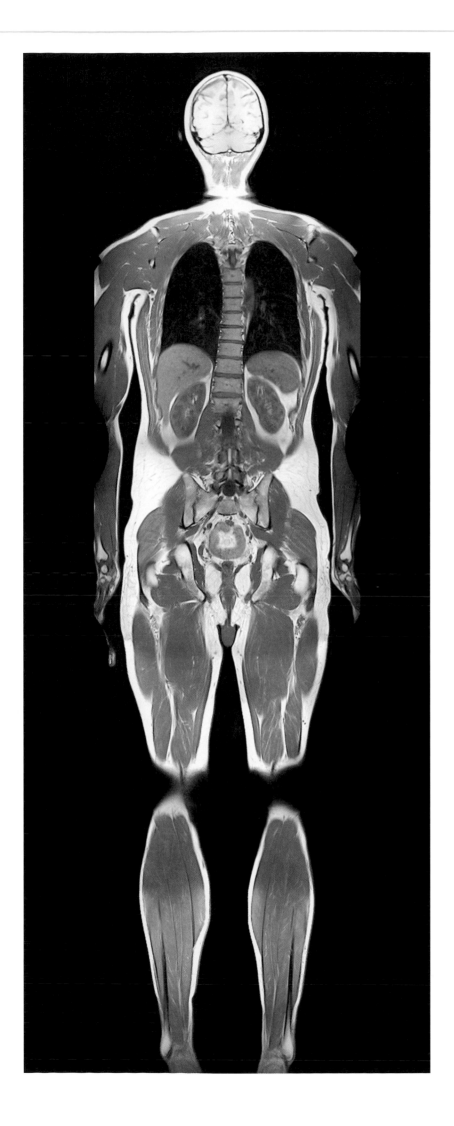

Cranial

Right
Lateral

Left
Lateral

Caudal

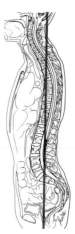

1 Semispinalis capitis muscle
2 Trapezius muscle
3 Levator scapulae muscle
4 Rhomboid minor muscle
5 Scapula (spine)
6 Iliocostalis cervicis muscle
7 Erector spinae muscle
8 Subscapularis muscle
9 Infraspinatus muscle
10 Deltoid muscle
11 Teres major muscle
12 Triceps brachii muscle
13 Right lung
14 Serratus anterior muscle
15 Diaphragm
16 Latissimus dorsi muscle
17 Liver
18 Spleen
19 Iliocostalis lumborum muscle
20 Intercostal muscle
21 Humerus
22 Cephalic vein
23 Flexor digitorum superficialis muscle
24 Longissimus lumborum muscle
25 Sacro-iliac joint
26 Multifidus lumborum muscle
27 Flexor carpi ulnaris muscle
28 Ilium
29 Piriformis muscle
30 Sacrum (lateral mass)
31 Levator ani muscle
32 Anus
33 Obturator internus muscle
34 Gluteus maximus muscle
35 Semitendinosus muscle
36 Ischium
37 Biceps femoris muscle (long head)
38 Semimembranosus muscle

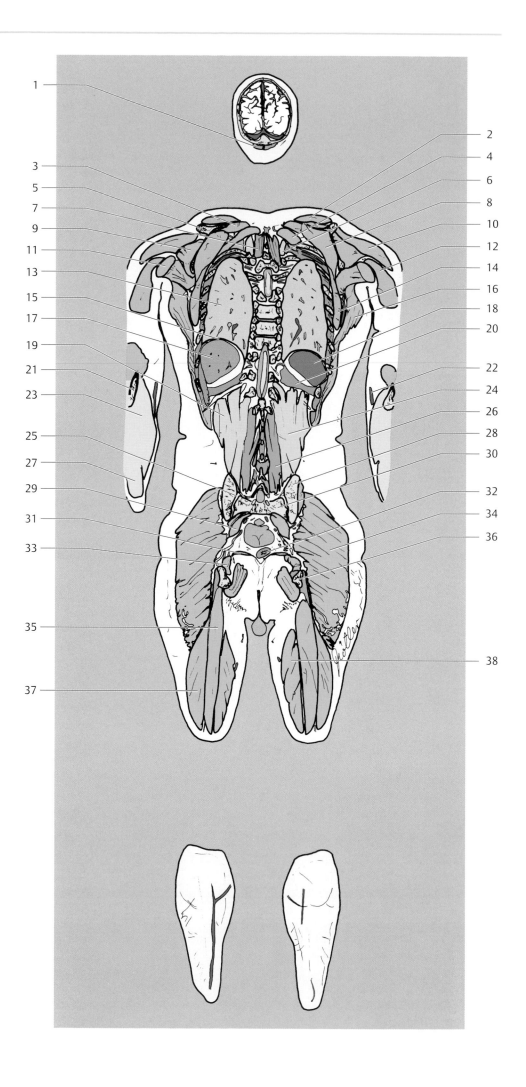

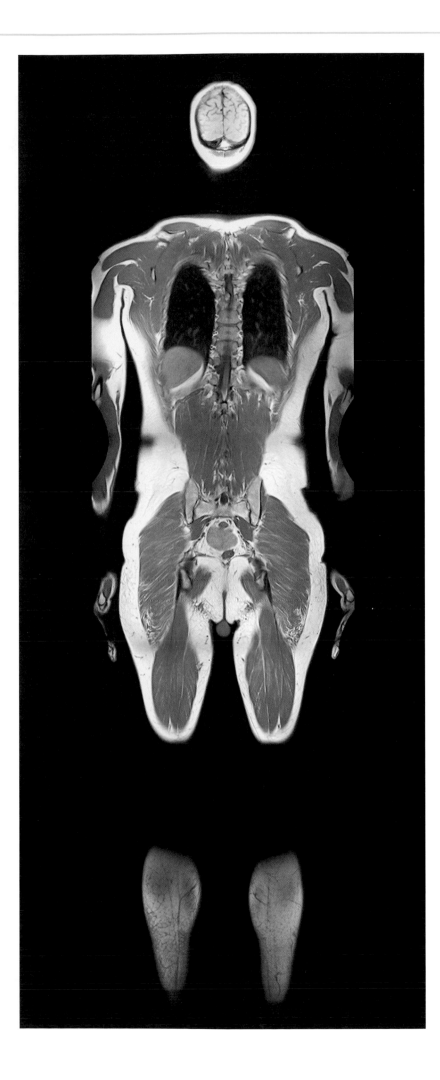

Cranial

Right
Lateral

Left
Lateral

Caudal

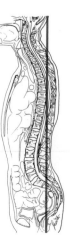

1 Trapezius muscle
2 Levator scapulae muscle
3 Scapula (spine)
4 Rhomboid minor muscle
5 Serratus posterior muscle
6 Erector spinae muscle
7 Deltoid muscle
8 Infraspinatus muscle
9 Subscapularis muscle
10 Teres major muscle
11 Serratus anterior muscle
12 Triceps brachii muscle
13 Right lung
14 Latissimus dorsi muscle
15 Diaphragm
16 Spinal cord (thoracic part)
17 Liver
18 Intercostal muscles and ribs
19 Iliocostalis lumborum muscle
20 Longissimus lumborum muscle
21 Interspinales lumborum muscles
22 Interspinal ligament
23 Ilium
24 Sacro-iliac joint
25 Sacrum (lateral mass)
26 Rectum
27 Piriformis muscle
28 Gluteus maximus muscle
29 Biceps femoris muscle (long head)
30 Semitendinosus muscle
31 Semimembranosus muscle

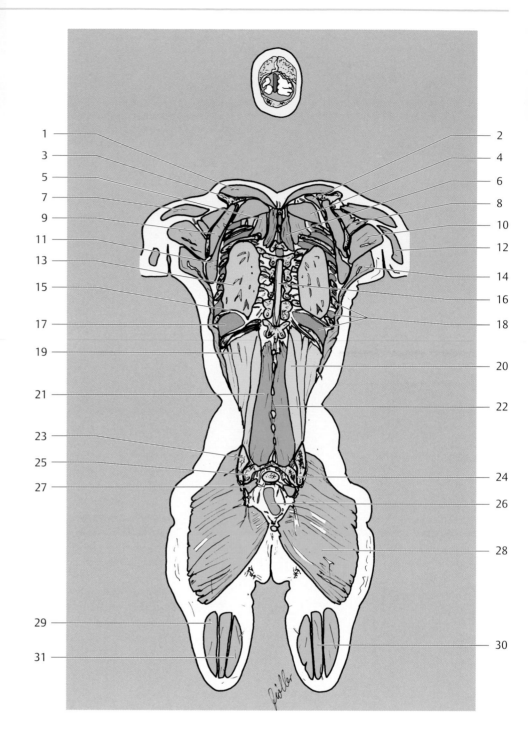

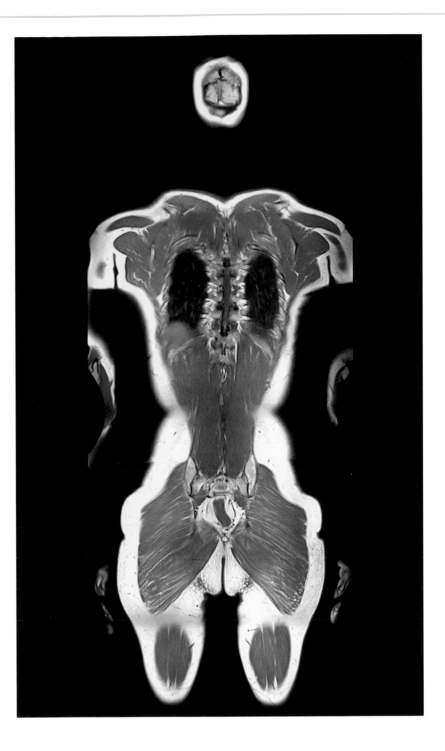

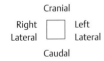

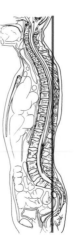

Anatomic Structures Color Code: Temporomandibular Joint

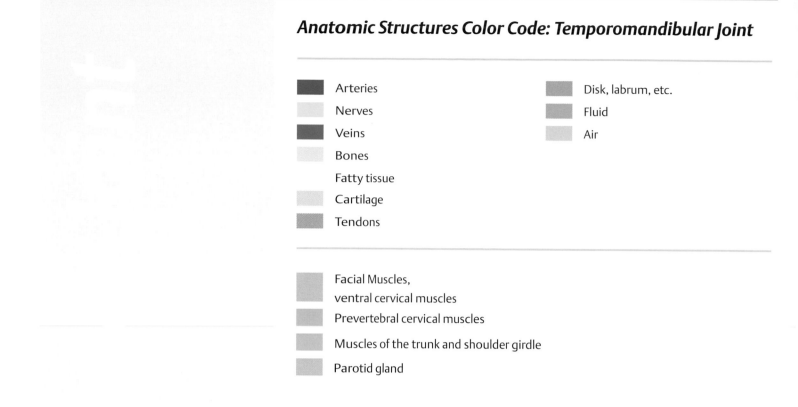

■ Arteries	■ Disk, labrum, etc.
■ Nerves	■ Fluid
■ Veins	■ Air
■ Bones	
Fatty tissue	
■ Cartilage	
■ Tendons	

■ Facial Muscles,
ventral cervical muscles

■ Prevertebral cervical muscles

■ Muscles of the trunk and shoulder girdle

■ Parotid gland

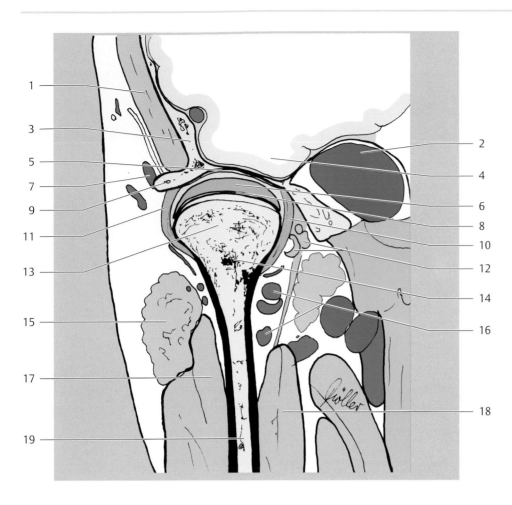

1 Temporal muscle
2 Internal carotid artery (petrous part)
3 Temporal bone
4 Temporal lobe
5 Upper joint space
6 Articular disk (posterior ligament)
7 Superficial temporal artery
8 Lower joint space
9 Zygomatic process
10 Medial joint capsule
11 Lateral joint capsule
12 Lateral pterygoid muscle
13 Mandible (head)
14 Mandible (neck)
15 Parotid gland
16 Maxillary veins
17 Masseter muscle
18 Medial pterygoid muscle
19 Ramus of mandible

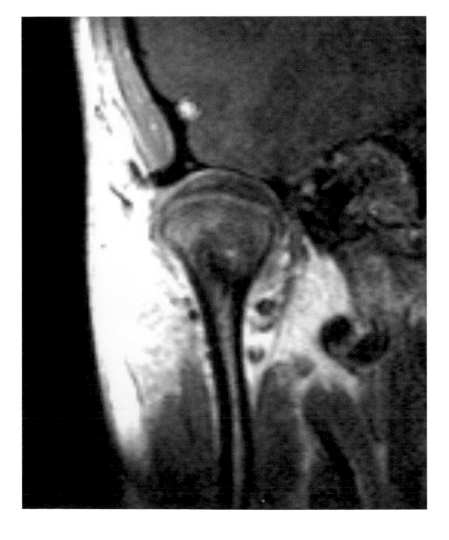

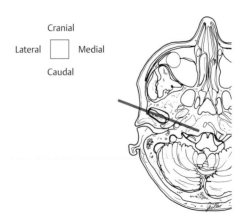

Cranial
Lateral ☐ Medial
Caudal

1 Temporal muscle
2 Temporal lobe and temporal bone
3 Upper joint space
4 Articular fossa
5 Articular disk (posterior ligament)
6 Bilaminar zone (upper retrodiskal layer)
7 Lower joint space
8 Bilaminar zone (lower retrodiskal layer)
9 Articular tubercle
10 Mandible (head)
11 Articular disk (intermediate zone)
12 Mastoid
13 Lateral pterygoid muscle (upper head)
14 Retroarticular tissue
15 Articular disk (anterior ligament)
16 External acoustic meatus
17 Maxillary artery and vein
18 Mandible (neck)
19 Lateral pterygoid muscle (lower head)
20 Sternocleidomastoid muscle
21 Inferior alveolar artery and nerve
22 Parotid gland
23 Masseter muscle
24 Parotid vein
25 Mandibular canal
26 Mandible (ramus)
27 Inferior alveolar nerve

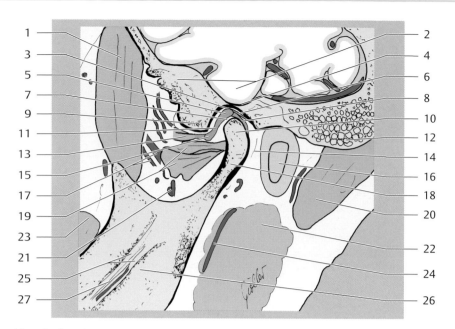

Mouth closed

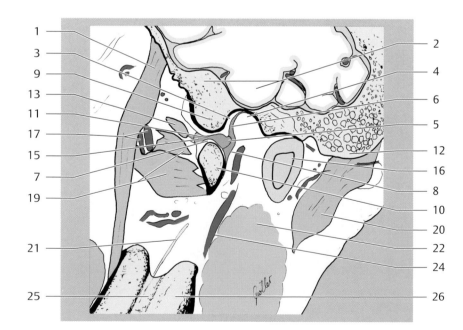

Mouth open

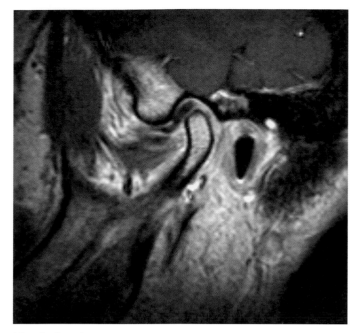

Mouth closed

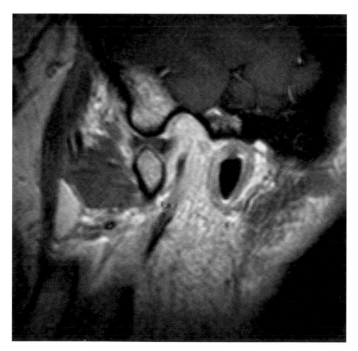

Mouth open

Cranial

Ventral ☐ Dorsal

Caudal

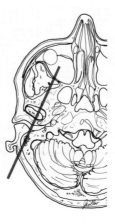

Anatomic Structures Color Code: Spine

Arteries

Nerves

Veins

Bones

Fatty tissue

Cartilage

Tendon

Disk, intervertebral cartilage

Fluid, cerebrospinal fluid

Lymph nodes

Esophagus

Liver

Air

Intestine

Muscles of Face and Ventral Cervical Muscles
Digastric muscle
Stylohyoid
Sternohyoid

Short Muscles of Neck and Head Joints
Rectus capitis posterior major and minor
Obliquus capitis superior and inferior

Prevertebral Cervical Muscles
Longus capitis and longus colli
Rectus capitis lateralis and anterior

Erector Spinae Muscles (Lateral Tract)
Iliocostalis
Longissimus
Splenius capitis and splenius cervicis
Intertransversarii
Levatores costarum

Erector Spinae Muscles (Medial Tract)
Spinal system:
interspinous muscles
Transversospinal system:
rotatores breves and longi
Multifidus cervicis, thoracis, and lumborum
Semispinalis capitis, cervicis, and thoracis

Muscles of Thoracic Cage
External, internal, and innermost intercostals
Transversus thoracis
Subcostal
Scalenus anterior, medius, minimus, and posterior

Peroneus

Muscles of the Trunk— Shoulder Girdle—Arm
Rhomboideus major and minor
Sternocleidomastoid
Levator scapulae
Serratus anterior and posterior
Pectoralis major and minor
Trapezius

Muscles of the Trunk— Leg—Abdomen
Latissimus dorsi
Psoas
Quadratus lumborum
Piriformis
Gluteus medius

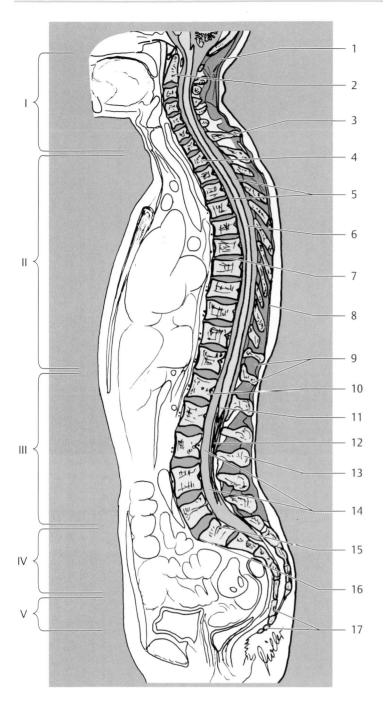

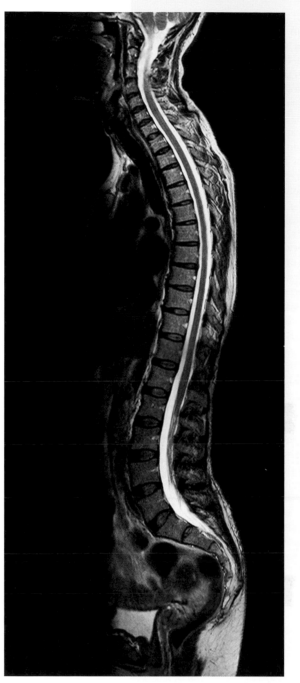

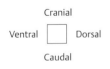

Cranial

Ventral ☐ Dorsal

Caudal

I Cervical vertebrae C 1–7
II Thoracic vertebrae Th 1–12
III Lumbar vertebrae L 1–5
IV Sacrum (sacral vertebrae 1–5)
V Coccyx (coccygeal vertebrae 1–3 or 1–4)

1 Nuchal ligament
2 Dens axis, C 2
3 Vertebra prominens, C 7
4 Body of thoracic vertebra T1
5 Vertebral canal
6 Spinal cord (thoracic part)
7 Intervertebral disk
8 Supraspinous ligament
9 Interspinous ligaments
10 Body of lumbar vertebra L 1
11 Conus medullaris
12 Cauda equina
13 Spinous process
14 Thecal sac
15 Sacrum (S 1)
16 Promontory
17 Coccyx

1 Occipital condyle
2 Semispinalis capitis muscle
3 Internal carotid artery
4 Suboccipital fatty tissue
5 Atlanto-occipital joint
6 Rectus capitis posterior minor muscle
7 Atlas (lateral mass)
8 Rectus capitis posterior major muscle
9 Vertebral artery
10 Spinal nerve C 2
11 Deep cervical veins
12 Obliquus capitis inferior muscle
13 Intervertebral foramen
14 Trapezius muscle (descending part)
15 Longus capitis muscle
16 Splenius capitis muscle
17 Vertebral artery (spinal and radicular branches)
18 Inferior articular process
19 Spinal ganglion C 8
20 Zygapophyseal joint
21 Longus colli muscle
22 Superior articular process
23 First thoracic vertebral body
24 Spinalis cervicis muscle and multifidus muscle
25 Posterior intercostal artery (spinal and radicular branches of dorsal branch)
26 Ligamentum flavum
27 Posterior intercostal vein
28 Trapezius muscle (transverse part)
29 Posterior intercostal artery (dorsal branch)

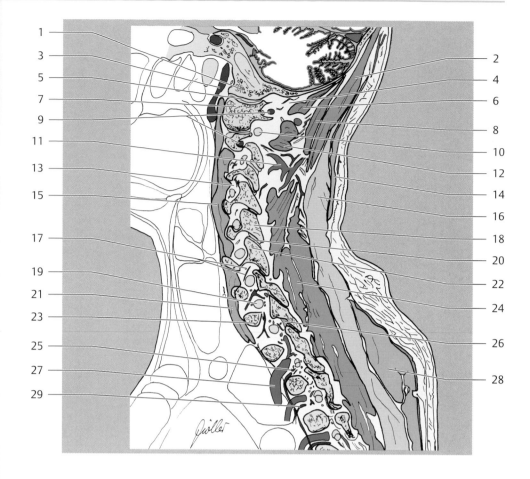

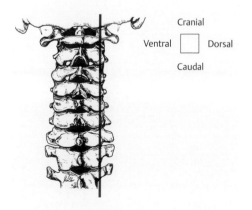

Cranial

Ventral ☐ Dorsal

Caudal

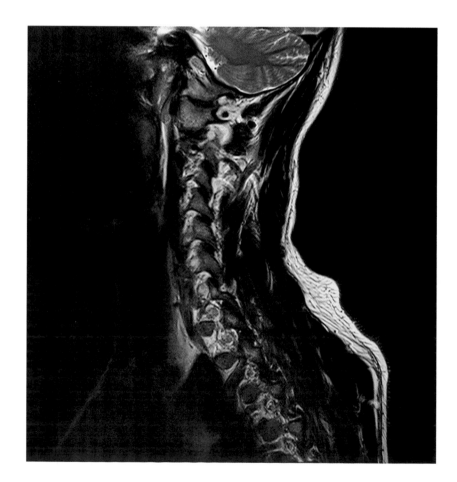

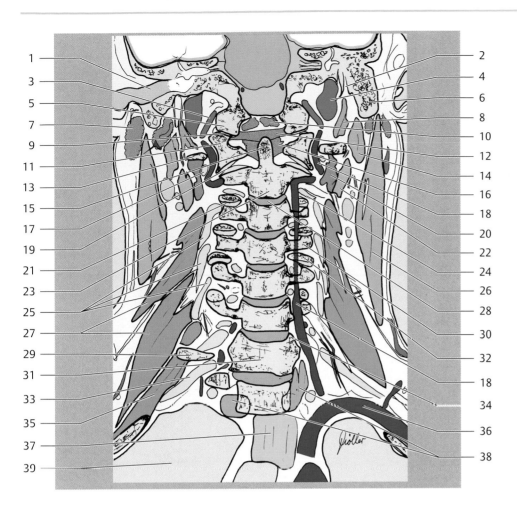

1 External auditory canal
2 Stylomastoid foramen
3 Vertebral vein
4 Internal jugular vein
5 Occipital condyle
6 Mastoid process
7 Parotid gland
8 Rectus capitis lateralis muscle
9 Atlanto-occipital joint
10 Tectorial membrane
11 Atlas (lateral mass)
12 Transverse ligament
13 Atlas (transverse process)
14 Digastric muscle (posterior belly)
15 Axis (dens)
16 Alar ligaments
17 Spinal nerve C 2
18 Vertebral artery
19 Lateral atlanto-axial joint
20 Obliquus capitis inferior muscle
21 Zygapophyseal joint
22 Levator scapulae muscle
23 Axis (vertebral body)
24 Spinal ganglion C 3
25 Cervical plexus
26 Sternocleidomastoid muscle
27 Scalenus medius muscle
28 Intervertebral disk (C 2 / C 3)
29 Transverse process C 7
30 Superior articular process C 4
31 Cervical vertebral body C 7
32 Inferior articular process
33 Spinal nerve C 8
34 Uncinate process C 7
35 Scalenus posterior muscle
36 Subclavian artery
37 Esophagus
38 Longus colli muscle
39 Lung

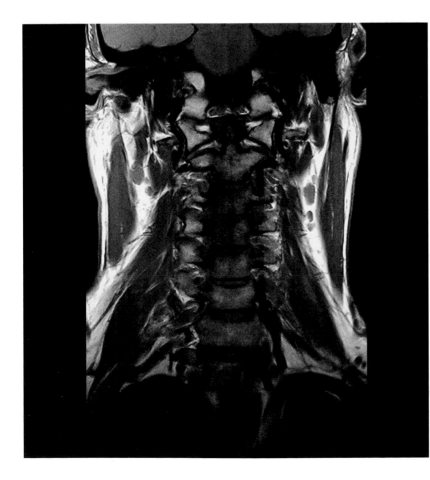

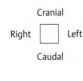

Cranial

Right ☐ Left

Caudal

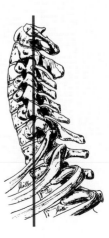

1 Medulla oblongata
2 Sigmoid sinus
3 Mastoid process
4 Foramen magnum
5 Vertebral artery
6 Splenius capitis muscle
7 Digastric muscle (posterior belly)
8 Obliquus capitis superior muscle
9 Atlas (posterior arch)
10 Obliquus capitis inferior muscle
11 Vertebral artery
12 Sternocleidomastoid muscle
13 Spinal ganglion C 2
14 Levator scapulae muscle
15 Axis (vertebral arch)
16 Splenius cervicis muscle
17 Spinal cord (cervical pulp with central canal)
18 Scalenus medius muscle
19 Posterior intercostal artery (spinal and radicular branches of dorsal branch)
20 Inferior articulate process C 6
21 Semispinalis cervicis muscle
22 Zygapophyseal joint
23 Cerebrospinal fluid in spinal canal
24 Superior articular process C 7
25 Spinal dura mater
26 Scalenus posterior muscle
27 Posterior longitudinal ligament
28 First rib (neck)
29 Spinal nerve C 8
30 Thoracic vertebral body T1
31 Spinal nerve T1
32 Intervertebral disk
33 Second rib (head)
34 Left lung
35 First rib (body)

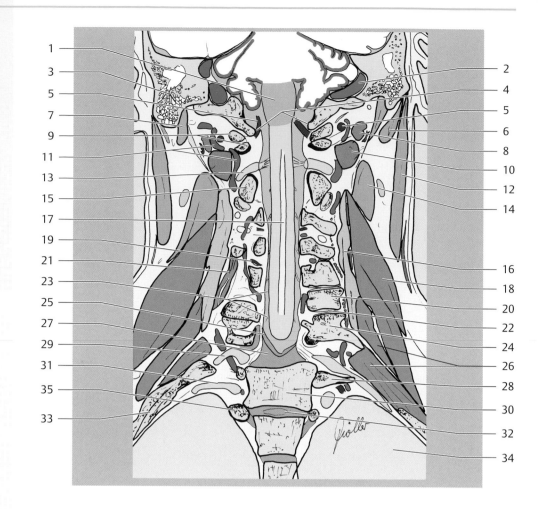

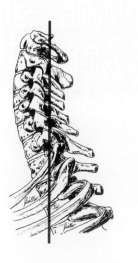

Cranial
Right ☐ Left
Caudal

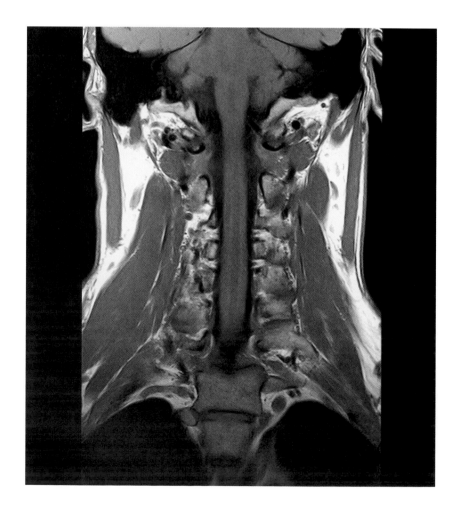

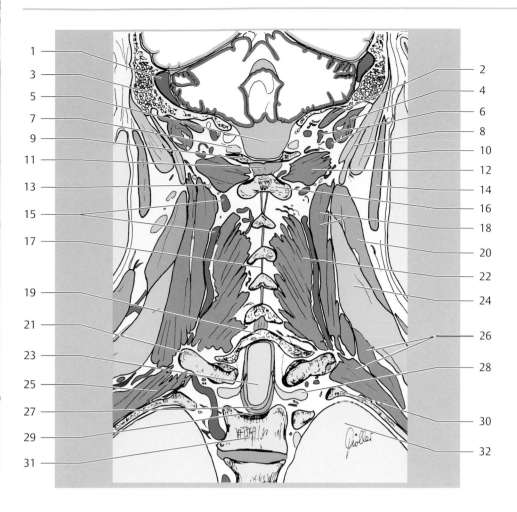

1 Sigmoid sinus
2 Rectus capitis posterior major muscle
3 Mastoid process
4 Obliquus capitis superior muscle
5 Cisterna magna
6 Suboccipital venous plexus
7 Suboccipital nerve
8 Longissimus capitis muscle
9 Atlas (posterior arch)
10 Splenius capitis muscle
11 Nuchal ligament
12 Obliquus capitis inferior muscle
13 Major occipital nerve
14 Sternocleidomastoid muscle
15 Deep cervical vein
16 Spinous process C 2
17 Interspinous ligament
18 Semispinalis cervicis muscle
19 Vertebral arch C 7
20 Levator scapulae muscle
21 First rib (neck and tubercle)
22 Spinalis cervicis muscle and multifidus muscle
23 Spinal cord (thoracic part)
24 Splenius cervicis muscle
25 Intercostal muscles
26 Scalenus posterior muscle
27 Cerebrospinal fluid in vertebral canal
28 Spinal ganglion T1
29 Spinal dura mater and posterior longitudinal ligament
30 Second rib
31 Second thoracic vertebral body
32 Left lung

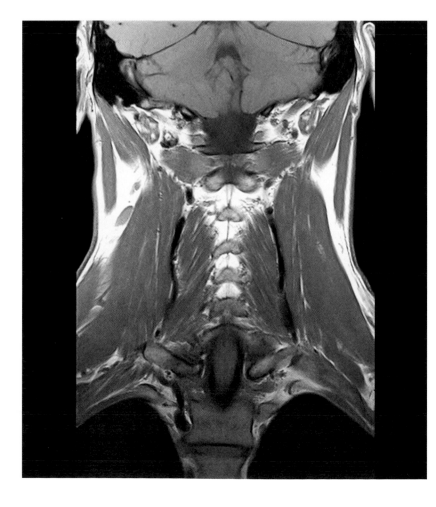

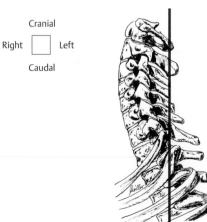

Cranial

Right Left

Caudal

1 Retromandibular vein
2 Mandible
3 Digastric muscle (posterior belly)
4 Internal jugular vein
5 Internal carotid artery
6 Longus capitis muscle
7 Median atlantoaxial joint
8 Atlas (anterior arch)
9 Hypoglossal nerve (XII)
10 Pterygoid venous plexus
11 Vagus nerve (X)
12 Stylohyoid muscle
13 Maxillary artery (mandibular part)
14 Parotid gland
15 Alar ligaments
16 Rectus capitis lateralis muscle
17 Lateral mass of atlas
18 Dens of axis
19 Vertebral artery
20 Cruciate ligament of atlas (longitudinal fascicles and transverse ligament of atlas)
21 Longissimus capitis muscle
22 Sternocleidomastoid muscle
23 Splenius capitis muscle
24 Deep cervical vein
25 Obliquus capitis superior muscle
26 Spinal cord
27 Atlas (posterior arch)
28 Semispinalis capitis muscle
29 Rectus capitis posterior major muscle
30 Rectus capitis posterior minor muscle
31 Trapezius muscle
32 Nuchal ligament

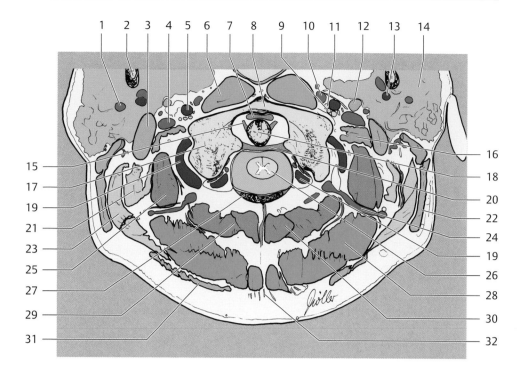

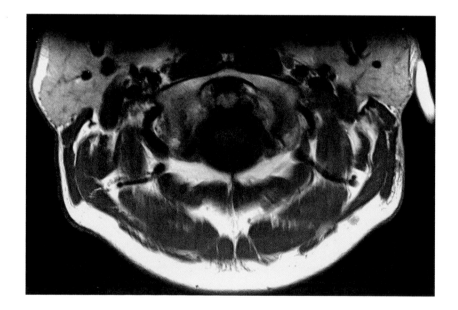

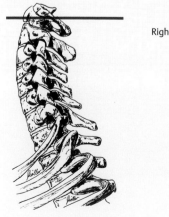

Ventral

Right   Left

Dorsal

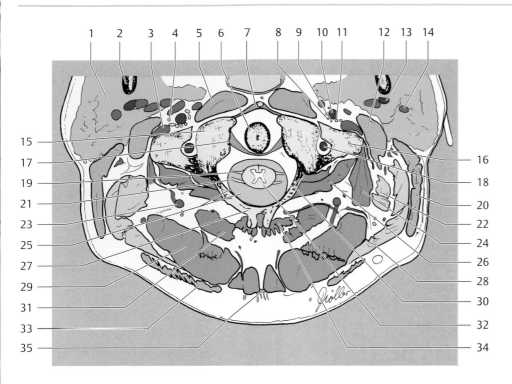

1 Parotid gland
2 Mandible (ramus)
3 Internal jugular vein
4 Glossopharyngeal nerve (IX)
5 Longus capitis muscle
6 Dens of axis
7 Anterior longitudinal ligament
8 Vagus nerve (X)
9 Hypoglossal nerve (XII)
10 Internal carotid artery
11 Accessory nerve (XI)
12 Digastric muscle (posterior belly)
13 Maxillary artery (mandibular part)
14 Retromandibular vein
15 Atlas (lateral mass)
16 Atlas (transverse process)
17 Transverse ligament of atlas
18 Vertebral artery
19 Ventral nerve root
20 Sternocleidomastoid muscle
21 Dorsal nerve root
22 Longissimus capitis muscle
23 Deep cervical vein
24 Obliquus capitis superior muscle
25 Dura mater and cerebrospinal fluid
   (subarachnoid space)
26 Obliquus capitis inferior muscle
27 Spinous process
28 Splenius capitis muscle
29 Semispinalis capitis muscle
30 Axis (posterior arch)
31 Rectus capitis posterior major muscle
32 Spinal cord
33 Trapezius muscle
34 Rectus capitis posterior minor muscle
35 Nuchal ligament

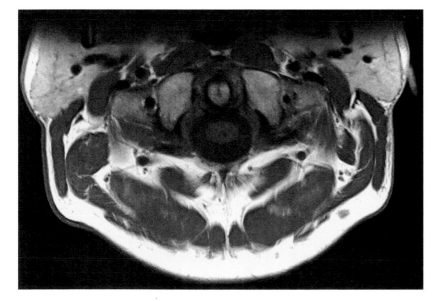

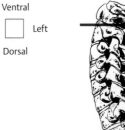

Ventral

Right ☐ Left

Dorsal

1 Medial pterygoid muscle
2 Vagus nerve (X)
3 Accessory nerve (XI)
4 Styloglossus muscle
5 Stylopharyngeus muscle
6 Longus capitis muscle
7 Longus colli muscle
8 Axis (body)
9 Superior constrictor muscle of pharynx
10 Atlas (articular process)
11 Internal carotid artery
12 External carotid artery
13 Mandible (ramus)
14 Digastric muscle (posterior belly)
15 Retromandibular vein
16 Parotid gland
17 Hypoglossal nerve (XII)
18 Internal jugular vein
19 Atlas (transverse process)
20 Axis (body)
21 Sternocleidomastoid muscle
22 Premedullary subarachnoid space
23 Vertebral artery
24 Ventral root of 2nd spinal nerve
25 Longissimus capitis muscle
26 Spinal cord
27 Splenius capitis muscle
28 Dorsal root of 2nd spinal nerve
29 Obliquus capitis inferior muscle
30 Deep cervical vein
31 Spinal ganglion (nerve root)
32 Trapezius muscle
33 Semispinalis capitis muscle
34 Rectus capitis posterior major muscle
35 Axis (posterior arch)

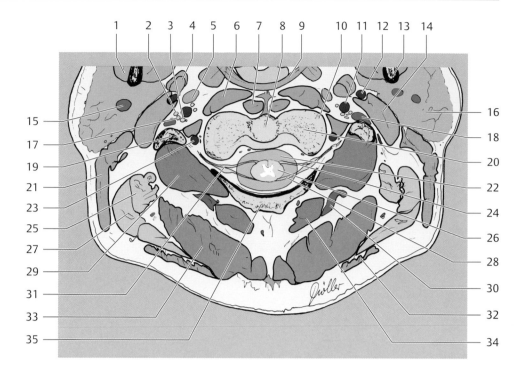

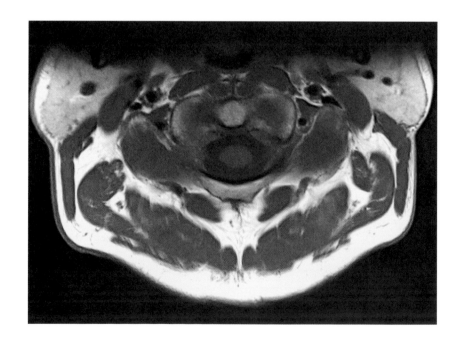

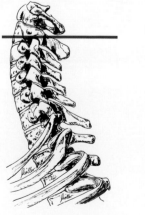

Ventral

Right ☐ Left

Dorsal

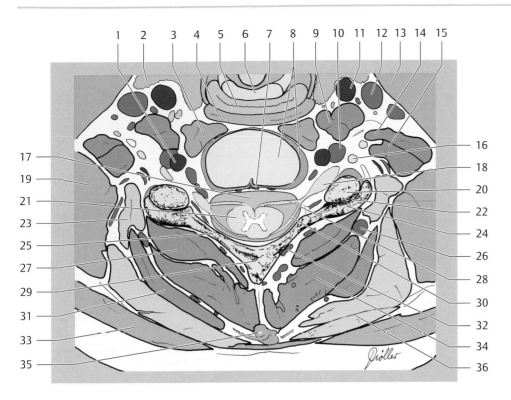

1 2 3 4 5 6 7 8 9 10 11 12 13 14 15

17
19
21
23
25
27
29
31
33
35

16
18
20
22
24
26
28
30
32
34
36

1 Vertebral artery
2 Thyroid gland
3 Longus colli muscle
4 Superior constrictor muscle of pharynx
5 Esophagus
6 Cricoid cartilage
7 Basivertebral veins
8 Cervical vertebral body C 5 and intervertebral space C 5 / C 6
9 Scalenus anterior muscle
10 Vertebral vein
11 Common carotid artery
12 Internal jugular vein
13 Sternocleidomastoid muscle
14 Scalenus medius muscle
15 Scalenus posterior muscle
16 Spinal nerve C 5
17 Premedullary subarachnoid space
18 Spinal ganglion (nerve root)
19 Levator scapulae muscle
20 Superior articular process
21 Spinal cord
22 Zygapophyseal joint
23 Longissimus cervicis muscle
24 Inferior articular process
25 Posterior vertebral arch C 5 (lamina)
26 Deep cervical vein
27 Spinalis cervicis muscle and multifidus
   muscle
28 Ventral nerve root C 6
29 Spinous process
30 Dorsal nerve root C 6
31 Semispinalis capitis muscle
32 Posterior external vertebral venous
   plexus
33 Trapezius muscle
34 Semispinalis cervicis muscle
35 Nuchal ligament
36 Splenius capitis muscle

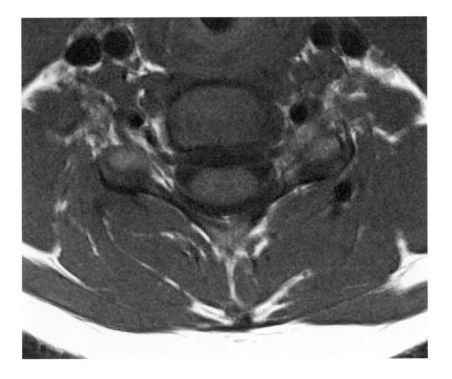

Ventral

Right ☐ Left

Dorsal

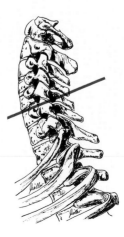

1 Transverse process
2 Pedicle of vertebral arch
3 Thyroid gland
4 Superior constrictor muscle of pharynx
5 Anterior internal vertebral venous plexus
6 Esophagus
7 Larynx
8 Cervical vertebral body C 6
9 Longus colli muscle
10 Common carotid artery
11 Internal jugular vein
12 Sternocleidomastoid muscle
13 Scalenus anterior muscle
14 Scalenus medius muscle
15 Ventral nerve root C 7
16 Vertebral artery
17 Articular process
18 Spinal nerve C 6
19 Levator scapulae muscle
20 Longissimus capitis muscle
21 Spinal cord
22 Deep cervical vein
23 Dorsal nerve root C 7
24 Longissimus cervicis muscle
25 Posterior vertebral arch C 6 (lamina)
26 Spinalis cervicis muscle and multifidus cervicis muscle
27 Semispinalis cervicis muscle
28 Splenius cervicis muscle
29 Posterior external vertebral venous plexus
30 Nuchal ligament
31 Splenius capitis muscle
32 Rhomboid minor muscle
33 Trapezius muscle

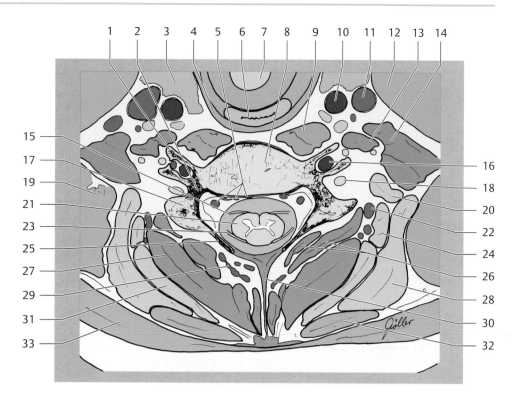

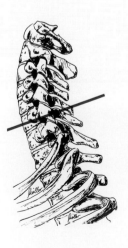

Ventral

Right ☐ Left

Dorsal

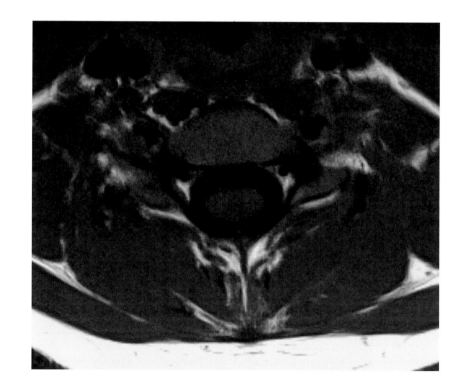

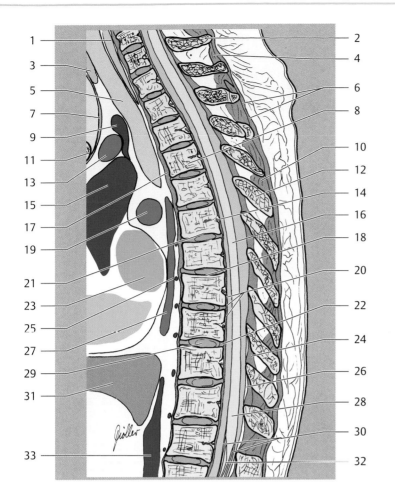

1 Esophagus
2 Vertebra prominens C 7
3 Thyroid gland
4 Interspinales cervices muscles
5 Trachea
6 Supraspinous ligament
7 Sternohyoid muscle
8 Thoracic vertebral body T4
9 Brachiocephalic trunk
10 Interspinous ligament
11 Sternum (manubrium)
12 Spinous process
13 Left brachiocephalic vein
14 Basivertebral vein
15 Ascending aorta
16 Spinal cord (thoracic part)
17 Anterior longitudinal ligament
18 Posterior intercostal artery
19 Pulmonary artery
20 Posterior longitudinal ligament
21 Inferior vertebral endplate T6
22 Intervertebral disk T9 / T10
   (anulus fibrosus)
23 Left atrium
24 Ligamentum flavum
25 Superior vertebral endplate T7
26 Epidural fatty tissue (retrospinal fat)
27 Azygos vein
28 Conus medullaris
29 Intervertebral disk T9 / T10
   (nucleus pulposus)
30 Cauda equina
31 Liver
32 Filum terminale
33 Descending aorta

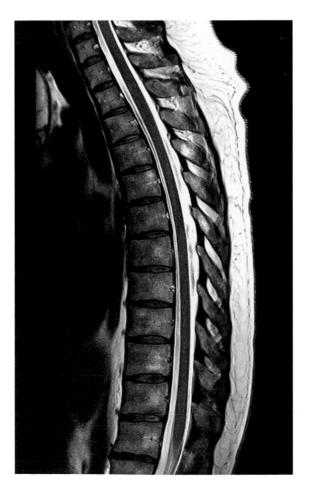

Cranial

Ventral   Dorsal

Caudal

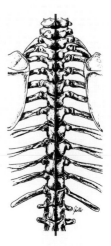

1 Trachea
2 Splenius cervicis muscle
3 Thyroid gland
4 Semispinalis capitis muscle
5 Sternohyoid muscle
6 Serratus posterior superior muscle
7 Esophagus
8 Rhomboid major muscle
9 Brachiocephalic trunk
10 Zygapophyseal joint T3 / T4
11 Left brachiocephalic vein
12 Inferior articular process T4
13 Sternum (manubrium)
14 Superior articular process T5
15 Left main bronchus
16 Trapezius muscle
17 Ascending aorta
18 Posterior intercostal artery (spinal branch)
19 Pulmonary artery
20 Intervertebral vein
21 Hemi-azygos vein
22 Erector spinae muscle
23 Intervertebral disk T7 / T8
24 Intervertebral foramen
25 Left atrium
26 Spinal ganglion (dorsal root)
27 Superior vertebral endplate T9
28 Spinal ganglion (ventral root)
29 Right atrium
30 Multifidus thoracis muscle and semispinalis thoracis muscle
31 Inferior vertebral endplate T9
32 Posterior external vertebral venous plexus
33 Thoracic vertebral body T10
34 Latissimus dorsi muscle
35 Descending aorta
36 Pedicle of vertebral arch (interarticular portion)
37 Liver
38 Ligamentum flavum

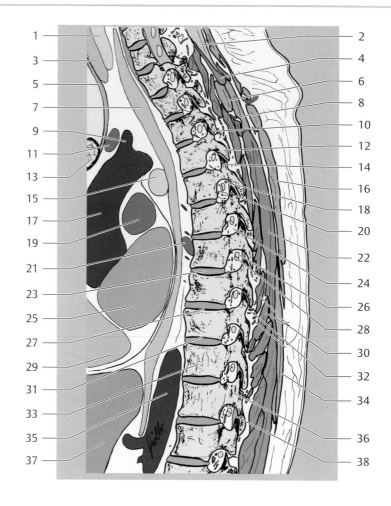

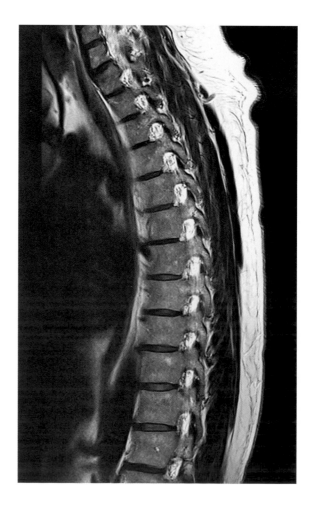

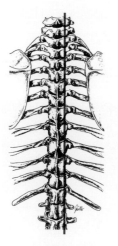

Cranial

Ventral ☐ Dorsal

Caudal

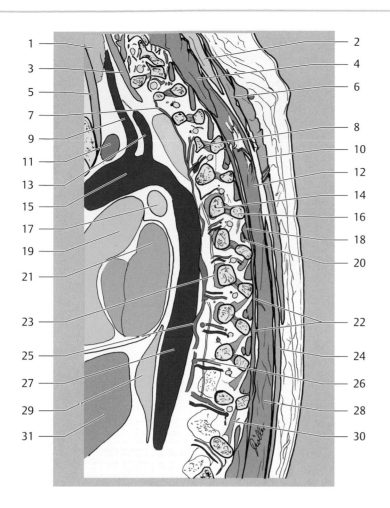

1 Thyroid gland
2 Splenius cervicis muscle
3 Longus capitis muscle
4 Spinalis cervicis muscle and multifidus muscle
5 Sternohyoid muscle
6 Rhomboid major muscle
7 Accessory hemi-azygos vein
8 Costotransverse ligament
9 Common carotid artery
10 Trapezius muscle
11 Left brachiocephalic vein
12 Spinalis thoracis muscle
13 Subclavian artery
14 Sixth rib (head)
15 Aortic arch
16 Transverse process T6
17 Left main bronchus
18 Intertransversarii muscles
19 Pulmonary trunk
20 Rotatores muscles
21 Left atrium
22 Multifidus thoracis muscle
23 Radiate ligament of head of rib T8
24 Latissimus dorsi muscle
25 Hemi-azygos vein
26 Posterior intercostal artery and vein (dorsal branch)
27 Descending aorta
28 Erector spinae muscle
29 Esophagus
30 Superior costotransverse ligament
31 Liver

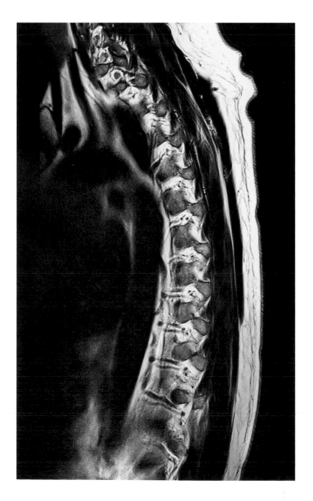

Cranial
Ventral ☐ Dorsal
Caudal

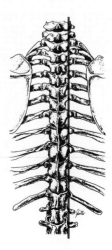

Thoracic Spine, Coronal

1 Trapezius muscle (ascending part)
2 Trapezius muscle (transverse part)
3 Scapula
4 Rhomboid major muscle
5 Interspinal ligament
6 Infraspinatus muscle
7 Longissimus thoracis muscle
8 Spine of vertebra
9 Latissimus dorsi muscle
10 Spinalis thoracis muscle

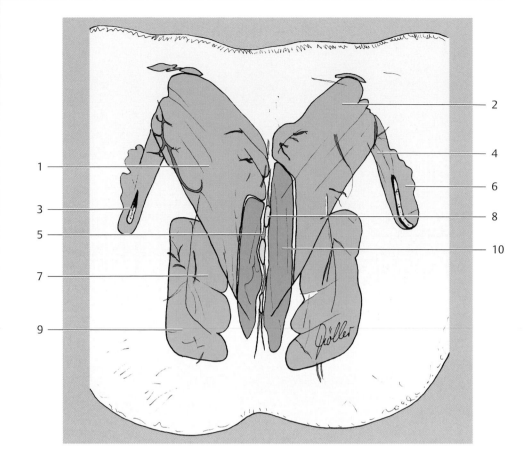

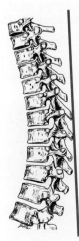

Cranial

Right
Lateral

Left
Lateral

Caudal

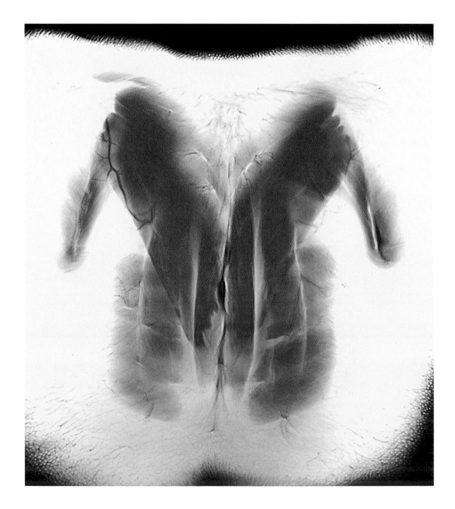

1 Trapezius muscle (transverse part)
2 Splenius cervicis muscle
3 Scapula (spine)
4 Longissimus capitis muscle
5 Rhomboid major muscle
6 Spine of vertebra
7 Infraspinatus muscle
8 Latissimus dorsi muscle
9 Scapula (lateral margin)
10 Interspinal ligament
11 Spinalis thoracis muscle
12 Iliocostalis lumborum muscle
13 Longissimus thoracis muscle

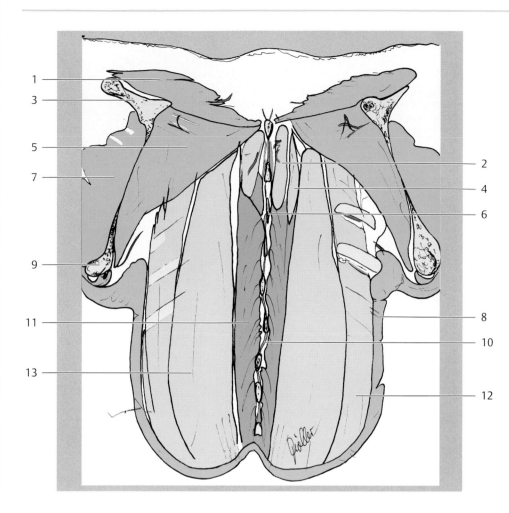

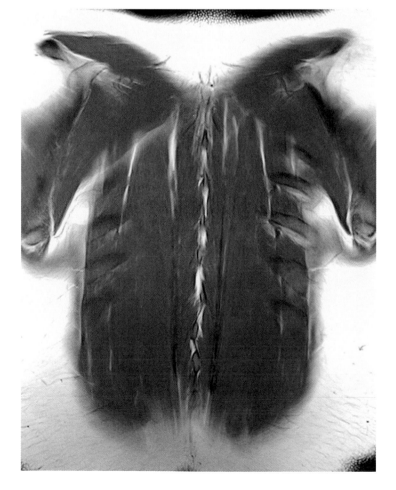

Cranial

Right Lateral | | Left Lateral

Caudal

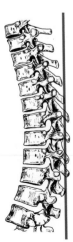

1 Trapezius muscle (transverse part)
2 Splenius cervicis muscle
3 Levator scapulae muscle
4 Supraspinatus muscle
5 Subscapularis muscle
6 Scapula (spine)
7 Semispinalis capitis muscle
8 Rhomboid minor muscle
9 Longissimus capitis muscle
10 Serratus posterior superior muscle
11 Intercostal muscle
12 Iliocostalis cervicis muscle
13 Rib
14 Longissimus cervicis muscle
15 Spinalis cervicis muscle
16 Costotransverse joint
17 Spinous process of vertebra
18 Interspinal ligament
19 Lung
20 Transverse process of vertebra
21 Costotransverse ligament
22 Posterior intercostal artery, vein, and nerve
23 Liver
24 Neck of rib
25 Spinal cord (conus)
26 Diaphragm
27 Lamina of posterior vertebral arch
28 Spinal cord (thoracic part)
29 Inferior articular process
30 Superior articular process
31 Longissimus thoracis muscle, lumbar part
32 Iliocostalis lumborum muscle
33 Posterior inferior serratus muscle
34 Transversus abdominis muscle and external and internal oblique abdominal muscles
35 Latissimus dorsi muscle
36 Spinalis thoracis muscle

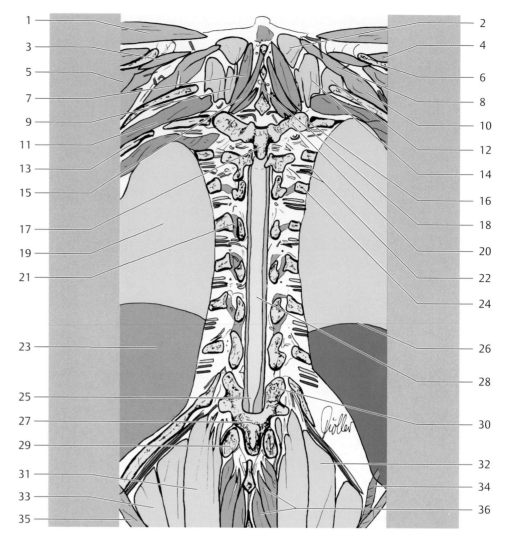

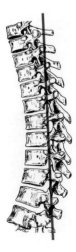

Cranial
Right
Lateral
Left
Lateral
Caudal

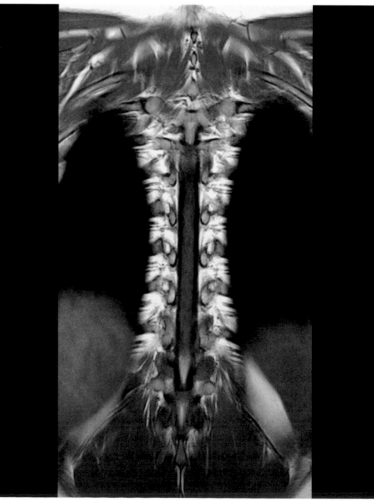

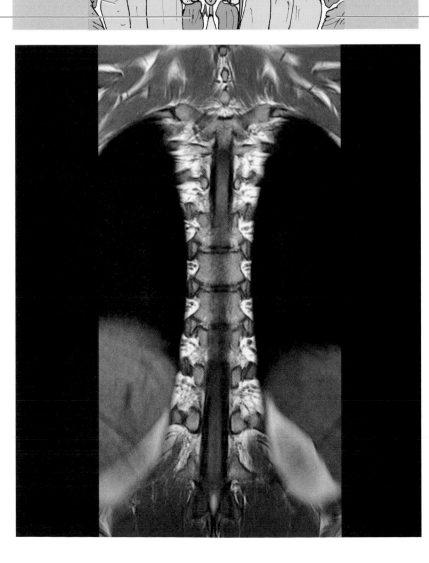

1 Trapezius muscle (transverse part)
2 Semispinalis capitis muscle
3 Splenius cervicis muscle
4 Supraspinatus muscle
5 Levator scapulae muscle
6 Scapula (spine)
7 Subscapularis muscle
8 Serratus posterior superior muscle
9 Longissimus capitis muscle
10 Spinous process of vertebra
11 Spinalis cervicis muscle
12 Rib
13 Costotransverse joint
14 Interspinal ligament
15 Intercostal muscle
16 Transverse process of vertebra
17 Posterior intercostal artery, vein, and nerve
18 Spinal cord (thoracic part)
19 Lung
20 Intervertebral space
21 Head of rib
22 Body of vertebra
23 Diaphragm
24 Longissimus thoracis muscle, lumbar part
25 Liver
26 Spinal cord (conus medullaris)
27 Iliocostalis lumborum muscle
28 Transversus abdominis muscle and external and internal oblique abdominal muscles
29 Serratus posterior inferior muscle
30 Latissimus dorsi muscle
31 Spinalis thoracis muscle

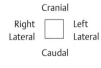

Cranial
Right Lateral   Left Lateral
Caudal

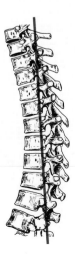

1 Trapezius muscle (transverse part)
2 Semispinalis cervicis muscle
3 Longissimus cervicis muscle
4 Levator scapulae muscle
5 Splenius cervicis muscle
6 Spinalis cervicis muscle
7 Interspinal ligament
8 Tubercle of rib
9 Costotransverse joint
10 Spinous process of vertebra
11 Transverse process of rib
12 Lamina of vertebral arch
13 Intercostal muscle
14 Spinal cord (thoracic part)
15 Posterior intercostal artery, vein, and nerve
16 Nerve root
17 Lateral costotransverse ligament
18 Head of rib
19 Body of vertebra
20 Intervertebral space
21 Lung
22 Spleen
23 Diaphragm
24 Kidney
25 Liver
26 Longissimus muscle, lumbar part
27 Superior joint process
28 Interarticular portion of thoracic vertebra
29 Spinalis thoracis muscle
30 Iliocostalis lumborum muscle

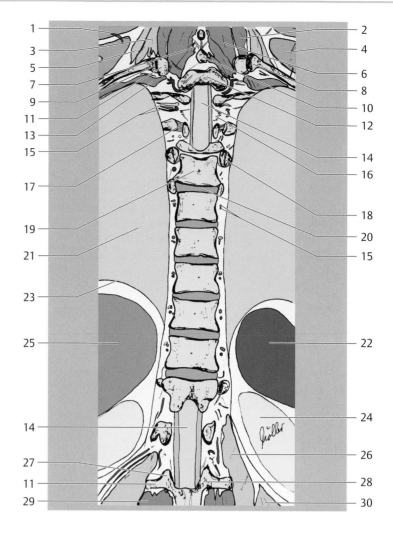

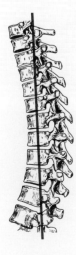

Cranial

Right
Lateral

Left
Lateral

Caudal

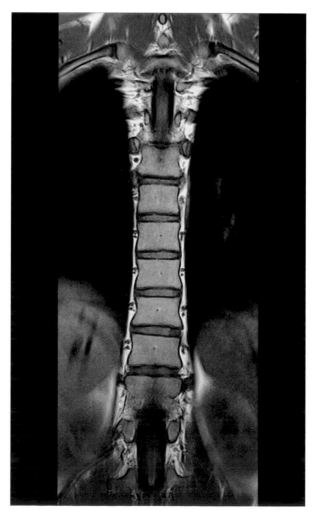

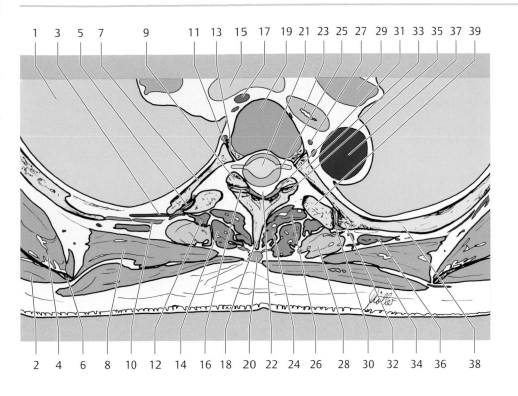

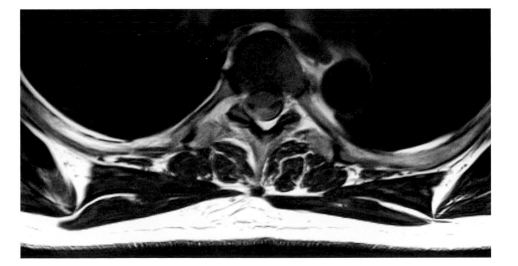

1 Right lung
2 Infraspinatus muscle
3 Intercostal artery
4 Subscapularis muscle
5 Costotransverse joint
6 Scapula
7 Rib (neck)
8 Rhomboid major muscle
9 Fifth rib (head)
10 Intercostal muscles
11 Radiate ligament of head of rib
12 Rotatores thoracis muscles
13 Joint of head of rib
14 Semispinalis thoracis muscle
15 Trachea (bifurcation)
16 Zygapophyseal joint T4/T5
17 Azygos vein
18 Spinous process
19 Intervertebral disk T4/T5
20 Supraspinous ligament
21 Spinal cord (thoracic part)
22 Retrospinal fatty triangle (epidural fat)
23 Esophagus
24 Spinalis thoracis muscle
25 Spinal ganglion
26 Multifidus thoracis muscle
27 Accessory hemi-azygos vein
28 Longissimus thoracis muscle
29 Left pulmonary artery
30 Costotransverse ligament (lateral)
31 Ligamentum flavum
32 Fifth rib (tubercle)
33 Superior articular process T5
34 Trapezius muscle
35 Inferior articular process T4
36 Iliocostalis thoracis muscle
37 Descending aorta
38 Fifth rib (body)
39 Transverse process T5

Ventral

Right ☐ Left

Dorsal

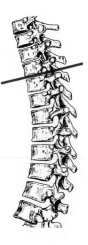

1 Spinal cord
2 Conus medullaris
3 Abdominal aorta
4 Ligamentum flavum
5 Lumbar vertebral body L 1
6 Spinous process L 1
7 Intervertebral disk L 1 / L 2
   (nucleus pulposus)
8 Interspinous ligament
9 Anterior longitudinal ligament
10 Supraspinous ligament
11 Intervertebral disk L 2 / L 3
   (anulus fibrosus)
12 Cauda equina
13 Basivertebral vein
14 Epidural fatty tissue
15 Left common iliac vein
16 Posterior longitudinal ligament
17 Sacral spinal canal
18 Thecal sac (lumbar cistern)
19 Promontory of sacrum
20 Dura mater
21 Sacrum (S 1)
22 Median sacral crest

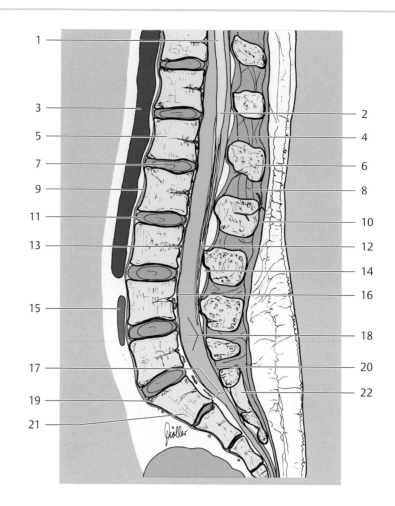

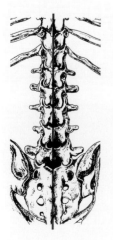

Cranial
Ventral ☐ Dorsal
Caudal

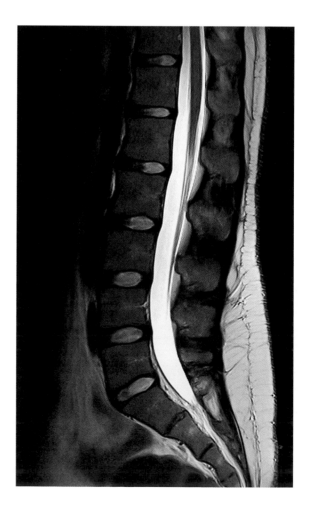

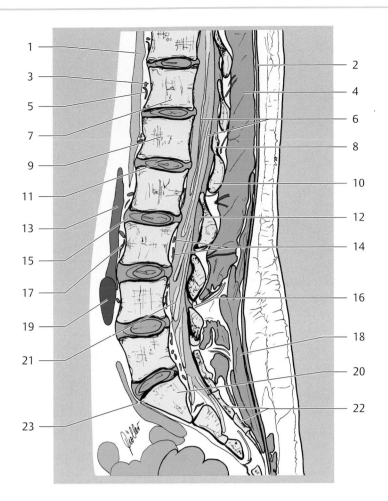

1 Diaphragm (lumbar part)
2 Thoracolumbar fascia
3 Anterior external vertebral venous plexus
4 Erector spinae muscle (spinalis muscle)
5 Posterior intercostal artery
6 Nerve filaments
7 Thoracic vertebral body T12
8 Superior articular process
9 Lumbar vertebral body L1
10 Posterior vertebral arch (lamina)
11 Intervertebral disk L1/L2 (nucleus pulposus)
12 Ligamentum flavum
13 Inferior vena cava
14 Anterior internal vertebral venous plexus
15 Intervertebral disk L2/L3 (anulus fibrosus)
16 Lumbar artery and nerve (medial cutaneous branch of dorsal branch)
17 Lumbar artery
18 Multifidus lumborum muscle
19 Common iliac artery
20 Sacrum (S1)
21 Spinal ganglion
22 Median sacral crest
23 Promontory of sacrum

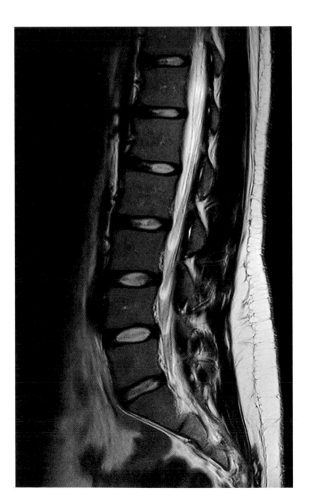

Cranial
Ventral Dorsal
Caudal

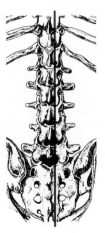

1 Thoracic vertebral body T12
2 Mamillary process
3 Diaphragm (lumbar part)
4 Erector spinae muscle (spinalis thoracis muscle)
5 Lumbar vertebral body L2
6 Thoracolumbar fascia
7 Inferior vena cava
8 Spinal branch of lumbar artery (dorsal branch)
9 Posterior intercostal artery
10 Spinal ganglion L2
11 Intervertebral disk L3/L4 (nucleus pulposus)
12 Posterior vertebral arch (lamina)
13 Ligamentum flavum
14 Intervertebral foramen
15 Superior articular process
16 Inferior articular process
17 Common iliac artery
18 Zygapophyseal joint
19 Promontory of sacrum
20 Multifidus lumborum muscle
21 Sacrum (S1)
22 Gluteus maximus muscle

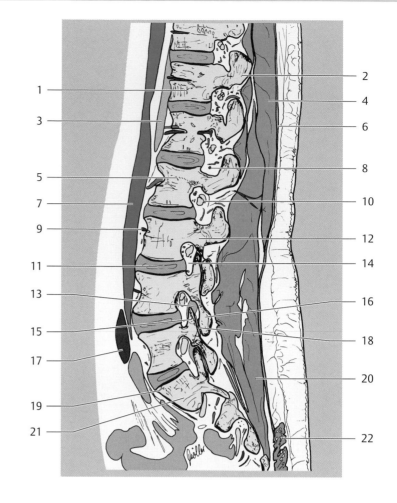

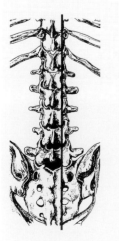

Cranial

Ventral | | Dorsal

Caudal

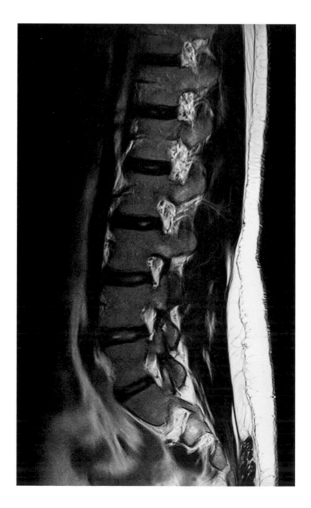

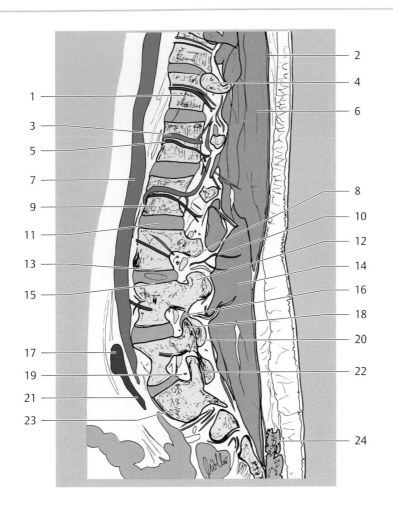

1 Thoracic vertebral body T12
2 Thoracolumbar fascia
3 Lumbar vein
4 Rib (head)
5 Lumbar artery
6 Erector spinae muscle (spinalis muscle)
7 Inferior vena cava
8 Spinal nerve L3
9 Lumbar vertebral body L2
10 Lumbar artery (dorsal branch)
11 Intervertebral disk
12 Transverse process
13 Inferior vertebral endplate
14 Multifidus lumborum muscle
15 Superior vertebral endplate (L4)
16 Ligamentum flavum
17 Common iliac artery
18 Superior articular process
19 Intervertebral foramen
20 Inferior articular process
21 Internal iliac artery
22 Zygapophyseal joint
23 Sacrum (S1)
24 Gluteus maximus muscle

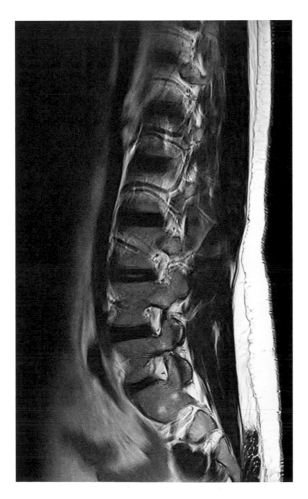

Cranial

Ventral ☐ Dorsal

Caudal

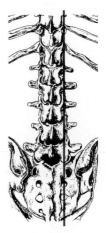

1 Diaphragm (lumbar part)
2 Posterior intercostal artery and vein
3 Thoracic vertebral body T12
4 Left kidney
5 Superior vertebral endplate L 1
6 Psoas major muscle
7 Inferior vertebral endplate L 1
8 Anterior external vertebral venous plexus
9 Intervertebral disk L 1 / L 2 (anulus fibrosus)
10 Transverse process L 4
11 Lumbar artery and vein
12 Iliacus muscle
13 Lumbar plexus
14 Ilium
15 Thecal sac (lumbar cistern)
16 Iliolumbar artery and vein
17 Lumbar vertebral body L 5
18 Internal iliac artery and vein
19 Promontory of sacrum
20 Gluteus medius muscle
21 Median sacral artery and vein

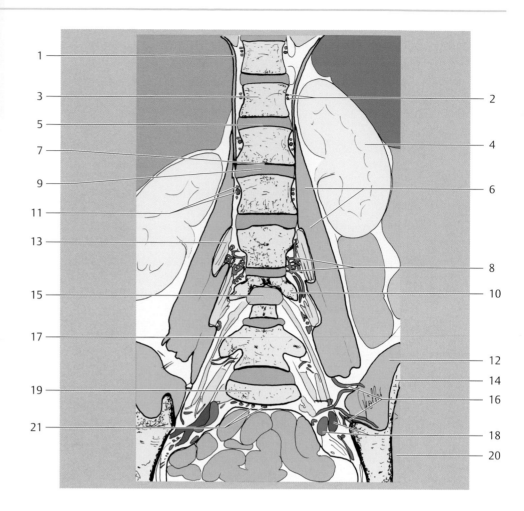

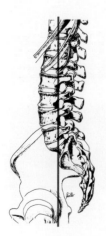

Cranial

Right ☐ Left

Caudal

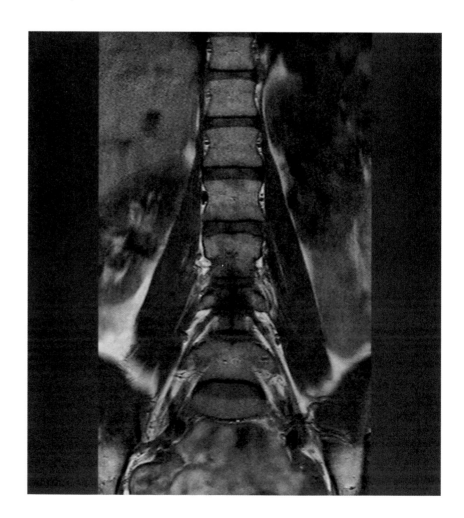

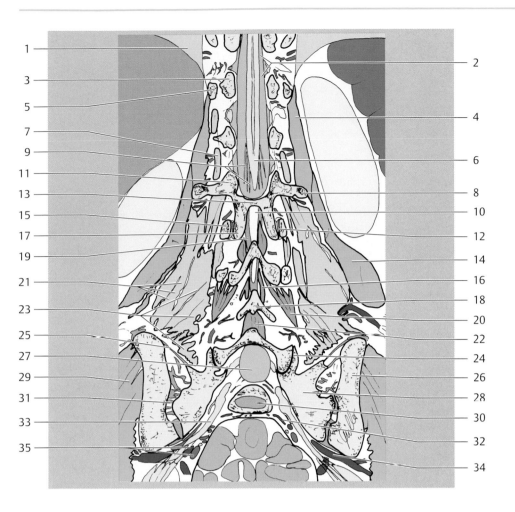

1 Right lung
2 Cerebrospinal fluid in thecal sac (lumbar cistern)
3 Pedicle of vertebral arch T12
4 Psoas major muscle
5 Twelfth rib (head)
6 Conus medullaris
7 Intertransversarii muscles
8 Transverse process L2
9 Cauda equina
10 Posterior epidural fat (retrospinal fat, dorsal fat)
11 Posterior vertebral arch L2 (lamina)
12 Zygapophyseal joint
13 Pedicle of vertebral arch L2
14 Quadratus lumborum muscle
15 Superior articular process L3
16 Interspinales (lumborum) muscles
17 Inferior articular process L2
18 Spinous process L4
19 Ligamentum flavum
20 Multifidus muscle
21 Iliocostalis lumborum muscle
22 Interspinous ligament
23 Longissimus muscle
24 Lumbosacral zygapophyseal joint L5 / S1
25 Sacro-iliac ligaments
26 Ilium
27 Thecal sac (lumbar cistern)
28 Sacrum (lateral mass)
29 Gluteus medius muscle
30 Intervertebral space S1 / S2
31 Sacro-iliac joint
32 Lateral sacral artery and vein
33 Sacral plexus
34 Superior gluteal artery
35 Internal iliac artery and vein

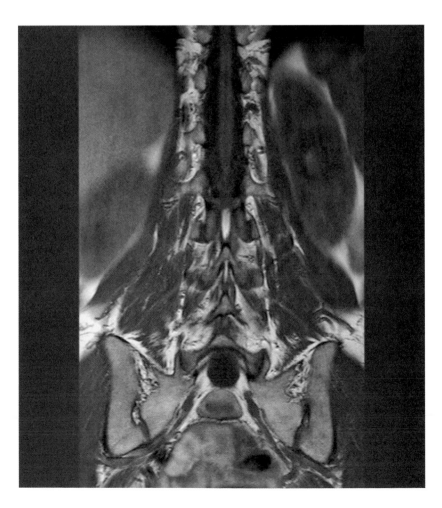

Cranial

Right ☐ Left

Caudal

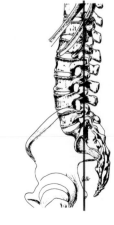

1 Interspinous ligament
2 Spinalis thoracis muscle and rotatores thoracis muscle
3 Serratus anterior muscle
4 Levatores costarum muscles
5 Inferior articular process T12
6 Posterior intercostal artery and vein
7 Superior articular process L 1
8 Intercostal muscles
9 Eleventh rib
10 Zygapophyseal joint
11 Spinous process L 2
12 Iliocostalis lumborum muscle
13 Latissimus dorsi muscle
14 Quadratus lumborum muscle
15 Lumbar artery and vein
16 Longissimus thoracis muscle, lumbar part
17 Posterior vertebral arch S 1 (lamina)
18 Interspinales lumborum muscles
19 Cerebrospinal fluid in thecal sac (lumbar cistern)
20 Multifidus lumborum muscle
21 Sacro-iliac ligaments
22 Ilium
23 Sacrum
24 Gluteus medius muscle
25 Median sacral artery and vein
26 Lateral sacral artery and vein
27 Superior gluteal artery and vein
28 Sacro-iliac joint
29 Piriformis muscle

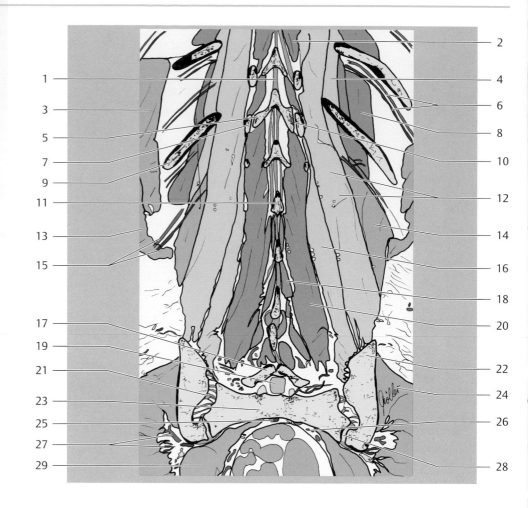

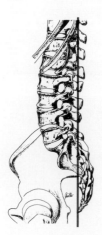

Cranial

Right ☐ Left

Caudal

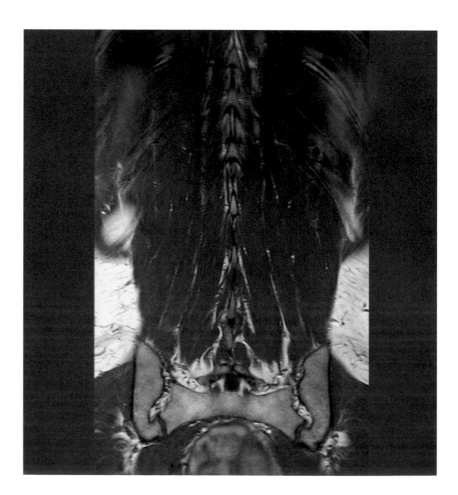

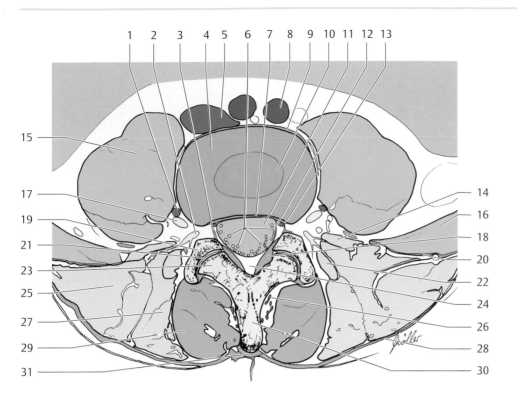

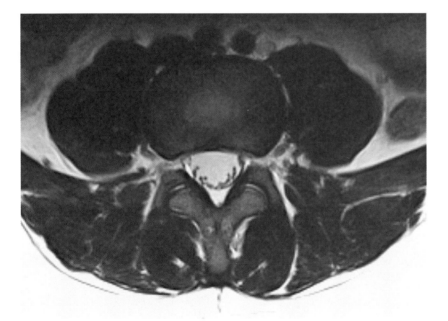

1 Lumbar vein
2 Spinal nerve (dorsal ramus)
3 Neural foraminal ligament
4 Intervertebral disk L 3 / L 4 (anulus fibrosus)
5 Inferior vena cava (confluence)
6 Nerve filaments
7 Posterior longitudinal ligament
8 Left common iliac artery
9 Anterior longitudinal ligament
10 Intervertebral disk L 3 / L 4 (nucleus pulposus)
11 Thecal sac (lumbar cistern)
12 Spinal dura mater
13 Internal vertebral venous plexus
14 Erector spinae muscle (lateral tract: intertransversarii laterales lumborum muscles)
15 Psoas major muscle
16 Quadratus lumborum muscle
17 Spinal ganglion L 3
18 Ligamentum flavum
19 Inferior articular process
20 Thoracolumbar fascia (anterior layer)
21 Zygapophyseal joint
22 Erector spinae muscle (lateral tract: intertransversarii mediales lumborum muscles)
23 Superior articular process
24 Epidural fatty tissue (retrospinal/dorsal fatty triangle)
25 Erector spinae muscle (lateral tract: iliocostalis lumborum muscle)
26 Posterior external vertebral venous plexus
27 Erector spinae muscle (lateral tract: longissimus muscle)
28 Thoracolumbar fascia (posterior layer)
29 Erector spinae muscle (medial tract: multifidus muscle)
30 Spinous process
31 Supraspinous ligament

Ventral

Right ☐ Left

Dorsal

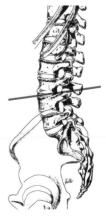

1 Costal process
2 Nerve filaments
3 Lumbar artery
4 Spinal ganglion in lateral recess L4
5 Anterior internal vertebral venous plexus
6 Inferior vena cava (confluence)
7 Nutrient foramen
8 Lumbar vertebral body L4
9 Anterior longitudinal ligament
10 Left common iliac artery
11 Basivertebral vein
12 Ascending lumbar vein
13 Posterior longitudinal ligament
14 Thecal sac (lumbar cistern)
15 Interarticular portion L4
16 Spinal ganglion L3
17 Psoas major muscle
18 Spinal dura mater
19 Zygapophyseal joint
20 Quadratus lumborum muscle
21 Superior articular process
22 Thoracolumbar fascia (anterior layer)
23 Inferior articular process
24 Ligamentum flavum
25 Posterior vertebral arch (lamina)
26 Epidural fatty tissue (retrospinal/dorsal fatty triangle)
27 Posterior external vertebral venous plexus
28 Erector spinae muscle (lateral tract: iliocostalis lumborum muscle)
29 Erector spinae muscle (medial tract: multifidus lumborum muscle)
30 Erector spinae muscle (lateral tract: longissimus muscle)
31 Interspinous ligament
32 Thoracolumbar fascia (posterior layer)
33 Supraspinous ligament

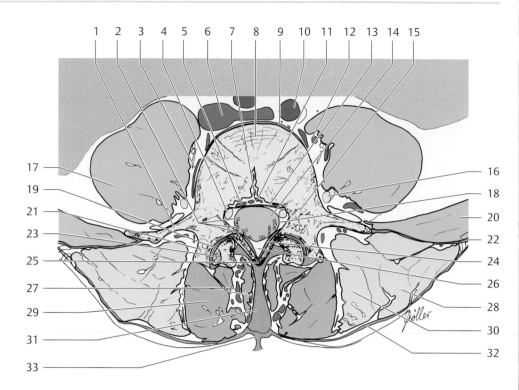

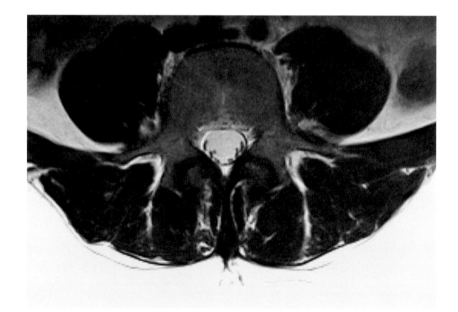

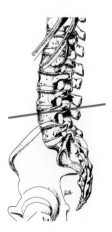

Ventral

Right ☐ Left

Dorsal

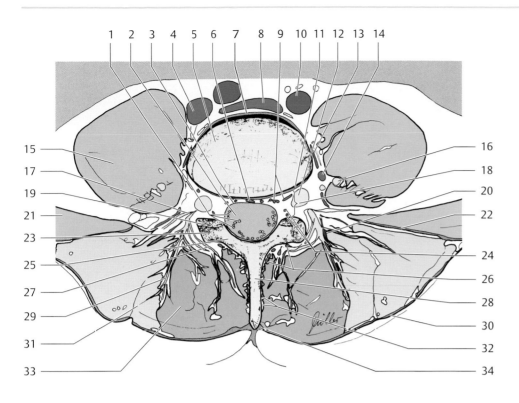

1 2 3 4 5 6 7 8 9 10 11 12 13 14

15
17
19
21
23
25
27
29
31
33

16
18
20
22
24
26
28
30
32
34

1 Nerve filaments
2 Cerebrospinal fluid in thecal sac (lumbar cistern)
3 Spinal dura mater
4 Right common iliac vein
5 Lumbar vertebral body L 4
6 Basivertebral vein
7 Anterior longitudinal ligament
8 Left common iliac vein
9 Anterior internal vertebral venous plexus
10 Left common iliac artery
11 Posterior longitudinal ligament
12 Spinal ganglion L 4
13 Lumbar artery
14 Ascending lumbar vein
15 Psoas major muscle
16 Spinal ganglion L 3
17 Spinal nerve (dorsal branch)
18 Intervertebral foramen
19 Zygapophyseal joint
20 Lumbar artery (lateral cutaneous branch of dorsal branch)
21 Quadratus lumborum muscle
22 Thoracolumbar fascia (anterior layer)
23 Inferior articular process
24 Radicular artery and vein
25 Posterior vertebral arch (lamina)
26 Posterior external vertebral venous plexus
27 Spinal nerve (medial dorsal branch)
28 Spinous process
29 Spinal nerve (lateral dorsal branch)
30 Thoracolumbar fascia (posterior layer)
31 Erector spinae muscle (lateral tract: iliocostalis lumborum and longissimus muscles)
32 Paraspinal fatty tissue
33 Erector spinae muscle (medial tract: multifidus lumborum muscle)
34 Supraspinous ligament

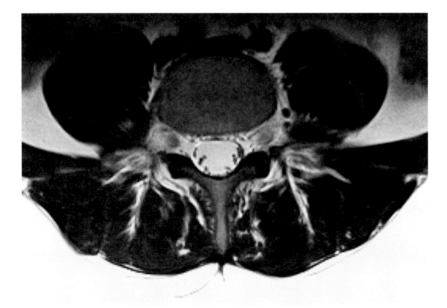

Ventral
Right ☐ Left
Dorsal

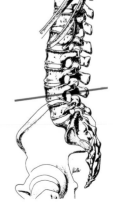

1 Rectus abdominis muscle
2 Ileum
3 External oblique (abdominal) muscle
4 Psoas major muscle
5 Internal oblique (abdominal) muscle
6 Ilium (wing)
7 Transversus abdominis muscle
8 Iliacus muscle
9 Iliac arteries
10 Femoral nerve
11 Common iliac artery and vein
12 Sacral plexus
13 Promontory
14 Sacrum (body of first sacral vertebra)
15 Gluteus medius muscle
16 Sacrum (lateral mass)
17 Sacro-iliac joint
18 Median sacral artery
19 Gluteus maximus muscle
20 Inferior gluteal artery
21 Piriformis muscle
22 Coccygeus muscle
23 Sacrospinous ligament
24 Rectum
25 Coccyx

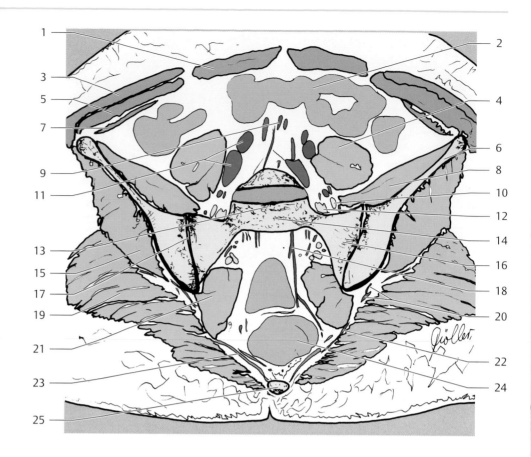

Cranial
Ventral

Right
Lateral   □   Left
Lateral

Caudal
Dorsal

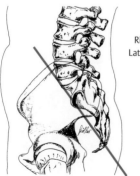

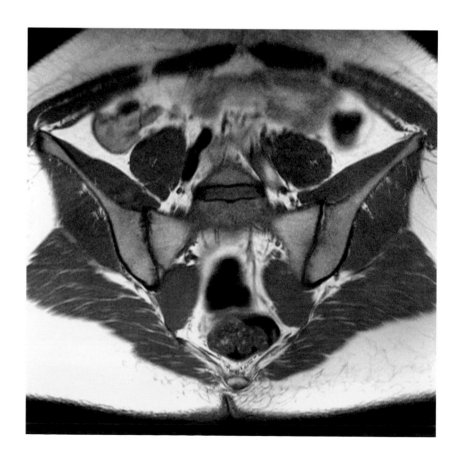

Anatomic Structures Color Code: Upper Extremity

Arteries		Cartilage	
Nerves		Tendon	
Veins		Disk, labrum etc.	
Bones		Fluid	
Fatty tissue			

Shoulder and Muscles of Upper Arm

Muscles of Trunk
Serratus anterior and serratus posterior
Omohyoid
Trapezius
Subclavius
Intercostal

Muscles of Shoulder
Deltoid
Supraspinatus
Infraspinatus
Pectoralis major and minor
Subscapularis
Coracobrachialis
Latissimus dorsi
Teres major and minor

Volar Muscles of Upper Arm
Biceps brachii
Brachialis

Dorsal Muscles of Upper Arm
Triceps brachii
Anconeus

Muscles of Lower Arm

Dorsal Muscles of Lower Arm (superficial layer)
Extensor digitorum
Extensor digiti minimi
Extensor carpi ulnaris

Dorsal Muscles of Lower Arm
Supinator
Extensor pollicis longus and brevis
Extensor indicis

Radial Muscles of Lower Arm
Brachioradialis
Extensor carpi radialis longus
and brevis

Volar Muscles of Lower Arm (superficial layer)
Pronator teres
Flexor digitorum superficialis
Flexor carpi radialis et ulnaris
Palmaris longus et brevis

Volar Muscles of Lower Arm (deep layer)
Flexor digitorum profundus
Flexor pollicis longus
Pronator quadratus

Muscles of Hand

Dorsal and palmar interosseous
Lumbrical

Muscles of Thumb
Abductor pollicis longus and brevis
Opponens pollicis
Flexor pollicis brevis
Adductor pollicis

Muscles of Little (Fifth) Finger
Abductor digiti minimi
Flexor digiti minimi brevis
Opponens digiti minimi

1 Trapezius muscle
2 Deltoid muscle (clavicular part)
3 Clavicle
4 Coracoclavicular ligament
5 Acromioclavicular joint
6 Suprascapular artery and vein
7 Acromion
8 Subclavius muscle
9 Deltoid muscle (acromial part)
10 Omohyoid muscle
11 Supraspinatus muscle (central tendon)
12 Rib
13 Deltoid muscle (spinal part)
14 Serratus anterior muscle
15 Supraspinatus muscle (dorsal ligament)
16 Supraspinatus muscle (ventral ligament)
17 Scapula (spine)

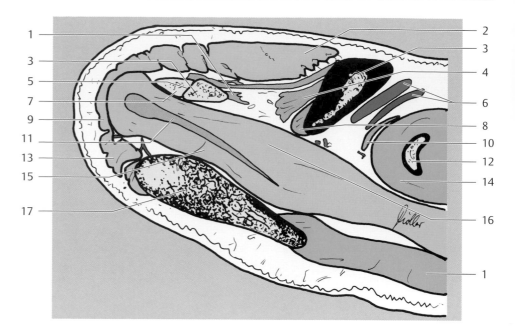

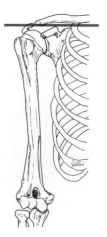

Ventral

Lateral   Medial

Dorsal

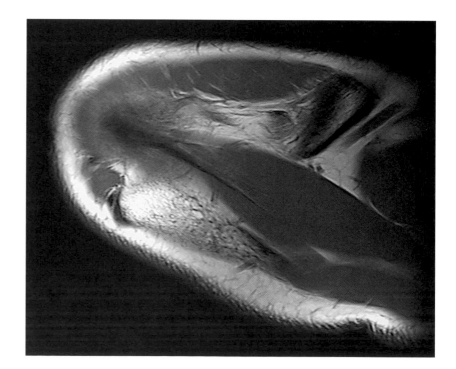

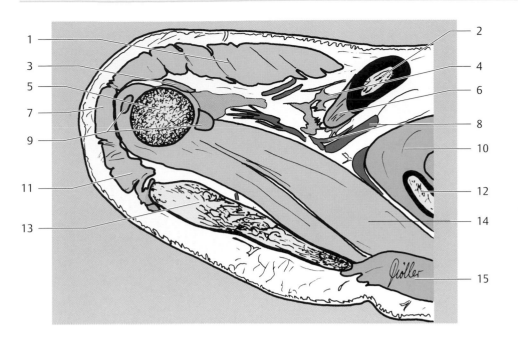

1 Deltoid muscle (clavicular part)
2 Clavicle
3 Coraco-acromial ligament
4 Coracoclavicular ligament
5 Humerus (head)
6 Subclavius muscle
7 Deltoid muscle (acromial part)
8 Suprascapular artery and vein
9 Supraspinatus muscle (tendon)
10 Serratus anterior muscle
11 Deltoid muscle (spinal part)
12 Rib
13 Scapula (spine)
14 Supraspinatus muscle
15 Trapezius muscle

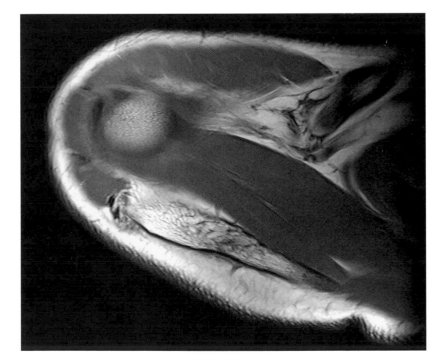

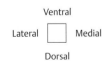

Ventral

Lateral ☐ Medial

Dorsal

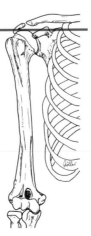

1 Coracohumeral ligament
2 Deltoid muscle (clavicular part)
3 Middle glenohumeral ligament
4 Coracoid process
5 Supraspinatus muscle (tendon)
6 Clavicle
7 Humerus (greater tubercle)
8 Subclavius muscle
9 Deltoid muscle (acromial part)
10 Coracoclavicular ligament
11 Humerus (head)
12 Serratus anterior muscle
13 Superior glenoid labrum
14 Rib
15 Glenoid
16 Internal intercostal muscle
17 Deltoid muscle (spinal part)
18 External intercostal muscle
19 Infraspinatus muscle
20 Supraspinatus muscle
21 Scapula (spine)

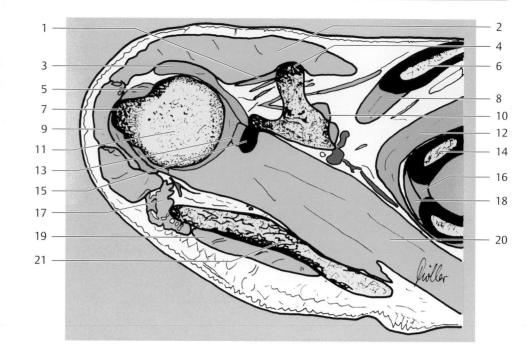

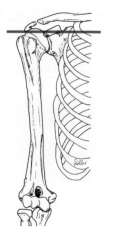

Ventral

Lateral ☐ Medial

Dorsal

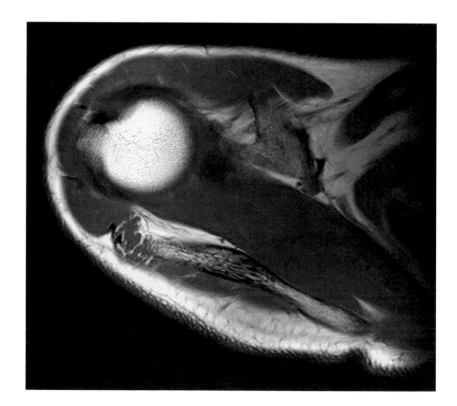

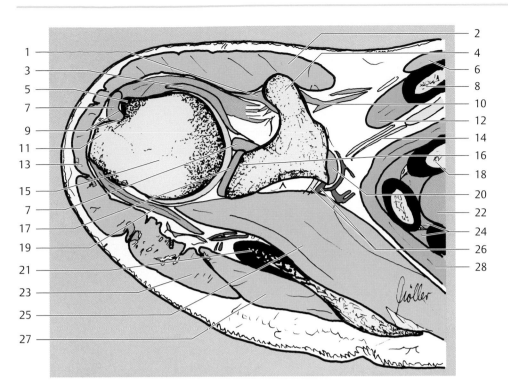

1 Coracohumeral ligament
2 Deltoid muscle (clavicular part)
3 Middle glenohumeral ligament
4 Coracoid process
5 Humerus (lesser tubercle)
6 Pectoralis major muscle
7 Biceps brachii muscle
   (long head, tendon)
8 Clavicle
9 Intertubercular sulcus (bicipital groove)
10 Pectoralis minor muscle (tendon)
11 Humerus (greater tubercle)
12 Subclavius muscle
13 Deltoid muscle (acromial part)
14 Brachial plexus
15 Humerus (head)
16 Glenoid
17 Superior glenoid labrum
18 Rib
19 Infraspinatus muscle (tendon attachment)
20 Coracoclavicular ligament
21 Scapula (spine)
22 Lung
23 Deltoid muscle (spinal part)
24 Internal and external intercostal muscles
25 Supraspinatus muscle
26 Suprascapular artery and vein
27 Infraspinatus muscle
28 Serratus anterior muscle

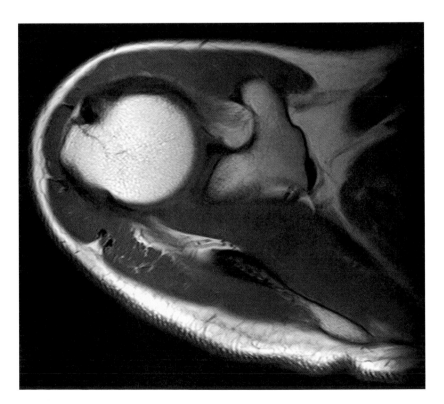

Ventral

Lateral ☐ Medial

Dorsal

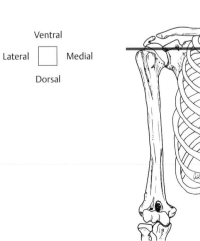

1 Deltoid muscle (clavicular part)
2 Pectoralis major muscle
3 Coracobrachialis muscle (and tendon)
4 Cephalic vein
5 Biceps brachii muscle
(short head, tendon)
6 Subclavius muscle
7 Humerus (lesser tubercle)
8 Pectoralis minor muscle
9 Biceps brachii muscle
(long head, tendon)
10 Axillary artery and vein
11 Humerus (greater tubercle)
12 Brachial plexus and subscapular nerve
13 Middle glenohumeral ligament
14 Subscapularis muscle
15 Deltoid muscle (acromial part)
16 Internal intercostal muscle
17 Anterior glenoid labrum
18 Serratus anterior muscle
19 Humerus (head)
20 Rib
21 Humeroscapular joint
22 Intercostal artery, vein, and nerve
23 Posterior glenoid labrum
24 Glenoid
25 Infraspinatus muscle
26 Suprascapular artery, vein, and nerve
27 Scapula
28 External intercostal muscle
29 Deltoid muscle (spinal part)

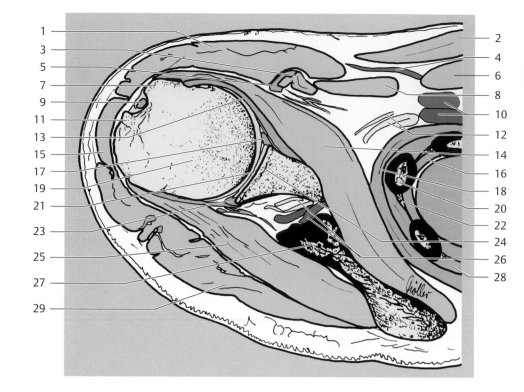

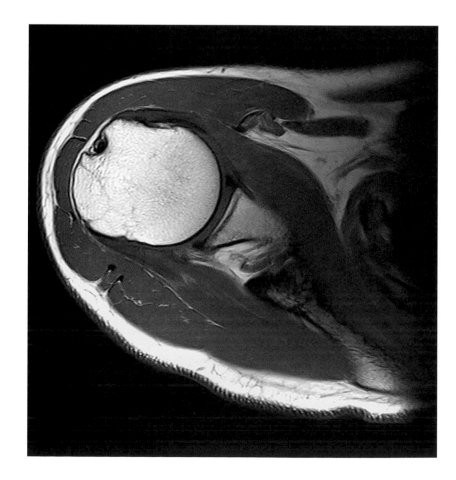

Ventral

Lateral ☐ Medial

Dorsal

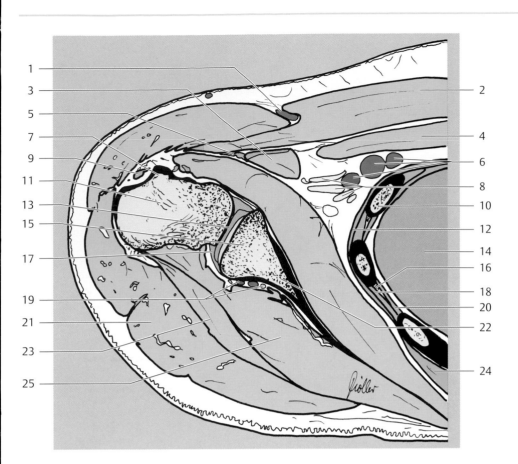

1 Cephalic vein
2 Pectoralis major muscle
3 Coracobrachialis muscle (and tendon)
4 Pectoralis minor muscle
5 Biceps brachii muscle
   (short head, tendon)
6 Axillary artery and vein
7 Humerus (lesser tubercle)
8 Brachial plexus
9 Biceps brachii muscle
   (long head, tendon)
10 Rib
11 Humerus
12 Serratus anterior muscle
13 Inferior glenoid labrum
14 Lung
15 Glenoid
16 Intercostal artery, vein, and nerve
17 Joint capsule
18 External intercostal muscle
19 Suprascapular artery, vein, and nerve
20 Internal intercostal muscle
21 Deltoid muscle
22 Scapula
23 Teres minor muscle
24 Serratus posterior muscle
25 Infraspinatus muscle

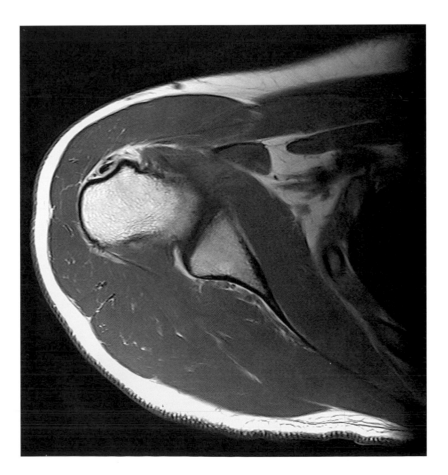

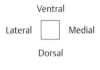

Ventral

Lateral Medial

Dorsal

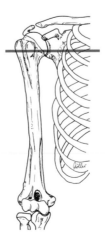

1 Cephalic vein
2 Pectoralis major muscle
3 Coracobrachialis muscle (and tendon)
4 Pectoralis minor muscle
5 Biceps brachii muscle
  (short head and tendon)
6 Axillary artery and vein
7 Biceps brachii muscle
  (long head, tendon)
8 Rib
9 Humerus (lesser tubercle)
10 Brachial plexus
11 Humerus
12 Subscapularis muscle
13 Joint capsule
14 Lung
15 Deltoid muscle
16 Internal and innermost intercostal
  muscles
17 Scapula (neck)
18 Intercostal artery, vein, and nerve
19 Circumflex scapular artery and vein
20 External intercostal muscle
21 Infraspinatus muscle
22 Serratus anterior muscle
23 Teres minor muscle

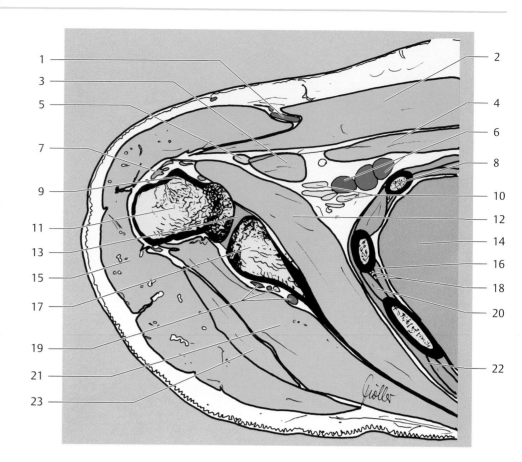

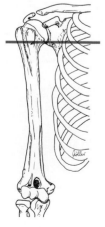

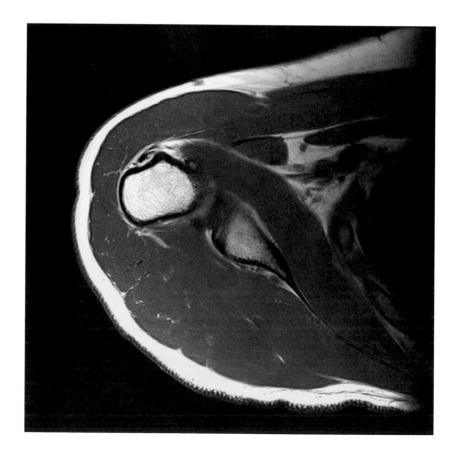

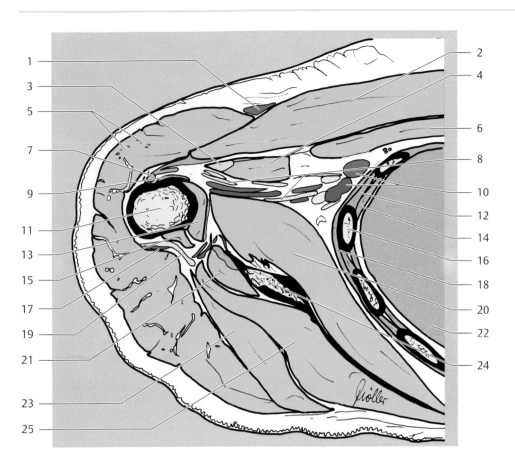

1 Cephalic vein
2 Pectoralis major muscle
3 Biceps brachii muscle (short head)
4 Coracobrachialis muscle (and tendon)
5 Deltoid muscle
6 Pectoralis minor muscle
7 Biceps brachii muscle
   (long head, tendon)
8 Brachial plexus
9 Latissimus dorsi muscle
   (tendon attachment)
10 Axillary artery and vein
11 Humerus
12 External intercostal muscle
13 Teres major muscle
14 Internal and innermost intercostal
   muscles
15 Triceps brachii muscle (lateral head)
16 Rib
17 Posterior circumflex humeral artery
   and vein
18 Serratus anterior muscle
19 Axillary nerve
20 Subscapularis muscle
21 Triceps brachii muscle
   (long head, insertion)
22 Lung
23 Teres minor muscle
24 Scapula
25 Infraspinatus muscle

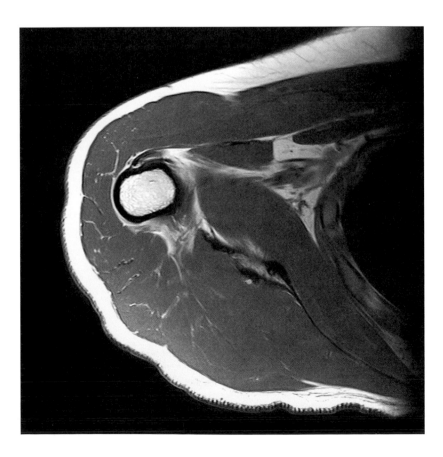

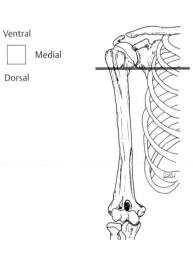

Ventral
Lateral ☐ Medial
Dorsal

1 Cephalic vein
2 Pectoralis major muscle
3 Biceps brachii muscle
  (short head, tendon)
4 Pectoralis minor muscle
5 Biceps brachii muscle
  (long head, tendon)
6 Coracobrachialis muscle
7 Humerus
8 Long thoracic nerve
9 Latissimus dorsi muscle and teres
  major muscle
10 Axillary artery and vein and brachial
  plexus
11 Deltoid muscle
12 Rib
13 Triceps brachii muscle (lateral head)
14 Anterior circumflex humeral artery
  and vein
15 Axillary nerve
16 Subscapularis muscle
17 Posterior circumflex humeral artery
  and vein
18 Lung
19 Triceps brachii muscle (long head)
20 Internal intercostal muscle and
  innermost intercostal muscle
21 Circumflex scapular artery
22 External intercostal muscle
23 Teres minor muscle
24 Serratus anterior muscle
25 Infraspinatus muscle
26 Scapula

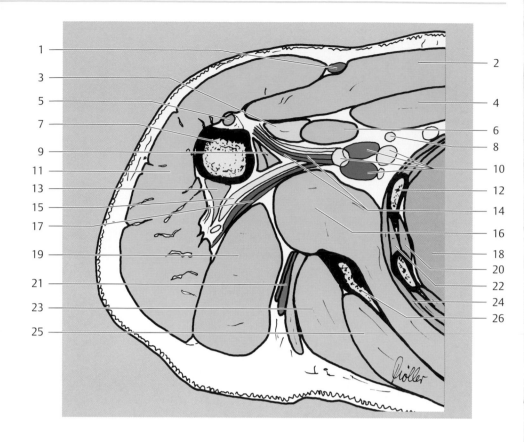

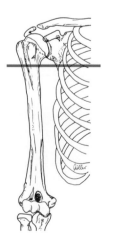

Ventral

Lateral   ☐   Medial

Dorsal

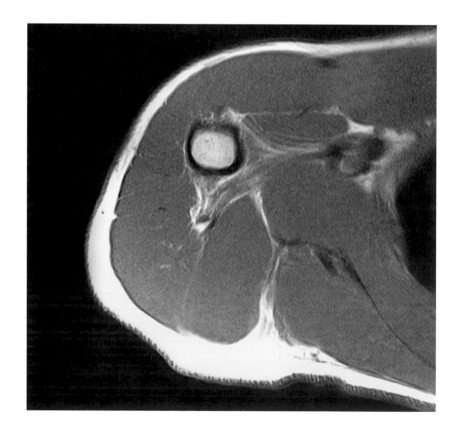

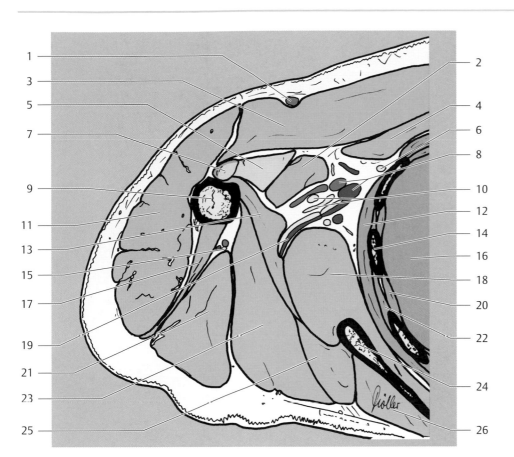

1 Cephalic vein
2 Coracobrachialis muscle
3 Pectoralis major muscle
4 Pectoralis minor muscle
5 Biceps brachii muscle (short head)
6 Long thoracic nerve
7 Biceps brachii muscle
   (long head and tendon)
8 Axillary artery and vein
9 Humerus
10 Brachial plexus
11 Deltoid muscle
12 Serratus anterior muscle
13 Latissimus dorsi muscle
14 Rib
15 Radial nerve (muscular branch)
16 Lung
17 Triceps brachii muscle (lateral head)
18 Subscapularis muscle
19 Subscapular artery
20 Internal and innermost intercostal
    muscles
21 Triceps brachii muscle (long head)
22 External intercostal muscle
23 Teres major muscle
24 Scapula
25 Teres minor muscle
26 Infraspinatus muscle

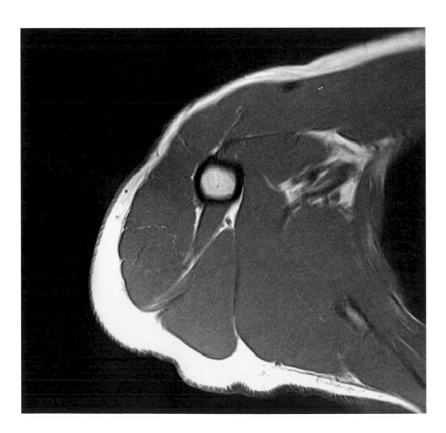

Ventral

Lateral ☐ Medial

Dorsal

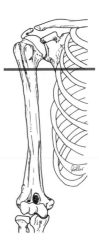

1 Pectoralis major muscle
2 Pectoralis minor muscle
3 Cephalic vein
4 Serratus anterior muscle
5 Biceps brachii muscle
6 Lateral thoracic artery and vein
7 Coracobrachialis muscle
8 Axillary artery and vein
9 Deltoid muscle
10 Lung
11 Humerus
12 Rib
13 Deep artery and vein of arm
14 Internal and innermost intercostal
   muscles
15 Radial nerve
16 External intercostal muscle
17 Triceps brachii muscle (lateral head)
18 Subscapularis muscle
19 Teres major muscle
20 Scapula
21 Triceps brachii muscle (long head)
22 Infraspinatus muscle
23 Teres major muscle and latissimus
   dorsi muscle

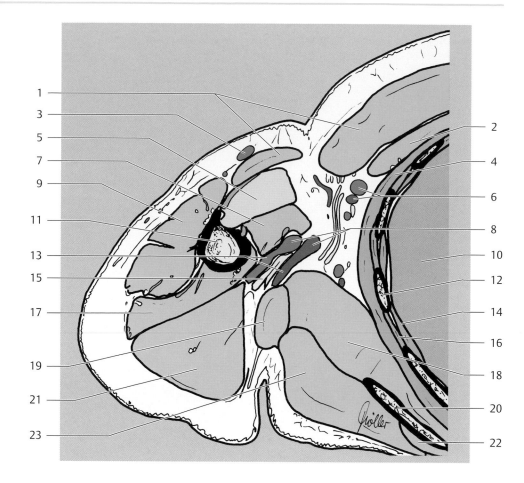

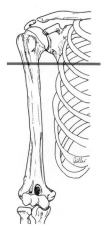

Ventral

Lateral ☐ Medial

Dorsal

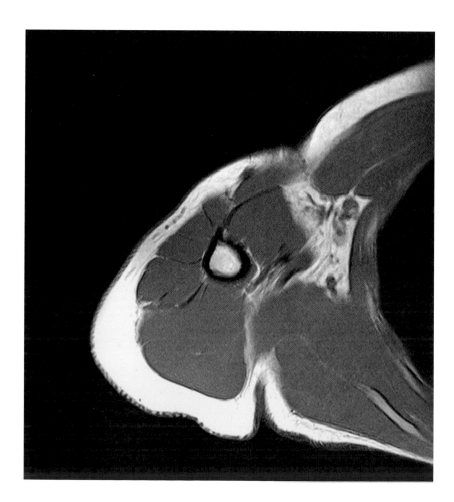

1 Cephalic vein
2 Pectoralis major muscle
3 Biceps brachii muscle
4 Pectoralis minor muscle
5 Coracobrachialis muscle
6 Lung
7 Musculocutaneous nerve
8 Rib
9 Deltoid muscle
10 Intercostal artery, vein, and nerve
11 Humerus (shaft)
12 Brachial artery and vein
13 Radial nerve
14 Median nerve
15 Triceps brachii muscle (medial head)
16 Thoracodorsal artery and nerve
17 Ulnar nerve
18 Serratus anterior muscle
19 Triceps brachii muscle (lateral head)
20 Internal and innermost intercostal muscles
21 Triceps brachii muscle (lateral head)
22 External intercostal muscle
23 Teres major muscle and latissimus dorsi muscle
24 Infraspinatus muscle

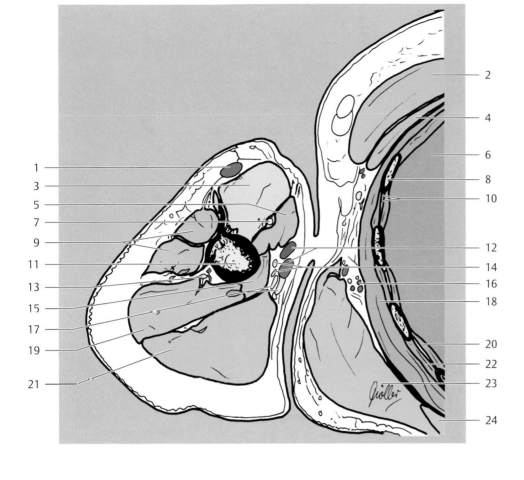

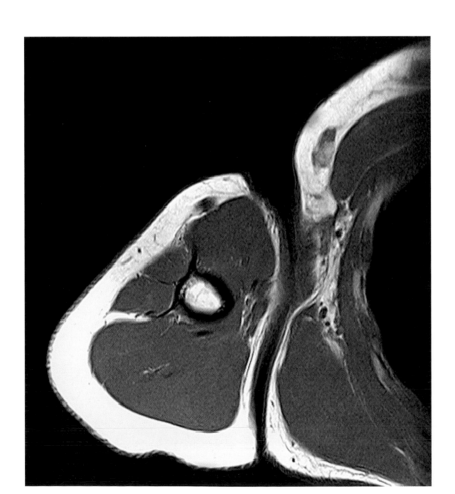

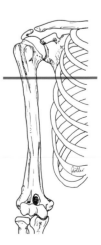

1 Cephalic vein
2 Biceps brachii muscle (short head)
3 Biceps brachii muscle (long head)
4 Musculocutaneous nerve
5 Brachialis muscle
6 Median nerve
7 Deep artery and vein of the arm
8 Brachial artery and vein
9 Brachioradialis muscle
10 Basilic vein
11 Radial nerve
12 Ulnar nerve
13 Posterior cutaneous nerve of forearm (branch)
14 Humerus (shaft)
15 Triceps brachii muscle (lateral head)
16 Triceps brachii muscle (medial head)
17 Triceps brachii muscle (long head)

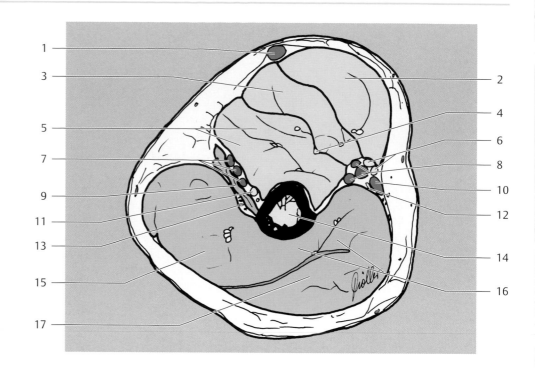

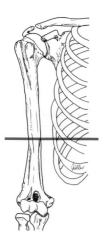

Ventral

Lateral ☐ Medial

Dorsal

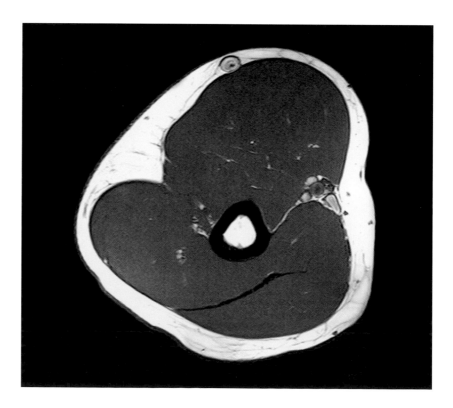

1 Cephalic vein
2 Biceps brachii muscle (short head)
3 Biceps brachii muscle (long head)
4 Musculocutaneous nerve
5 Brachialis muscle
6 Median nerve
7 Deep artery and vein of arm
8 Brachial artery and vein
9 Brachioradialis muscle
10 Basilic vein
11 Radial nerve
12 Ulnar nerve, artery, and vein
13 Posterior cutaneous nerve of forearm
14 Triceps brachii muscle (medial head)
15 Triceps brachii muscle (lateral head)
16 Triceps brachii muscle (tendon)
17 Humerus (shaft)
18 Triceps brachii muscle (long head)

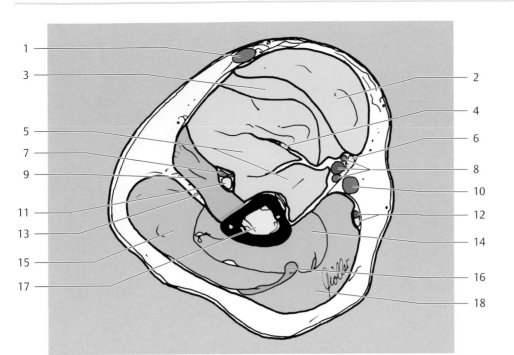

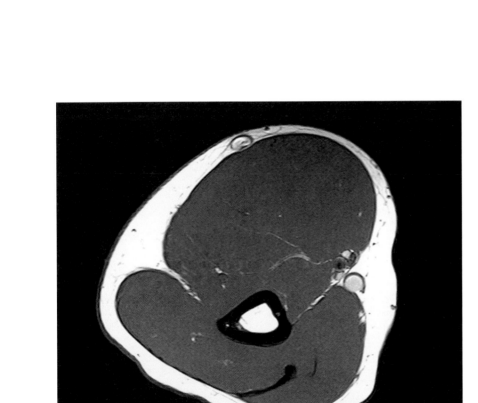

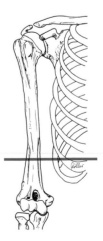

1 Cephalic vein
2 Biceps brachii muscle (short head)
3 Biceps brachii muscle (long head)
4 Musculocutaneous nerve
5 Brachioradialis muscle
6 Brachial artery and vein
7 Radial nerve
8 Median nerve
9 Deep brachial artery and vein
10 Brachialis muscle
11 Extensor carpi radialis longus muscle
12 Basilic vein
13 Posterior cutaneous nerve of forearm
14 Humerus (shaft)
15 Triceps brachii muscle
16 Ulnar nerve, artery, and vein

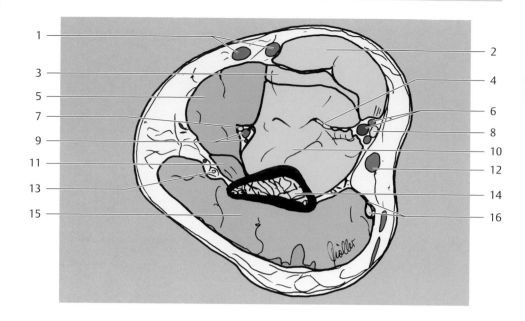

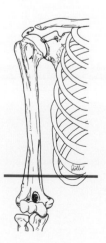

Ventral

Lateral   Medial

Dorsal

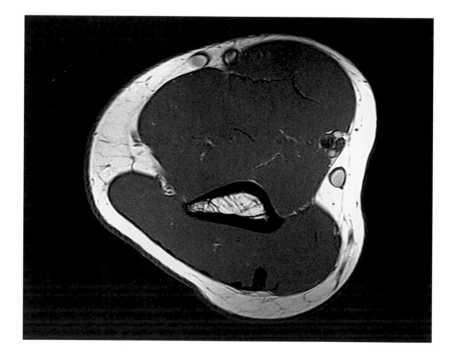

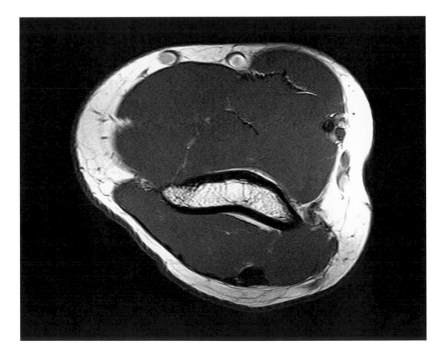

1 Cephalic vein
2 Biceps brachii muscle (short head)
3 Brachioradialis muscle
4 Biceps brachii muscle
   (long head, tendon)
5 Radial nerve
6 Brachial artery and vein
7 Deep brachial artery and nerve
8 Median nerve
9 Extensor carpi radialis longus muscle
10 Basilic vein
11 Medial collateral artery
12 Brachialis muscle
13 Posterior cutaneous nerve of forearm
14 Ulnar nerve
15 Humerus (shaft)
16 Ulnar artery and vein
17 Triceps brachii muscle (lateral head)
18 Triceps brachii muscle (medial head)
19 Triceps brachii muscle (tendon)

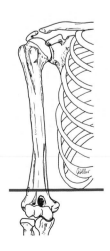

Ventral

Lateral Medial

Dorsal

1 Median cubital vein
2 Cutaneous nerve of forearm
3 Cephalic vein
4 Biceps brachii muscle (and tendon)
5 Brachioradialis muscle
6 Brachial artery and vein
7 Radial nerve
8 Median nerve
9 Lateral cutaneous nerve of forearm
10 Brachialis muscle
11 Extensor carpi radialis longus muscle
12 Coronoid fossa
13 Collateral radial artery and vein
14 Pronator teres muscle
15 Lateral humeral epicondyle
16 Basilic vein
17 Olecranon fossa
18 Medial cutaneous nerve of forearm
19 Anconeus muscle
20 Tendon attachment of anterior
   superficial muscles of forearm and
   collateral ligaments
21 Olecranon
22 Medial epicondyle of humerus
23 Triceps brachii muscle (and tendon)
24 Ulnar nerve
25 Superior ulnar collateral artery
   and vein

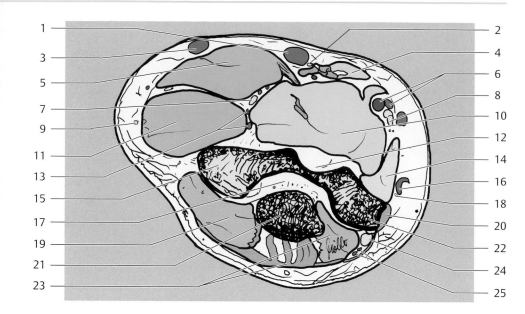

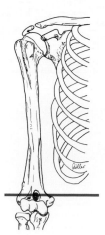

Ventral

Lateral | | Medial

Dorsal

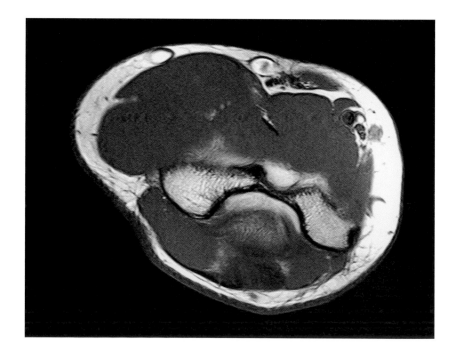

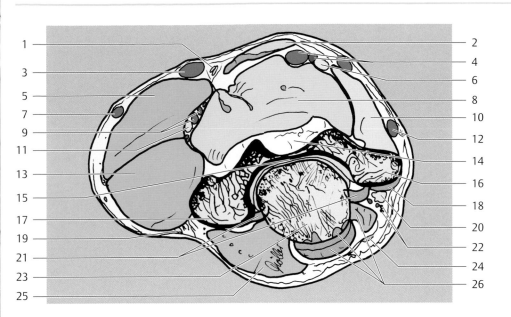

1 Cutaneous nerve of forearm
2 Biceps brachii muscle (and tendon)
3 Median cubital vein
4 Brachial artery and vein
5 Brachioradialis muscle
6 Median nerve
7 Cephalic vein
8 Brachialis muscle
9 Radial collateral artery and vein
10 Pronator teres muscle
11 Radial nerve
12 Basilic vein
13 Extensor carpi radialis longus muscle
14 Coronoid fossa
15 Humero-ulnar joint
16 Medial epicondyle of humerus
17 Lateral epicondyle of humerus
18 Tendon attachment of ventral
   superficial muscles of forearm and
   collateral ligaments
19 Posterior cutaneous nerve of forearm
   (radial nerve)
20 Ulnar nerve
21 Joint capsule
22 Superior collateral ulnar artery and vein
23 Olecranon
24 Subcutaneous olecranon bursa
25 Anconeus muscle
26 Triceps brachii muscle (and tendon)

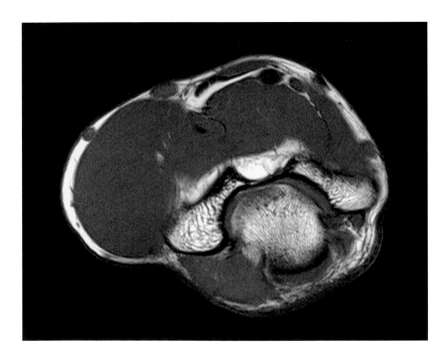

Ventral

Lateral | | Medial

Dorsal

1 Cutaneous nerve of forearm
2 Bicipital aponeurosis
3 Median cubital vein
4 Brachial artery and vein
5 Biceps brachii muscle (tendon)
6 Median nerve
7 Brachioradialis muscle
8 Pronator teres muscle
9 Cephalic vein
10 Brachialis muscle (and tendon)
11 Radial nerve
12 Articular capsule of elbow
13 Radial collateral artery and vein
14 Basilic vein
15 Humerus (capitulum)
16 Flexor carpi radialis muscle (tendon attachment)
17 Extensor carpi radialis longus muscle
18 Palmaris longus muscle (tendon attachment)
19 Lateral collateral ligament
20 Medial epicondyle of humerus
21 Posterior cutaneous nerve of forearm (radial nerve)
22 Ulnar nerve
23 Humero-ulnar joint
24 Superior collateral ulnar artery and vein
25 Anconeus muscle
26 Triceps brachii muscle (and tendon)
27 Olecranon
28 Subcutaneous olecranon bursa

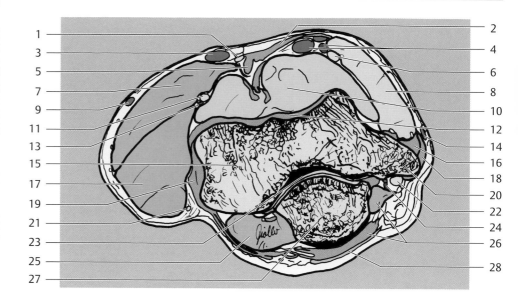

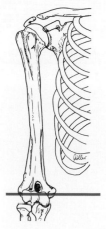

Ventral

Lateral [ ] Medial

Dorsal

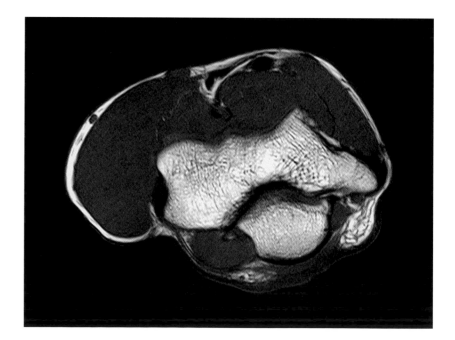

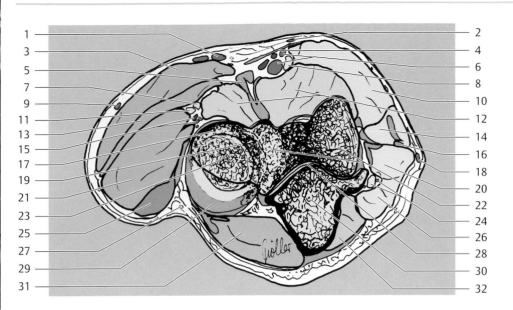

1 Median cubital vein
2 Cutaneous nerve of forearm
3 Brachioradialis muscle
4 Aponeurosis of biceps brachii muscle
5 Biceps brachii muscle (tendon)
6 Brachial artery and vein
7 Radial nerve (superficial branch)
8 Median nerve
9 Cephalic vein
10 Pronator teres muscle
11 Radial nerve (deep branch)
12 Brachialis muscle (and tendon)
13 Extensor carpi radialis longus muscle
14 Flexor carpi radialis muscle
15 Collateral radial artery and vein
16 Palmaris longus muscle
17 Humerus (capitulum)
18 Basilic vein
19 Humeroradial joint
20 Flexor digitorum superficialis muscle
21 Extensor carpi radialis brevis muscle
22 Humerus (trochlea)
23 Radius (head)
24 Ulnar nerve and superior ulnar collateral artery and vein
25 Extensor digitorum muscle
26 Flexor carpi ulnaris muscle
27 Posterior cutaneous nerve of forearm
28 Humero-ulnar joint
29 Anular ligament of radius
30 Olecranon
31 Anconeus muscle
32 Flexor digitorum profundus muscle

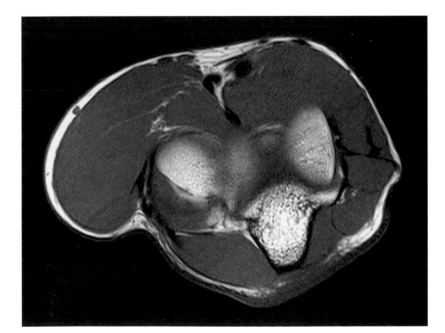

Ventral

Radial ☐ Ulnar

Dorsal

1 Median cubital vein
2 Bicipital aponeurosis
3 Brachioradialis muscle
4 Brachial artery and vein
5 Biceps brachii muscle (tendon)
6 Median nerve
7 Extensor carpi radialis longus muscle
8 Pronator teres muscle
9 Cephalic vein
10 Brachialis muscle (and tendon)
11 Radial nerve (superficial branch)
12 Flexor carpi radialis muscle
13 Radial nerve (deep branch)
14 Palmaris longus muscle
15 Supinator muscle (tendon)
16 Flexor digitorum superficialis muscle
17 Extensor carpi radialis brevis muscle
18 Basilic vein
19 Radius (head)
20 Ulnar nerve
21 Anular ligament of radius
22 Superior ulnar collateral artery
   and vein
23 Extensor digitorum muscle
24 Flexor carpi ulnaris muscle
25 Extensor carpi ulnaris muscle
26 Proximal radio-ulnar joint
27 Recurrent interosseous artery
28 Flexor digitorum profundus muscle
29 Anconeus muscle
30 Ulna

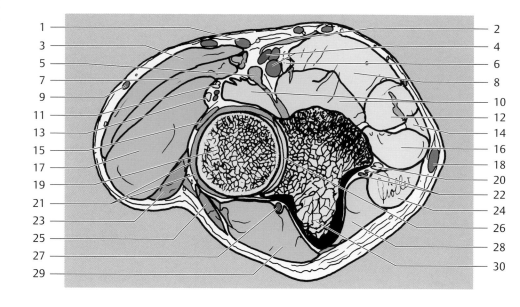

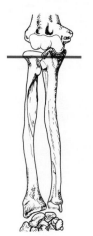

Ventral

Radial ☐ Ulnar

Dorsal

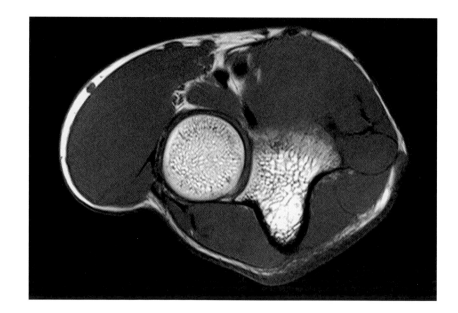

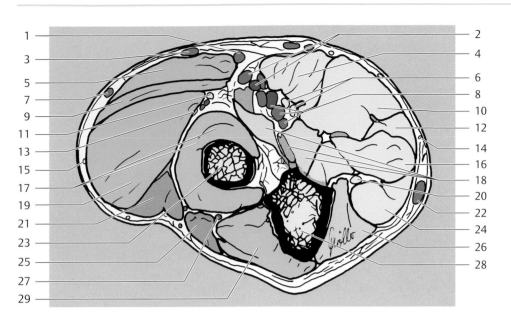

1 Median cubital vein
2 Radial artery and vein
3 Accessory cephalic vein
4 Pronator teres muscle
5 Brachioradialis muscle
6 Median nerve
7 Cephalic vein
8 Ulnar artery and vein
9 Extensor carpi radialis longus muscle
10 Flexor carpi radialis muscle
11 Radial nerve (superficial branch)
12 Palmaris longus muscle
13 Radial nerve (deep branch)
14 Medial cutaneous nerve of forearm
15 Posterior cutaneous nerve of forearm
16 Flexor digitorum superficialis muscle
17 Supinator muscle
18 Brachialis muscle (and tendon attachment)
19 Extensor carpi radialis brevis muscle
20 Ulnar nerve
21 Extensor digitorum muscle
22 Basilic vein
23 Radius
24 Flexor carpi ulnaris muscle
25 Extensor carpi ulnaris muscle
26 Flexor digitorum profundus muscle
27 Recurrent interosseous artery and vein
28 Ulna
29 Anconeus muscle

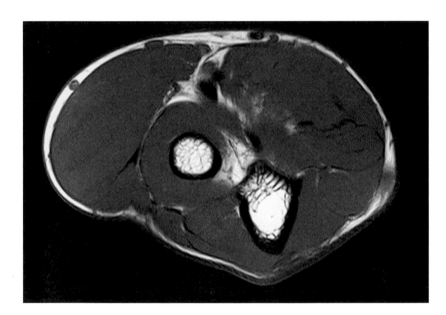

Ventral
Radial ☐ Ulnar
Dorsal

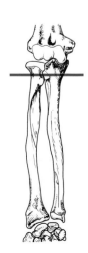

1 Median cubital vein
2 Pronator teres muscle
3 Radial artery and vein
4 Flexor carpi radialis muscle
5 Brachioradialis muscle
6 Anterior interosseous artery and vein
7 Cephalic vein
8 Ulnar artery and vein
9 Radial nerve (superficial branch)
10 Palmaris longus muscle
11 Extensor carpi radialis longus muscle
12 Median nerve
13 Lateral cutaneous nerve of forearm
14 Medial cutaneous nerve of forearm
15 Radial nerve (deep branch)
16 Flexor digitorum superficialis muscle
17 Biceps brachii muscle (tendon)
18 Brachialis muscle (and tendon attachment)
19 Extensor carpi radialis brevis muscle
20 Ulnar nerve
21 Supinator muscle
22 Pronator teres muscle (ulnar head, tendon attachment)
23 Radius
24 Flexor carpi ulnaris muscle
25 Extensor digitorum muscle
26 Basilic vein
27 Extensor digiti minimi muscle
28 Flexor digitorum profundus muscle
29 Recurrent interosseous artery and vein
30 Ulna
31 Extensor pollicis longus muscle
32 Extensor carpi ulnaris muscle

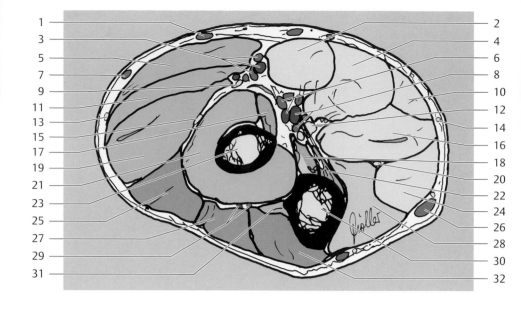

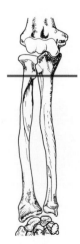

Ventral

Radial   ☐   Ulnar

Dorsal

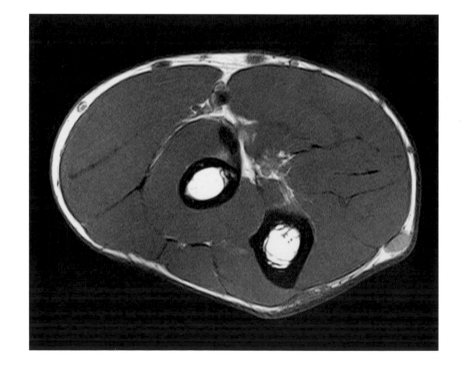

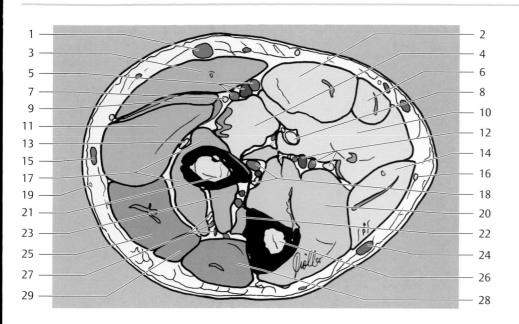

1   Median cubital vein
2   Flexor carpi radialis muscle
3   Brachioradialis muscle
4   Pronator teres muscle
5   Radial artery and vein
6   Palmaris longus muscle
7   Radial nerve (superficial branch)
8   Median nerve
9   Extensor carpi radialis longus muscle
    (and tendon)
10   Flexor digitorum superficialis muscle
11   Extensor carpi radialis brevis muscle
12   Ulnar artery, vein, and nerve
13   Radial nerve (deep branch)
14   Flexor carpi ulnaris muscle
15   Cephalic vein
16   Medial cutaneous nerve of forearm
17   Supinator muscle
18   Anterior interosseous artery and vein
19   Lateral cutaneous nerve of forearm
20   Flexor digitorum profundus muscle
21   Radius
22   Extensor pollicis longus muscle
23   Abductor pollicis longus muscle
24   Basilic vein
25   Extensor digitorum muscle
26   Ulna
27   Posterior interosseous artery, vein,
    and nerve
28   Extensor carpi ulnaris muscle
29   Extensor digiti minimi muscle

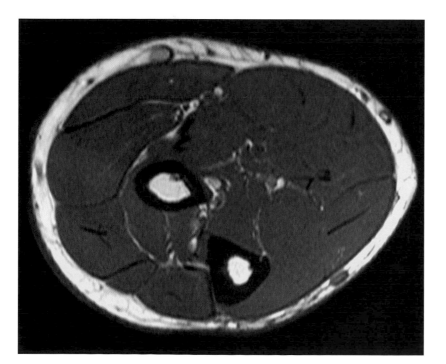

Ventral

Radial ☐ Ulnar

Dorsal

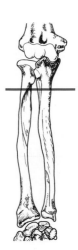

1 Median cubital vein
2 Flexor carpi radialis muscle
3 Brachioradialis muscle
4 Palmaris longus muscle
5 Radial artery and vein
6 Flexor digitorum superficialis muscle
7 Radial nerve (superficial branch)
8 Median nerve
9 Extensor carpi radialis longus muscle
   (and tendon)
10 Ulnar artery and vein
11 Pronator teres muscle
12 Ulnar nerve
13 Extensor carpi radialis brevis muscle
14 Flexor carpi ulnaris muscle
15 Flexor pollicis longus muscle
16 Posterior interosseous artery, vein, and
   nerve
17 Radial nerve (deep branch)
18 Flexor digitorum profundus muscle
19 Radius
20 Cephalic vein
21 Supinator muscle
22 Ulna
23 Abductor pollicis longus muscle
24 Extensor pollicis longus muscle
25 Extensor digitorum muscle
26 Extensor carpi ulnaris muscle
27 Posterior interosseous artery, vein,
   and nerve
28 Extensor digiti minimi muscle

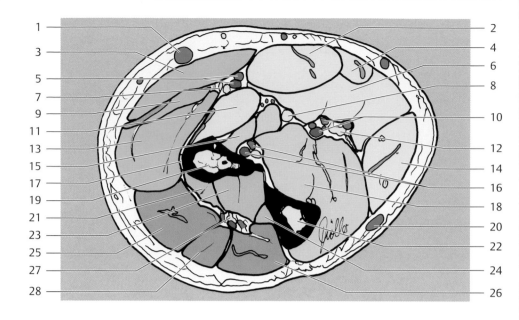

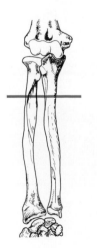

Ventral

Radial ☐ Ulnar

Dorsal

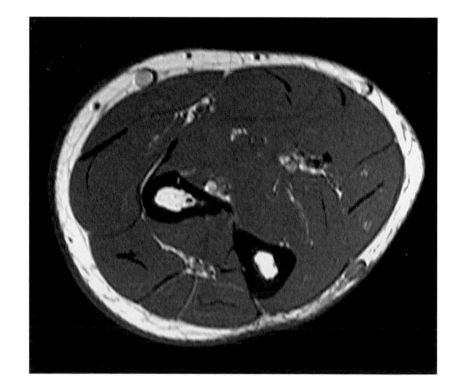

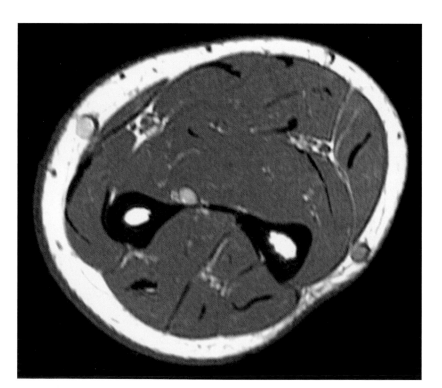

1 Flexor carpi radialis muscle
2 Medial cutaneous nerve of forearm (anterior branch)
3 Lateral cutaneous nerve of forearm (musculocutaneous nerve)
4 Palmaris longus muscle
5 Brachioradialis muscle
6 Flexor digitorum superficialis muscle
7 Radial artery and vein
8 Median nerve
9 Cephalic vein
10 Ulnar artery, vein, and nerve
11 Radial nerve (superficial branch)
12 Flexor carpi ulnaris muscle
13 Flexor pollicis longus muscle
14 Flexor digitorum profundus muscle
15 Extensor carpi radialis longus muscle (and tendon)
16 Interosseous membrane of forearm
17 Pronator teres muscle and anterior interosseous artery, vein, and nerve
18 Ulna
19 Radius
20 Basilic vein
21 Extensor carpi radialis brevis muscle
22 Extensor pollicis brevis muscle
23 Abductor pollicis longus muscle
24 Extensor pollicis longus muscle
25 Posterior interosseous artery, vein, and nerve
26 Extensor carpi ulnaris muscle
27 Extensor digitorum muscle
28 Extensor digiti minimi muscle

Ventral
Radial ☐ Ulnar
Dorsal

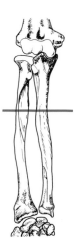

1 Flexor carpi radialis muscle
2 Median basilic vein
3 Median nerve
4 Palmaris longus muscle
5 Median artery and median antibrachial vein
6 Flexor digitorum superficialis muscle
7 Brachioradialis muscle (tendon)
8 Ulnar artery and vein
9 Radial artery and vein
10 Ulnar nerve
11 Radial nerve (superficial branch)
12 Medial cutaneous nerve of forearm
13 Cephalic vein
14 Flexor carpi ulnaris muscle
15 Flexor pollicis longus muscle
16 Flexor digitorum profundus muscle
17 Anterior interosseous artery, vein, and nerve
18 Basilic vein
19 Extensor carpi radialis longus muscle (and tendon)
20 Ulna
21 Lateral cutaneous nerve of forearm
22 Extensor indicis muscle
23 Extensor carpi radialis brevis muscle
24 Extensor pollicis longus muscle
25 Radius
26 Extensor pollicis brevis muscle
27 Interosseous membrane of forearm
28 Extensor carpi ulnaris muscle
29 Abductor pollicis longus muscle
30 Posterior interosseous artery, vein, and nerve
31 Extensor digitorum muscle
32 Extensor digiti minimi muscle

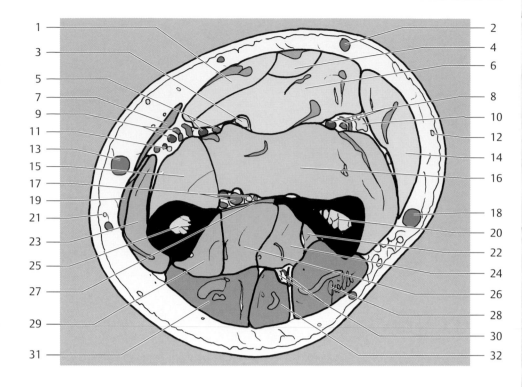

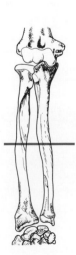

Ventral

Radial ☐ Ulnar

Dorsal

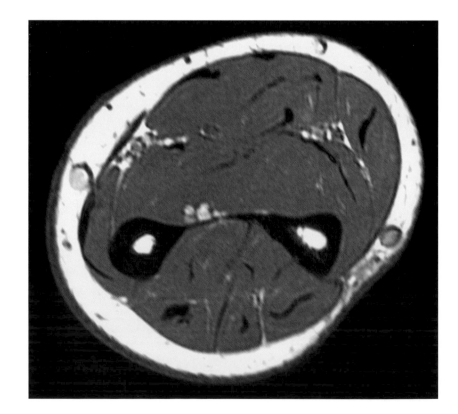

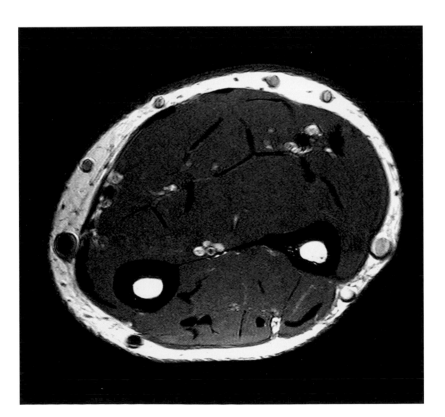

1 Flexor carpi radialis muscle
2 Median basilic vein
3 Median nerve
4 Palmaris longus muscle
5 Radial artery and veins
6 Flexor digitorum superficialis muscle
7 Brachioradialis muscle (tendon)
8 Ulnar artery, vein, and nerve
9 Radial nerve (superficial branch)
10 Flexor carpi ulnaris muscle
11 Lateral cutaneous nerve of forearm
12 Flexor digitorum profundus muscle
13 Anterior interosseous artery, vein, and nerve
14 Medial cutaneous nerve of forearm
15 Cephalic vein
16 Ulna
17 Flexor pollicis longus muscle
18 Basilic vein
19 Extensor carpi radialis longus muscle (tendon)
20 Interosseous membrane of forearm
21 Extensor carpi radialis brevis muscle (and tendon)
22 Extensor pollicis longus muscle
23 Radius
24 Extensor indicis muscle
25 Extensor pollicis brevis muscle
26 Extensor carpi ulnaris muscle
27 Abductor pollicis longus muscle
28 Extensor digiti minimi muscle
29 Extensor digitorum muscle

Ventral

Radial ☐ Ulnar

Dorsal

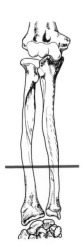

1 Palmaris longus muscle (and tendon)
2 Flexor digitorum superficialis muscle
3 Subcutaneous vein
4 Ulnar artery, vein, and nerve
5 Flexor carpi radialis muscle (tendon)
6 Flexor carpi ulnaris muscle
7 Median nerve
8 Flexor digitorum profundus muscle
9 Radial artery and veins
10 Pronator quadratus muscle
11 Flexor pollicis longus muscle
12 Basilic vein
13 Radial nerve (superficial branch)
14 Ulna
15 Cephalic vein
16 Anterior interosseous artery, vein, and nerve
17 Brachioradialis muscle (tendon)
18 Extensor indicis muscle
19 Abductor pollicis longus muscle
20 Extensor pollicis longus muscle
21 Extensor carpi radialis longus muscle (tendon)
22 Extensor carpi ulnaris muscle
23 Cephalic vein
24 Posterior interosseous artery and vein
25 Extensor carpi radialis brevis muscle (tendon)
26 Extensor digiti minimi muscle
27 Radius
28 Extensor digitorum muscle
29 Extensor pollicis brevis muscle

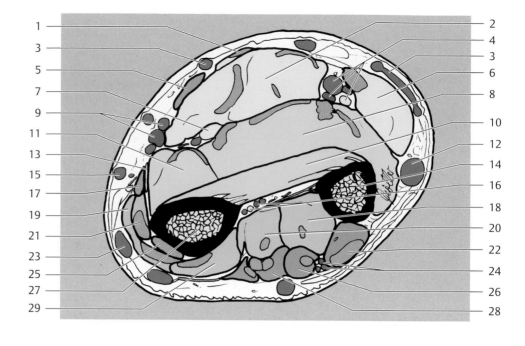

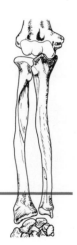

Ventral
Radial ☐ Ulnar
Dorsal

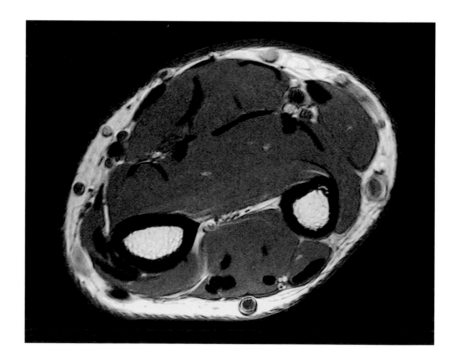

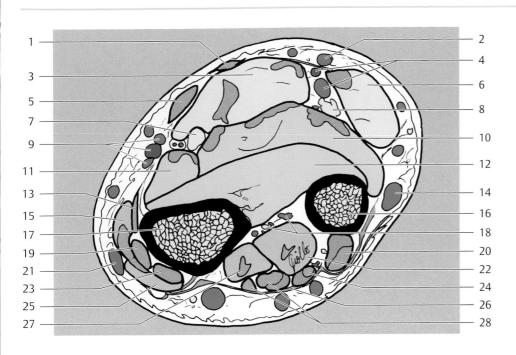

1 Palmaris longus muscle (tendon)
2 Subcutaneous vein
3 Flexor digitorum superficialis muscle
4 Ulnar artery and vein
5 Flexor carpi radialis muscle (tendon)
6 Flexor carpi ulnaris muscle
7 Median nerve
8 Ulnar nerve
9 Radial artery and veins
10 Flexor digitorum profundus muscle
11 Flexor pollicis longus muscle
12 Pronator quadratus muscle
13 Brachioradialis muscle (tendon)
14 Basilic vein
15 Abductor pollicis longus muscle
   (and tendon)
16 Ulna
17 Radius
18 Anterior interosseous artery, vein,
   and nerve
19 Extensor carpi radialis longus muscle
   (tendon)
20 Extensor carpi ulnaris muscle
21 Cephalic vein
22 Extensor indicis muscle
23 Extensor carpi radialis brevis muscle
   (tendon)
24 Extensor digiti minimi muscle
25 Extensor pollicis brevis muscle
26 Extensor retinaculum
27 Extensor pollicis longus muscle
28 Extensor digitorum muscle
   (and tendon)

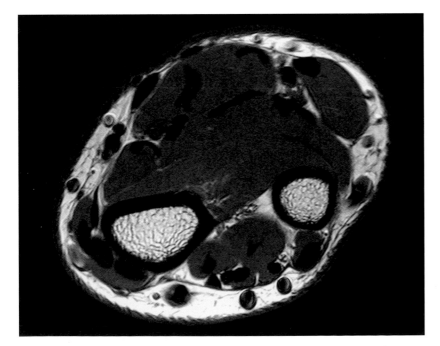

Ventral

Radial | | Ulnar

Dorsal

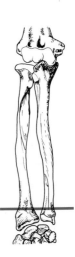

1 Fascia of forearm
2 Subcutaneous vein
3 Palmaris longus muscle (tendon)
4 Ulnar artery and vein
5 Flexor digitorum superficialis muscle
6 Flexor carpi ulnaris muscle
7 Flexor carpi radialis muscle (tendon)
8 Ulnar nerve
9 Median nerve
10 Flexor digitorum profundus muscle
11 Radial artery and veins
12 Pronator quadratus muscle
13 Flexor pollicis longus
14 Basilic vein
15 Cephalic vein
16 Ulna
17 Abductor pollicis longus muscle
18 Extensor carpi ulnaris muscle
19 Brachioradialis muscle
20 Extensor indicis muscle
21 Radius
22 Extensor digiti minimi muscle
23 Extensor pollicis brevis muscle
24 Extensor retinaculum
25 Extensor carpi radialis longus muscle (tendon)
26 Extensor digitorum muscle
27 Extensor carpi radialis brevis muscle (tendon)
28 Extensor pollicis longus muscle

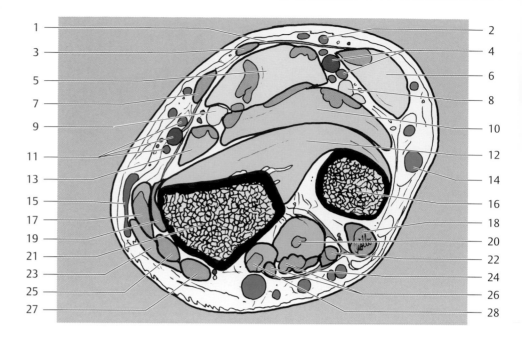

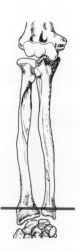

Ventral

Radial   Ulnar

Dorsal

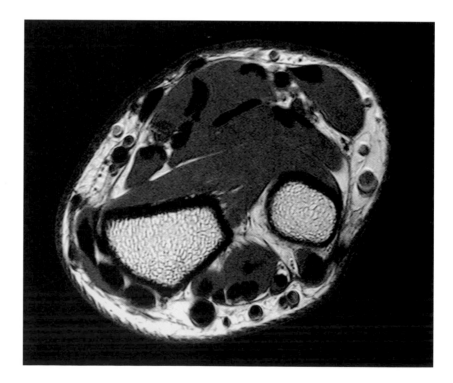

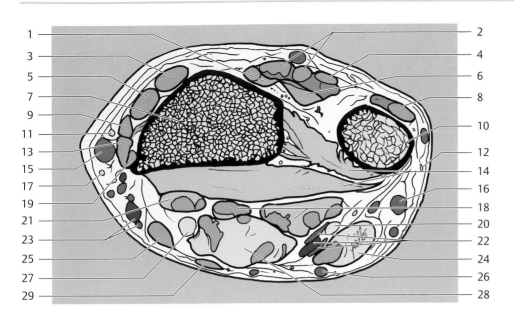

1 Extensor pollicis longus muscle
2 Extensor digitorum muscle
3 Extensor carpi radialis brevis muscle (tendon)
4 Extensor digiti minimi muscle
5 Extensor carpi radialis longus muscle (tendon)
6 Extensor indicis muscle
7 Radius
8 Extensor carpi ulnaris muscle
9 Extensor pollicis brevis muscle (tendon)
10 Ulna
11 Radial nerve (superficial branch)
12 Lateral cutaneous nerve of forearm
13 Abductor pollicis longus muscle (tendon)
14 Pronator quadratus muscle
15 Cephalic vein
16 Basilic vein
17 Lateral cutaneous nerve of forearm
18 Flexor digitorum profundus muscle
19 Brachioradialis muscle (tendon)
20 Ulnar nerve
21 Flexor pollicis longus muscle
22 Ulnar artery and veins
23 Radial artery and veins
24 Flexor carpi ulnaris muscle
25 Flexor carpi radialis muscle (tendon)
26 Subcutaneous vein
27 Median nerve
28 Flexor digitorum superficialis muscle
29 Palmaris longus muscle

According to the placement of the hand for MRI, from here onward the palm faces downward.

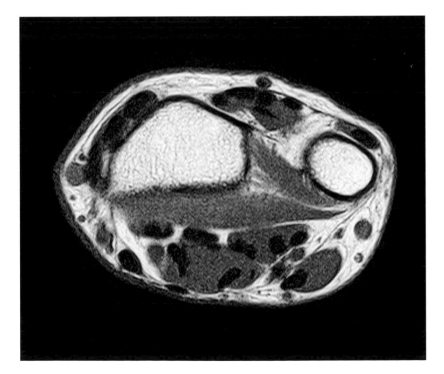

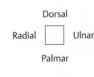

Dorsal
Radial · Ulnar
Palmar

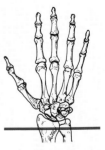

1 Subcutaneous vein
2 Extensor retinaculum
3 Extensor digitorum muscle
  (and tendons)
4 Extensor digiti minimi muscle (tendon)
5 Extensor indicis muscle (tendon)
6 Extensor carpi ulnaris muscle (tendon)
7 Extensor pollicis longus muscle
  (tendon)
8 Joint capsule
9 Accessory cephalic vein
10 Ulna
11 Extensor carpi radialis brevis muscle
  (tendon)
12 Basilic vein
13 Radial nerve (superficial branch)
14 Palmar ulnocarpal ligament
15 Extensor carpi radialis longus muscle
  (tendon)
16 Ulnar nerve (dorsal branch)
17 Radius
18 Flexor digitorum profundus muscle
19 Cephalic vein
20 Ulnar nerve
21 Extensor pollicis brevis muscle
  (tendon)
22 Flexor carpi ulnaris muscle
23 Abductor pollicis longus muscle
  (tendon)
24 Ulnar artery and veins
25 Flexor pollicis longus muscle
26 Antebrachial fascia
27 Radial artery and veins
28 Flexor digitorum superficialis muscle
29 Flexor carpi radialis muscle (tendon)
30 Median nerve
31 Palmaris longus muscle

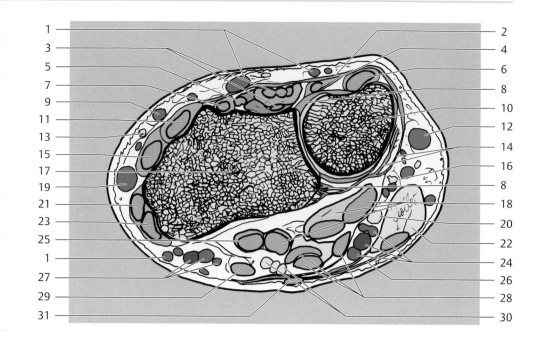

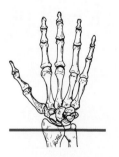

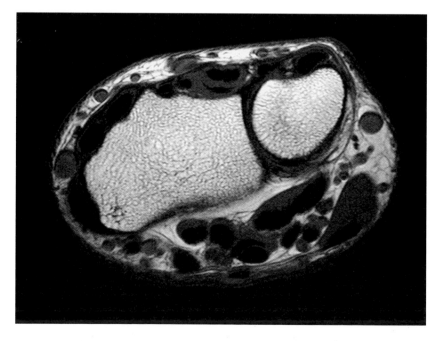

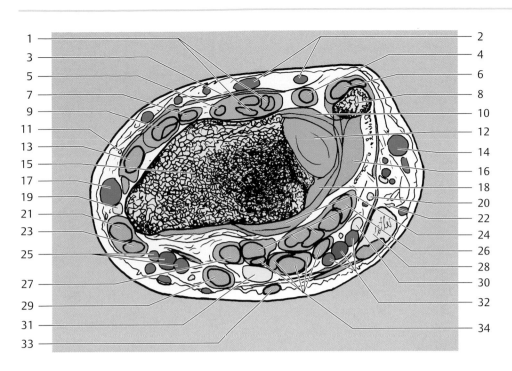

1 Extensor digitorum muscle (tendons)
2 Subcutaneous vein
3 Extensor retinaculum
4 Extensor digiti minimi muscle (tendon)
5 Extensor indicis muscle (tendon)
6 Extensor carpi ulnaris muscle (tendon)
7 Extensor pollicis longus muscle (tendon)
8 Ulna (styloid process)
9 Extensor carpi radialis brevis muscle (tendon)
10 Palmar radio-ulnar ligament
11 Posterior cutaneous nerve of forearm (radial nerve)
12 Triangular fibrocartilage (ulnar)
13 Extensor carpi radialis longus muscle (tendon)
14 Basilic vein
15 Radius
16 Palmar ulnocarpal ligament
17 Cephalic vein
18 Joint capsule
19 Radial nerve (superficial branch)
20 Ulnar nerve (dorsal branch)
21 Extensor pollicis brevis muscle (tendon)
22 Medial cutaneous nerve of forearm (ulnar nerve)
23 Abductor pollicis longus muscle (tendon)
24 Palmar radiocarpal ligament
25 Radial artery and veins
26 Flexor digitorum profundus muscle (tendons)
27 Flexor pollicis longus muscle
28 Flexor carpi ulnaris muscle
29 Flexor carpi radialis muscle (tendon)
30 Ulnar nerve
31 Median nerve
32 Ulnar artery and veins
33 Palmaris longus muscle
34 Flexor digitorum superficialis muscle (tendons)

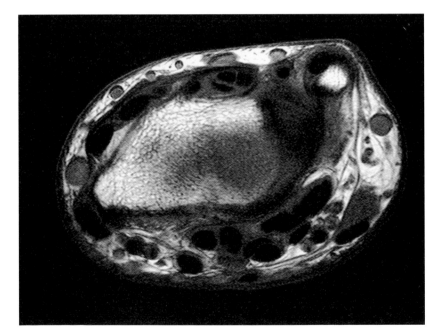

Dorsal

Radial   Ulnar

Palmar

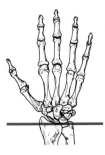

1 Extensor indicis muscle (tendon)
2 Extensor retinaculum
3 Extensor pollicis longus muscle (tendon)
4 Subcutaneous vein
5 Extensor carpi radialis brevis muscle (tendon)
6 Extensor digitorum muscle (tendon)
7 Joint capsule
8 Extensor carpi ulnaris muscle (tendon)
9 Extensor carpi radialis longus muscle (tendon)
10 Ulna (styloid process)
11 Posterior cutaneous nerve of forearm (radial nerve)
12 Extensor digiti minimi muscle (tendon)
13 Scaphoid
14 Dorsal radiocarpal ligament
15 Cephalic vein
16 Basilic vein
17 Radius
18 Palmar ulnocarpal ligament
19 Radial nerve (superficial branch)
20 Ulnar collateral ligament of wrist joint
21 Extensor pollicis brevis muscle (tendon)
22 Triangular fibrocartilage
23 Palmar radiocarpal ligament
24 Lunate
25 Abductor pollicis longus muscle (tendon)
26 Ulnar nerve (dorsal branch)
27 Radial artery and veins
28 Flexor digitorum profundus muscle (tendons)
29 Flexor pollicis longus muscle
30 Flexor carpi ulnaris muscle
31 Flexor carpi radialis muscle (tendon)
32 Ulnar nerve, artery, and veins
33 Median nerve
34 Flexor digitorum superficialis muscle (tendons)
35 Palmaris longus muscle
36 Flexor retinaculum

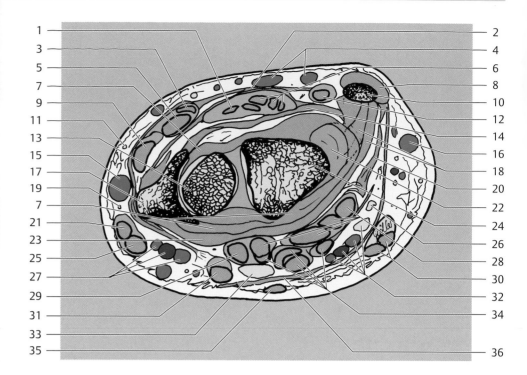

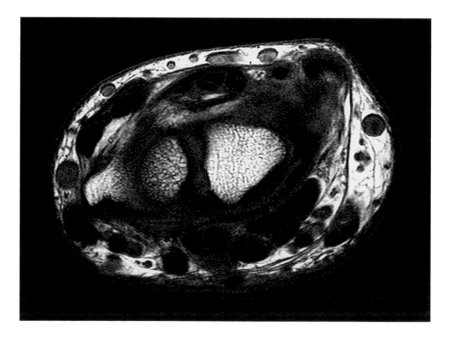

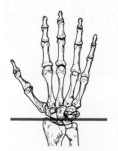

Dorsal

Radial | | Ulnar

Palmar

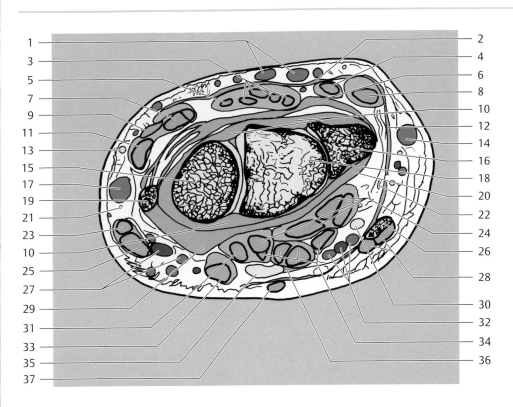

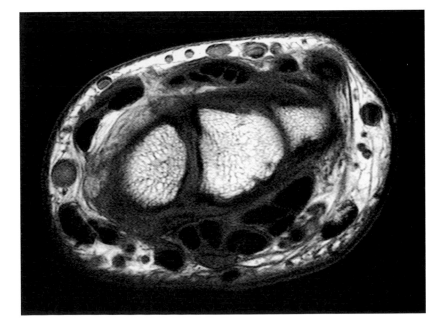

1 Subcutaneous vein
2 Extensor retinaculum
3 Extensor digitorum muscle (tendons)
4 Extensor digiti minimi muscle (tendon)
5 Extensor indicis muscle (tendon)
6 Dorsal radiocarpal ligament
7 Extensor carpi radialis brevis muscle (tendon)
8 Extensor carpi ulnaris muscle (tendon)
9 Extensor pollicis longus muscle (tendon)
10 Joint capsule
11 Extensor carpi radialis longus muscle (tendon)
12 Ulnar collateral ligament of wrist
13 Posterior cutaneous nerve of forearm (radial nerve)
14 Basilic vein
15 Scaphoid
16 Triquetrum
17 Cephalic vein
18 Lunate
19 Radius (styloid process)
20 Palmar ulnocarpal ligament
21 Radial nerve (superficial branch)
22 Ulnar nerve (dorsal branch)
23 Extensor pollicis brevis muscle (tendon)
24 Flexor digitorum profundus muscle (tendons)
25 Abductor pollicis longus muscle (tendon)
26 Pisiform
27 Radial artery and veins
28 Flexor carpi ulnaris muscle (tendon)
29 Palmar radiocarpal ligament
30 Ulnar nerve
31 Flexor pollicis longus muscle
32 Ulnar artery and veins
33 Flexor carpi radialis muscle (tendon)
34 Flexor digitorum superficialis muscle (tendons)
35 Median nerve
36 Flexor retinaculum
37 Palmaris longus muscle

Dorsal

Radial | | Ulnar

Palmar

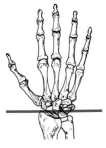

1 Extensor retinaculum
2 Subcutaneous vein
3 Extensor indicis muscle (tendon)
4 Extensor digitorum muscle (tendons)
5 Extensor carpi radialis brevis muscle (tendon)
6 Extensor digiti minimi muscle (tendon)
7 Joint capsule
8 Extensor carpi ulnaris muscle (tendon)
9 Extensor pollicis longus muscle (tendon)
10 Triquetrum
11 Extensor carpi radialis longus muscle (tendon)
12 Basilic vein
13 Capitate
14 Lunate
15 Posterior cutaneous nerve of forearm (radial nerve)
16 Palmar ulnocarpal ligament
17 Cephalic vein
18 Palmar intercarpal ligament
19 Scaphoid
20 Flexor digitorum profundus muscle (tendons)
21 Radial nerve (superficial branch)
22 Flexor digitorum superficialis muscle (tendons)
23 Extensor pollicis brevis muscle (tendon)
24 Pisiform
25 Abductor pollicis longus muscle (tendon)
26 Flexor carpi ulnaris muscle (tendon attachment)
27 Radial artery and veins
28 Ulnar nerve, artery, and veins
29 Ulnar radiocarpal ligament
30 Flexor retinaculum
31 Superficial palmar branch of radial artery and vein
32 Median nerve
33 Flexor carpi radialis muscle (tendon)
34 Palmaris longus muscle
35 Flexor pollicis longus muscle

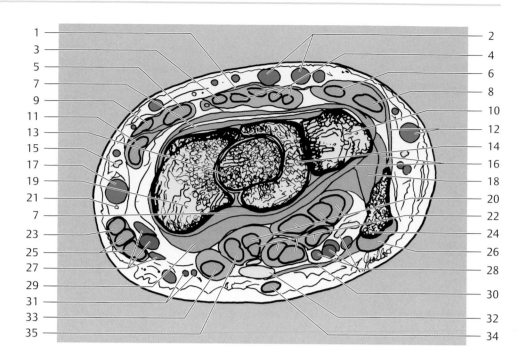

Dorsal

Radial | | Ulnar

Palmar

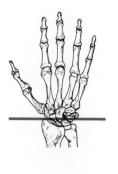

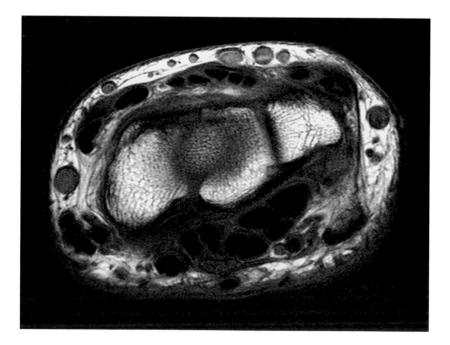

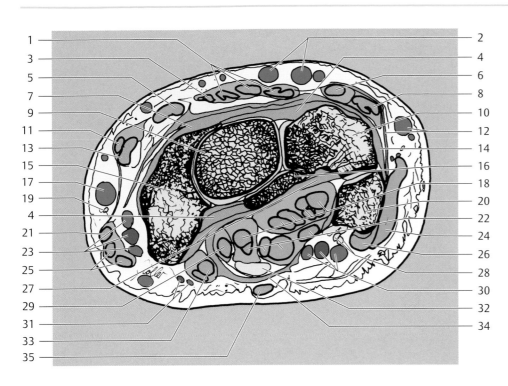

1 Extensor digitorum muscle (tendons)
2 Subcutaneous vein
3 Extensor indicis muscle (tendon)
4 Joint capsule
5 Extensor carpi radialis brevis muscle (tendon)
6 Extensor digiti minimi muscle (tendon)
7 Dorsal intercarpal ligament
8 Extensor carpi ulnaris muscle (tendon)
9 Capitate
10 Triquetrum
11 Extensor pollicis longus muscle (tendon)
12 Basilic vein
13 Extensor carpi radialis longus muscle (tendon)
14 Palmar ulnocarpal ligament
15 Scaphoid
16 Lunate
17 Cephalic vein
18 Flexor digitorum profundus muscle (tendons)
19 Radial nerve (superficial branch)
20 Pisiform
21 Extensor pollicis brevis muscle (tendon)
22 Flexor digitorum superficialis muscle (tendons)
23 Radial artery and veins
24 Abductor digiti minimi muscle
25 Abductor pollicis longus muscle (tendon)
26 Flexor carpi ulnaris muscle
27 Palmar radiocarpal ligament
28 Ulnar nerve
29 Flexor pollicis longus muscle
30 Ulnar artery and veins
31 Superficial palmar branch of radial artery and vein
32 Median nerve
33 Flexor carpi radialis muscle (tendon)
34 Flexor retinaculum
35 Palmaris longus muscle

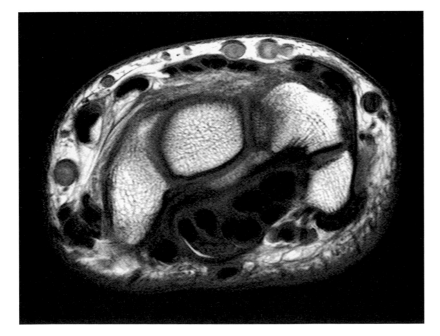

Dorsal

Radial Ulnar

Palmar

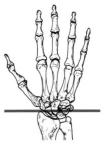

1 Extensor digitorum muscle (tendons)
2 Subcutaneous vein
3 Extensor indicis muscle (tendon)
4 Extensor digiti minimi muscle (tendon)
5 Extensor retinaculum
6 Extensor carpi ulnaris muscle (tendon)
7 Extensor carpi radialis brevis muscle (tendon)
8 Hamate
9 Dorsal intercarpal ligament
10 Basilic vein
11 Extensor pollicis longus muscle (tendon)
12 Palmar ulnocarpal ligament (tendon)
13 Extensor carpi radialis longus muscle (tendon)
14 Triquetrum
15 Capitate
16 Palmar radiocarpal ligament
17 Joint capsule
18 Flexor digitorum profundus muscle (tendons)
19 Cephalic vein
20 Abductor digiti minimi muscle
21 Scaphoid
22 Pisiform
23 Radial nerve (superficial branch)
24 Flexor digitorum superficialis muscle (tendons)
25 Radial artery and veins
26 Flexor carpi ulnaris muscle
27 Extensor pollicis brevis muscle (tendon)
28 Ulnar nerve
29 Abductor pollicis longus muscle (tendon)
30 Ulnar artery and veins
31 Trapezium with intercarpal ligament
32 Flexor retinaculum
33 Flexor carpi radialis muscle (tendon)
34 Median nerve
35 Flexor pollicis longus muscle
36 Palmaris longus muscle

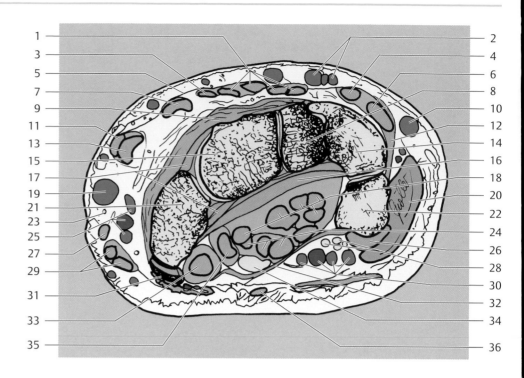

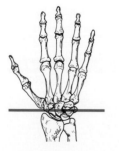

Dorsal

Radial ☐ Ulnar

Palmar

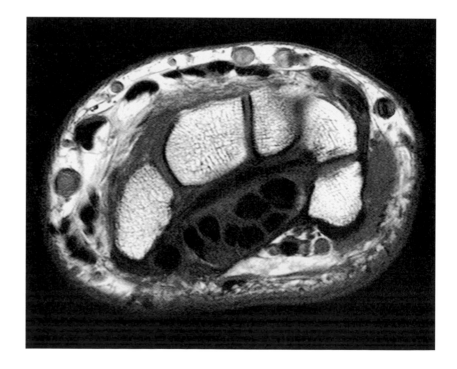

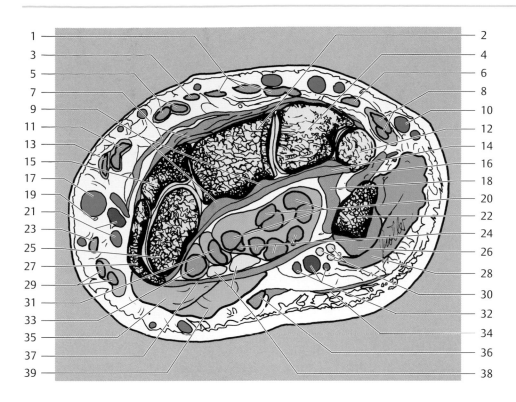

1 —
3 —
5 —
7 —
9 —
11 —
13 —
15 —
17 —
19 —
21 —
23 —
25 —
27 —
29 —
31 —
33 —
35 —
37 —
39 —

— 2
— 4
— 6
— 8
— 10
— 12
— 14
— 16
— 18
— 20
— 22
— 24
— 26
— 28
— 30
— 32
— 34
— 36
— 38

1 Extensor digitorum muscle (tendons)
2 Capitate
3 Extensor indicis muscle (tendon)
4 Hamate
5 Extensor carpi radialis brevis muscle (tendon)
6 Extensor digiti minimi muscle (tendon)
7 Dorsal intercarpal ligament
8 Extensor carpi ulnaris muscle (tendon)
9 Joint capsule
10 Basilic vein
11 Extensor carpi radialis longus muscle (tendon)
12 Triquetrum
13 Extensor pollicis longus muscle (tendon)
14 Palmar intercarpal ligament
15 Trapezoid
16 Pisometacarpal ligament
17 Cephalic vein
18 Pisohamate ligament
19 Radial nerve (superficial branch)
20 Flexor digitorum profundus muscle (tendons)
21 Radial artery and veins
22 Pisiform
23 Extensor pollicis brevis muscle (tendon)
24 Flexor digitorum superficialis muscle (tendons)
25 Scaphoid
26 Flexor carpi ulnaris muscle (tendon)
27 Trapezium
28 Abductor digiti minimi muscle
29 Abductor pollicis longus muscle (tendon)
30 Ulnar nerve
31 Flexor pollicis longus muscle (tendon)
32 Ulnar artery and veins
33 Flexor carpi radialis muscle (tendon)
34 Palmaris brevis muscle (tendon)
35 Opponens pollicis muscle
36 Palmaris longus muscle (tendon)
37 Flexor retinaculum
38 Median nerve
39 Abductor pollicis brevis muscle

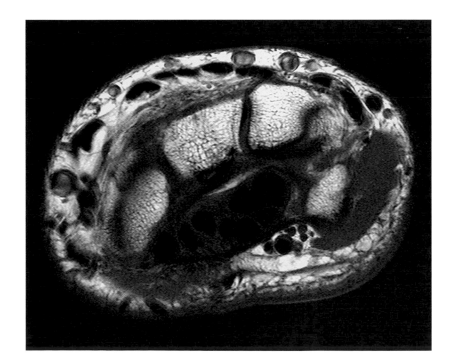

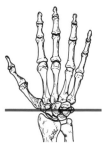

Dorsal

Radial ☐ Ulnar

Palmar

1 Intercarpal (capitohamate) joint
2 Extensor digitorum muscle (tendons)
3 Extensor indicis muscle (tendon)
4 Extensor digiti minimi muscle (tendon)
5 Extensor carpi radialis brevis muscle (tendon)
6 Hamate
7 Capitate
8 Extensor carpi ulnaris muscle (tendon)
9 Extensor carpi radialis longus muscle (tendon)
10 Metacarpal V (base)
11 Trapezoid
12 Pisometacarpal ligament
13 Extensor pollicis longus muscle (tendon)
14 Flexor digitorum profundus muscle (tendons)
15 Cephalic vein
16 Abductor digiti minimi muscle
17 Radial artery and veins
18 Hamate (hook)
19 Radial nerve (superficial branch)
20 Ulnar nerve (deep branch)
21 Palmar intercarpal ligament
22 Flexor digiti minimi muscle
23 Trapezium
24 Flexor digitorum superficialis muscle (tendons)
25 Extensor pollicis brevis muscle (tendon)
26 Ulnar nerve
27 Flexor carpi radialis muscle (tendon)
28 Palmaris brevis muscle
29 Abductor pollicis longus muscle (tendon)
30 Ulnar artery and veins
31 Flexor pollicis longus muscle
32 Flexor retinaculum
33 Opponens pollicis muscle
34 Median nerve
35 Abductor pollicis brevis muscle
36 Palmar aponeurosis

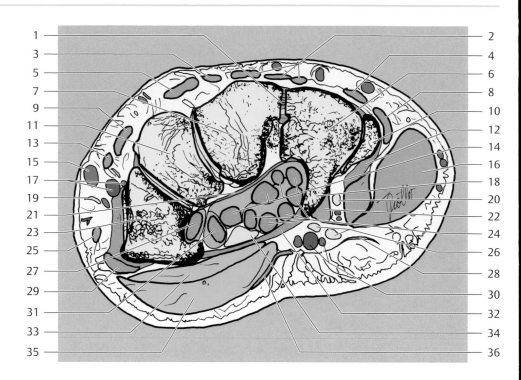

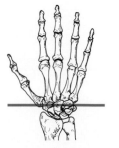

Dorsal

Radial ☐ Ulnar

Palmar

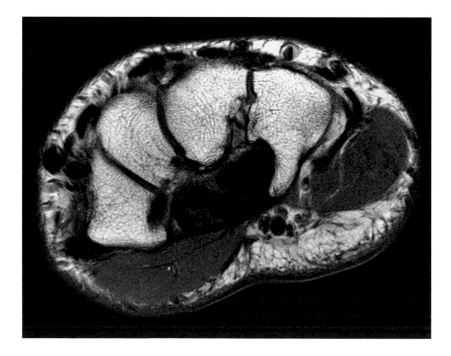

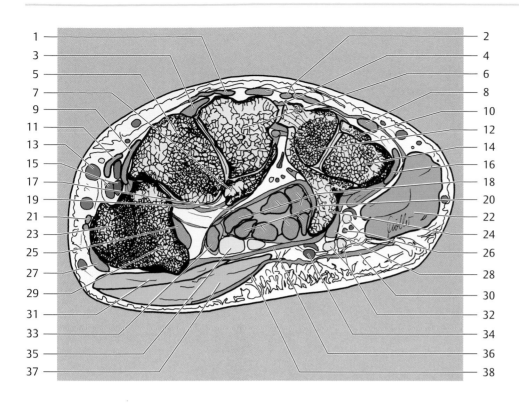

1 Extensor indicis muscle (tendon)
2 Extensor digitorum muscle (tendons)
3 Extensor carpi radialis brevis muscle (tendon attachment)
4 Dorsal metacarpal ligament
5 Metacarpal II (base)
6 Metacarpal III (base)
7 Capitate
8 Extensor digiti minimi muscle (tendon)
9 Extensor carpi radialis longus muscle (tendon)
10 Hamate
11 Extensor pollicis longus muscle (tendon)
12 Metacarpal IV (base)
13 Cephalic vein
14 Metacarpal V (base)
15 Radial artery and veins
16 Extensor carpi ulnaris muscle (tendon attachment)
17 Palmar intercarpal ligament
18 Flexor digitorum profundus muscle (tendons)
19 Joint capsule
20 Flexor digitorum superficialis muscle (tendons)
21 Extensor pollicis brevis muscle (tendon)
22 Abductor digiti minimi muscle
23 Metacarpal I (base)
24 Hamate (hook)
25 Flexor carpi radialis muscle (tendon attachment)
26 Ulnar nerve, artery, and vein (deep branch)
27 Abductor pollicis longus muscle (tendon attachment)
28 Flexor digiti minimi muscle
29 Trapezium
30 Palmaris brevis muscle
31 Opponens pollicis muscle
32 Ulnar nerve
33 Flexor pollicis longus muscle (tendon)
34 Ulnar artery and veins
35 Median nerve
36 Flexor retinaculum
37 Abductor pollicis brevis muscle
38 Palmar aponeurosis

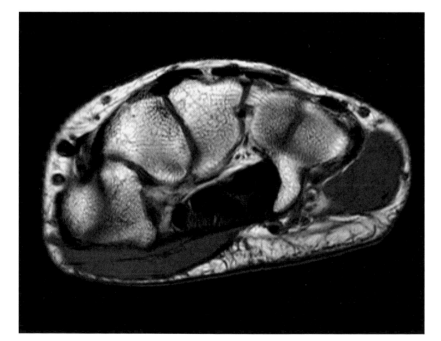

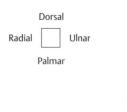

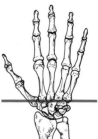

Dorsal

Radial   Ulnar

Palmar

1 Extensor indicis muscle (tendon)
2 Extensor digitorum muscle (tendons)
3 Dorsal metacarpal ligament
4 Metacarpal IV (base)
5 Metacarpal III (base)
6 Extensor digiti minimi muscle (tendon)
7 Metacarpal II (base)
8 Palmar intercarpal ligament
9 Radial artery and veins
10 Metacarpal V (base)
11 Cephalic vein
12 Flexor digitorum profundus muscle (tendons)
13 Extensor pollicis longus muscle (tendon)
14 Opponens digiti minimi muscle
15 Joint capsule
16 Abductor digiti minimi muscle
17 Adductor pollicis muscle (oblique head)
18 Hamate (hook)
19 Extensor pollicis brevis muscle (tendon)
20 Ulnar nerve, artery, and vein (deep branch)
21 Metacarpal I (base)
22 Flexor digiti minimi muscle
23 Flexor pollicis longus muscle (tendon)
24 Palmaris brevis muscle
25 Median nerve
26 Ulnar nerve
27 Opponens pollicis muscle
28 Ulnar artery and vein
29 Abductor pollicis brevis muscle
30 Flexor digitorum superficialis muscle (tendons)
31 Palmar aponeurosis
32 Flexor retinaculum

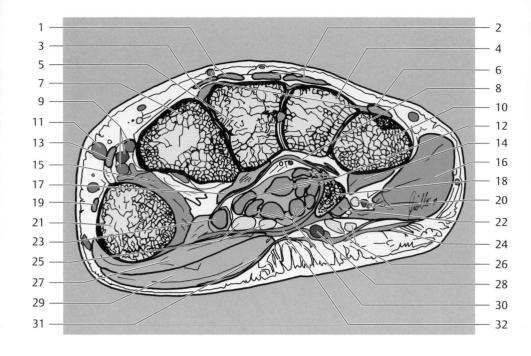

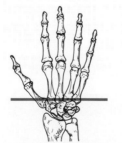

Dorsal

Radial   Ulnar

Palmar

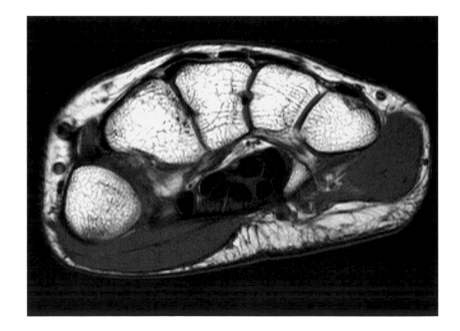

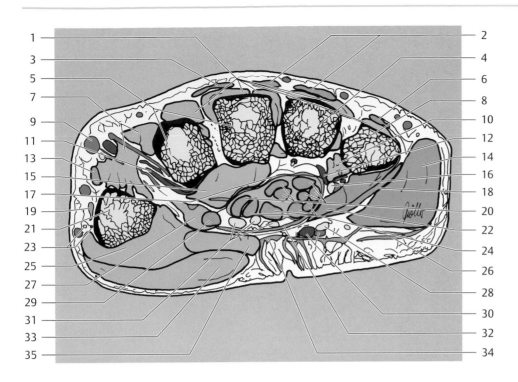

1 Dorsal interossei muscles
2 Extensor digitorum muscle (tendons)
3 Extensor indicis muscle (tendon)
4 Metacarpal IV (base)
5 Metacarpals II and III (bases)
6 Extensor digiti minimi muscle (tendon)
7 Dorsal interosseous muscle I
8 Metacarpal V
9 Cephalic vein
10 Palmar interossei muscles
11 Deep palmar arch (from radial artery)
12 Deep palmar arch (from deep ulnar artery)
13 Extensor pollicis longus muscle (tendon)
14 Abductor digiti minimi muscle
15 Adductor pollicis muscle (oblique head)
16 Ulnar nerve (deep branch)
17 Palmar intercarpal ligament
18 Flexor digiti minimi brevis muscle
19 Extensor pollicis brevis muscle (tendon)
20 Flexor digitorum profundus muscle (tendons)
21 Metacarpal I (head)
22 Opponens digiti minimi muscle
23 Dorsal nerve and artery of thumb
24 Flexor digitorum superficialis muscle (tendons)
25 Opponens pollicis muscle
26 Palmaris brevis muscle
27 Flexor pollicis brevis muscle (deep head)
28 Ulnar nerve
29 Flexor pollicis longus muscle (tendon)
30 Ulnar artery and veins
31 Median nerve
32 Flexor retinaculum
33 Abductor pollicis brevis muscle
34 Palmar aponeurosis
35 Flexor pollicis brevis muscle (superficial head)

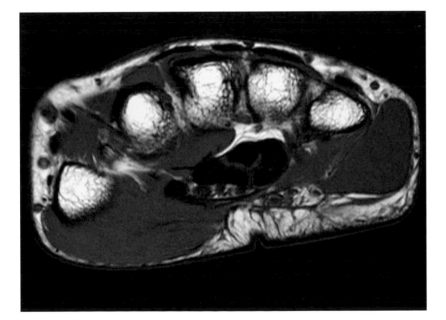

Dorsal

Radial ▢ Ulnar

Palmar

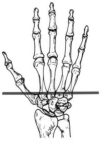

1 Extensor indicis muscle (tendon)
2 Extensor digitorum muscle (tendons)
3 Dorsal interossei muscles
4 Extensor digiti minimi muscle (tendon)
5 Deep palmar arch
6 Metacarpals II–V (shafts)
7 Adductor pollicis muscle (oblique head)
8 Palmar interossei muscles
9 Princeps pollicis artery and palmar
   digital nerve (of thumb)
10 Flexor digitorum profundus muscle
   (tendons)
11 Extensor pollicis longus muscle
   (tendon)
12 Opponens digiti minimi muscle
13 Cephalic vein (of thumb)
14 Flexor digiti minimi brevis muscle
15 Extensor pollicis brevis muscle
   (tendon)
16 Flexor digitorum superficialis muscle
   (tendons)
17 Metacarpal I (shaft)
18 Abductor digiti minimi muscle
19 Dorsal digital artery and nerve of thumb
20 Palmaris brevis muscle
21 Flexor pollicis brevis muscle
   (deep head)
22 Ulnar nerve, artery, and vein
23 Flexor pollicis brevis muscle
   (superficial head)
24 Palmar aponeurosis
25 Flexor pollicis brevis muscle
   (superficial head)
26 Median nerve
27 Opponens pollicis muscle
28 Abductor pollicis brevis muscle

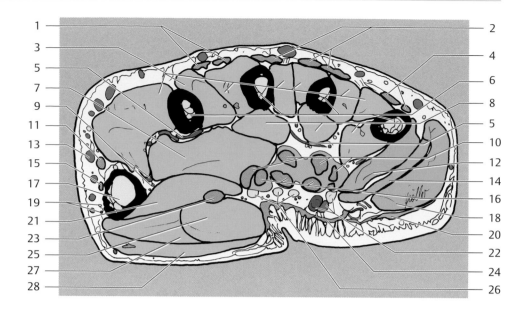

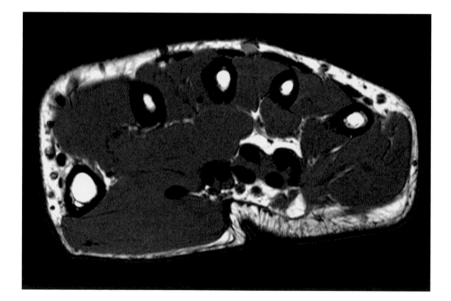

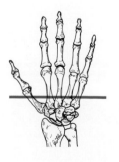

Dorsal

Radial ☐ Ulnar

Palmar

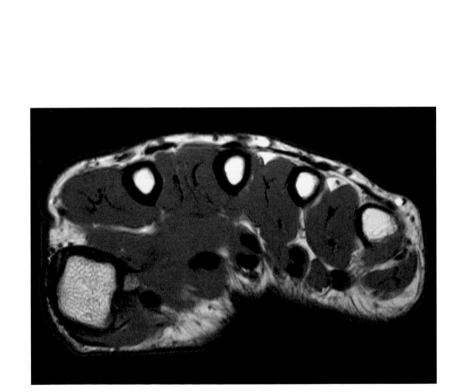

1 Extensor digitorum muscle (tendons)
2 Metacarpals II–IV (shafts)
3 Deep palmar arch
4 Dorsal interossei muscles
5 Lumbrical muscles
6 Extensor digiti minimi muscle (tendon)
7 Adductor pollicis muscle
   (transverse head)
8 Palmar interossei muscles
9 Dorsal digital nerve and artery of thumb
10 Metacarpal V (head)
11 Collateral ligament
12 Opponens digiti minimi muscle (tendon)
13 Extensor pollicis brevis muscle (tendon)
14 Flexor digiti minimi brevis muscle
15 Extensor pollicis brevis muscle (tendon)
16 Ulnar nerve (superficial branch)
17 Metacarpal I (head)
18 Abductor digiti minimi muscle
19 Sesamoid bones
20 Flexor digitorum profundus muscle
   (tendons)
21 Opponens pollicis muscle (and tendon
   attachment)
22 Flexor digitorum superficialis muscle
   (tendons)
23 Abductor pollicis brevis muscle
24 Common palmar digital nerves of
   median nerve
25 Flexor pollicis brevis muscle
   (superficial head)
26 Adductor pollicis muscle (oblique head)
27 Flexor pollicis longus muscle (tendon)
28 Flexor pollicis brevis muscle
   (deep head)

Dorsal

Radial ☐ Ulnar

Palmar

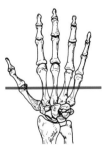

1 Extensor digitorum muscle (tendons)
2 Dorsal digital vein
3 Sagittal ligament
4 Collateral ligament
5 Dorsal digital artery and nerve
6 Extensor digiti minimi muscle (tendon)
7 Extensor indicis muscle (tendon)
8 Extensor hood
9 Metacarpals II–IV (shafts)
10 Interossei muscles (tendon)
11 Interossei muscles
12 Proximal phalanx V (base)
13 Palmar ligament
14 Flexor digitorum profundus muscle
   (tendons)
15 Extensor pollicis muscle (aponeurosis)
16 Flexor digitorum superficialis muscle
   (tendon)
17 Proximal phalanx I
18 Palmar digital arteries and nerves
19 Flexor pollicis longus muscle (tendon)
20 Anular ligament
21 Lumbrical muscle

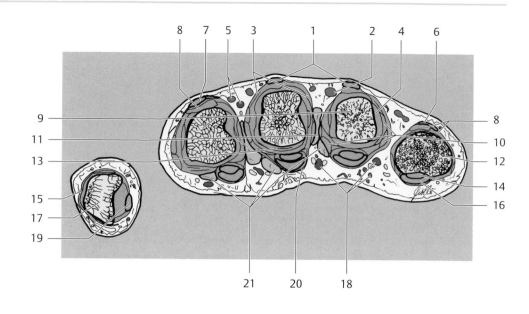

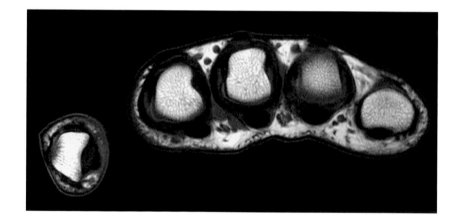

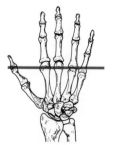

Dorsal

Radial ☐ Ulnar

Palmar

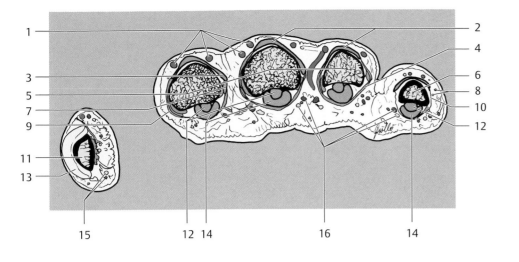

1 Dorsal digital vein
2 Extensor digitorum muscle (aponeurosis)
3 Lateral band
4 Anular ligament
5 Proximal phalanges II–IV (bases)
6 Proximal phalanx V (shaft)
7 Interossei muscles (tendons)
8 Dorsal digital artery and nerve
9 Sagittal ligament
10 Collateral ligament
11 Distal phalanx of thumb
12 Flexor digitorum profundus muscle (tendons)
13 Body of fingernail
14 Flexor digitorum superficialis muscle (tendons)
15 Palmar digital arteries and nerves of thumb
16 Palmar digital arteries and nerves

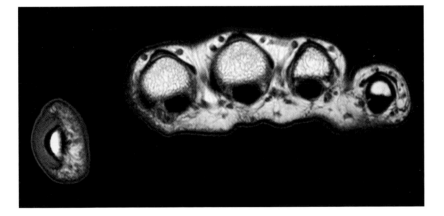

Dorsal

Radial ☐ Ulnar

Palmar

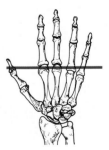
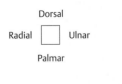

1 Digital artery and nerve
2 Extensor digitorum muscle (aponeurosis)
3 Digital vein
4 Proximal phalanges II–IV (shafts)
5 Interossei muscles (tendons)
6 Proximal phalanx V (head)
7 Anular ligament
8 Flexor digitorum profundus muscle (tendon)
9 Digital arteries and nerves
10 Flexor digitorum superficialis muscle (tendons)
11 Synovial sheath of finger

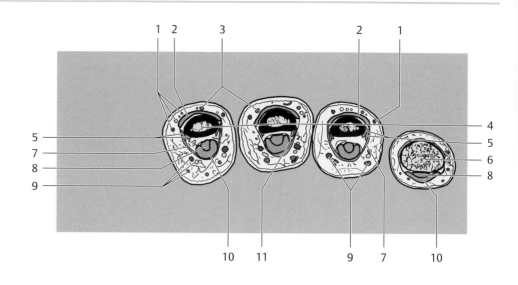

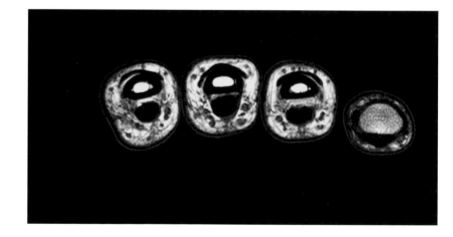

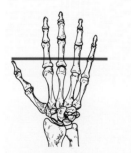

Dorsal

Radial   Ulnar

Palmar

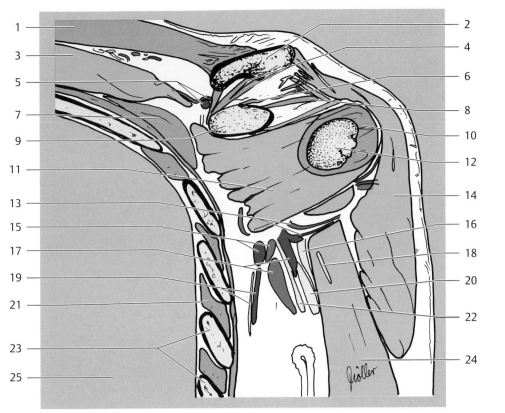

1 Trapezius muscle
2 Clavicle
3 Supraspinatus muscle
4 Coracoclavicular ligament
5 Suprascapular artery and vein
6 Coraco-acromial ligament
7 Serratus anterior muscle
8 Coracohumeral ligament
9 Coracoid
10 Joint capsule
11 Subscapularis muscle
12 Humerus (head)
13 Anterior circumflex humeral artery
   and vein
14 Deltoid muscle
15 Subscapular artery and vein
16 Radial nerve
17 Brachial artery and vein
18 Musculocutaneous nerve
   (muscular branches)
19 Thoracodorsal artery and nerve
20 Median nerve
21 Intercostal muscle
22 Ulnar nerve
23 Ribs
24 Coracobrachialis muscle
25 Lung

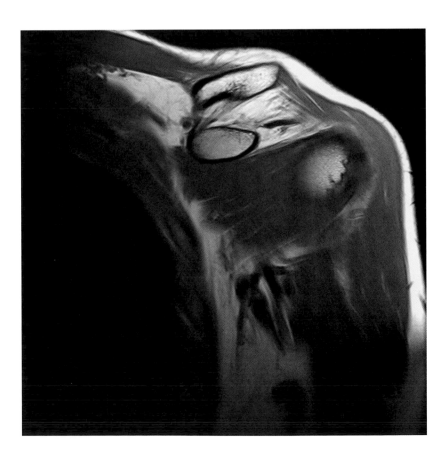

Cranial

Medial ☐ Lateral

Caudal

1 Trapezius muscle
2 Clavicle
3 Suprascapular artery and vein
4 Coraco-acromial ligament
5 Supraspinatus muscle
6 Coracohumeral ligament
7 Coracoclavicular ligament
8 Coracoid process
9 Scapula (superior border)
10 Humerus (head)
11 Serratus anterior muscle
12 Joint capsule
13 Subscapularis muscle
14 Anterior circumflex humeral artery and vein
15 Lung
16 Deltoid muscle
17 Intercostal muscle
18 Coracobrachialis muscle
19 Rib
20 Radial nerve
21 Thoracodorsal nerve
22 Median nerve
23 Suprascapular artery and vein
24 Brachial artery and vein
25 Latissimus dorsi muscle

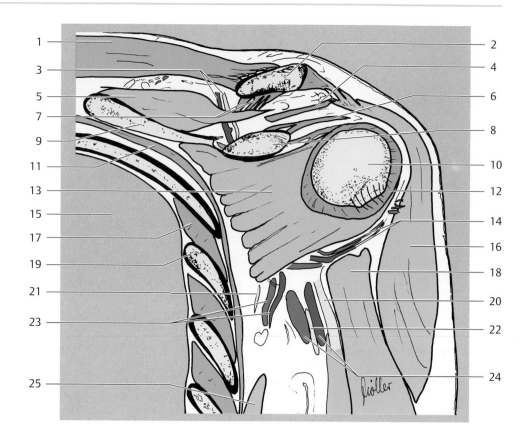

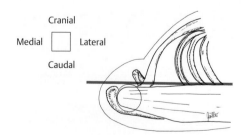

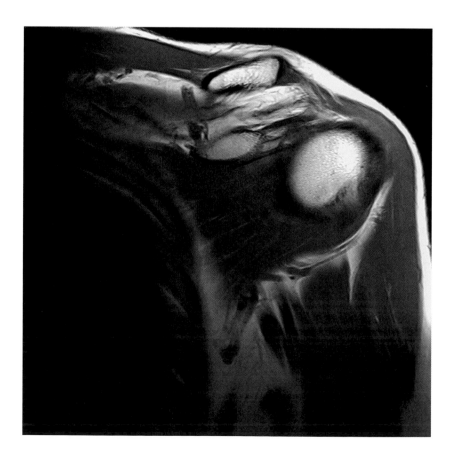

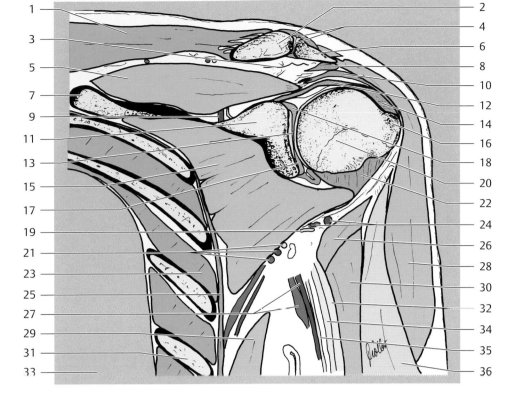

1 —
3 —
5 —
7 —
9 —
11 —
13 —
15 —
17 —
19 —
21 —
23 —
25 —
27 —
29 —
31 —
33 —

— 2
— 4
— 6
— 8
— 10
— 12
— 14
— 16
— 18
— 20
— 22
— 24
— 26
— 28
— 30
— 32
— 34
— 35
— 36

1 Trapezius muscle
2 Clavicle
3 Subacromial bursa
4 Acromioclavicular joint and acromioclavicular ligament
5 Supraspinatus muscle
6 Acromion
7 Scapula
8 Coraco-acromial ligament
9 Suprascapular artery and vein
10 Coracohumeral ligament
11 Glenoid
12 Biceps brachii muscle (long head, tendon)
13 Glenohumeral joint
14 Supraspinatus muscle (tendon attachment)
15 Subscapularis muscle
16 Greater tubercle
17 Glenoid labrum (inferior)
18 Glenoid labrum (superior)
19 Axillary nerve
20 Humerus (head)
21 Subscapular artery, vein, and nerve
22 Glenohumeral ligament
23 Intercostal muscle
24 Posterior circumflex humeral artery and vein
25 Serratus anterior muscle
26 Teres major muscle
27 Axillary artery and vein
28 Deltoid muscle
29 Latissimus dorsi muscle
30 Coracobrachialis muscle
31 Rib
32 Radial nerve
33 Lung
34 Median nerve
35 Ulnar nerve
36 Biceps muscle (long head)

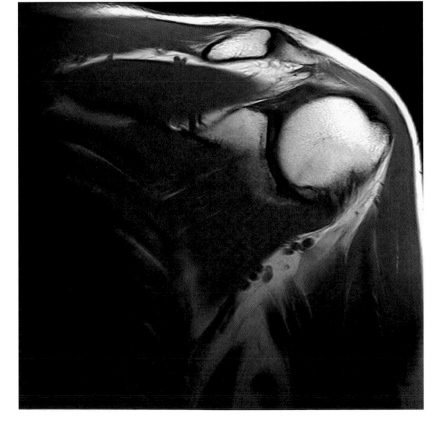

Cranial

Medial Lateral

Caudal

1 Clavicle
2 Acromioclavicular ligament
3 Trapezius muscle
4 Acromioclavicular joint
5 Superficial cervical vein
6 Acromion and subacromial bursa
7 Supraspinatus muscle
8 Biceps brachii muscle
(long head, tendon attachment)
9 Scapula
10 Supraspinatus muscle
(tendon attachment)
11 Suprascapular artery, vein, and nerve
12 Glenoid labrum (superior lip)
13 Joint socket
14 Greater tubercle
15 Shoulder joint
16 Subdeltoid bursa
17 Subscapularis muscle
18 Humerus (head)
19 Glenoid labrum (inferior lip)
20 Deltoid muscle
21 Axillary recess
22 Posterior circumflex humeral artery
and vein and axillary nerve
23 Intercostal muscle
24 Teres major muscle
25 Subscapular artery and vein
26 Ulnar, median, and radial nerves
27 Serratus anterior muscle
28 Coracobrachialis muscle
29 Lung
30 Brachial artery and vein
31 Ribs
32 Biceps brachii muscle (long head)
33 Latissimus dorsi muscle

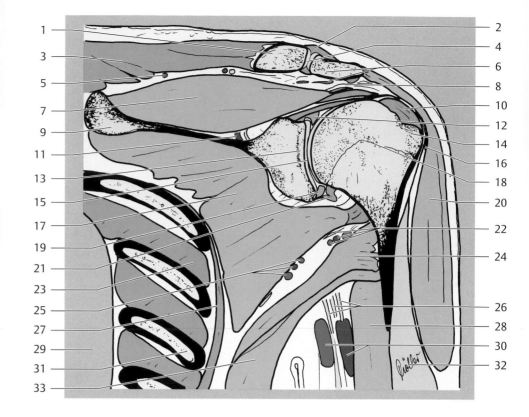

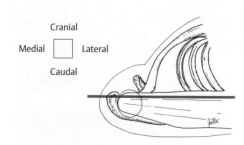

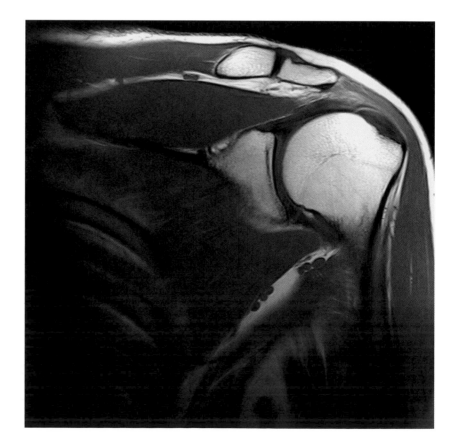

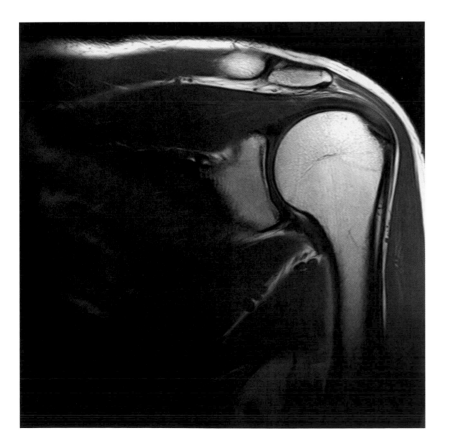

1 Clavicle
2 Acromioclavicular joint and acromioclavicular ligament
3 Trapezius muscle
4 Acromion
5 Supraspinatus muscle
6 Biceps brachii muscle (long head, tendon)
7 Scapula
8 Glenoid labrum (superior)
9 Suprascapular artery, vein, and nerve
10 Greater tubercle
11 Glenoid
12 Humerus (head)
13 Subscapularis muscle
14 Glenohumeral joint
15 Glenoid labrum (inferior)
16 Axillary recess
17 Intercostal muscle
18 Posterior circumflex humeral artery and vein and axillary nerve
19 Serratus anterior muscle
20 Deltoid muscle
21 Subscapular artery and vein
22 Humerus (shaft)
23 Teres major muscle
24 Coracobrachialis muscle
25 Rib
26 Biceps brachii muscle (long head)
27 Latissimus dorsi muscle
28 Ulnar, medial, and radial nerves
29 Brachial artery and vein

Cranial
Medial Lateral
Caudal

1 Acromion
2 Subacromial bursa
3 Trapezius muscle
4 Glenoid labrum (superior)
5 Supraspinatus muscle
6 Lesser tubercle
7 Scapula
8 Humerus (head)
9 Suprascapular artery, vein, and nerve
10 Shoulder joint
11 Joint socket
12 Glenoid labrum (inferior)
13 Neck of scapula
14 Axillary recess
15 Triceps brachii muscle
   (long head, tendon attachment)
16 Posterior circumflex humeral artery
   and vein, axillary nerve
17 Subscapular muscle
18 Deltoid muscle
19 Subscapular artery and vein
20 Humerus (shaft)
21 Teres major muscle
22 Triceps brachii muscle (lateral head)
23 Latissimus dorsi muscle
24 Ulnar, median, and radial nerves

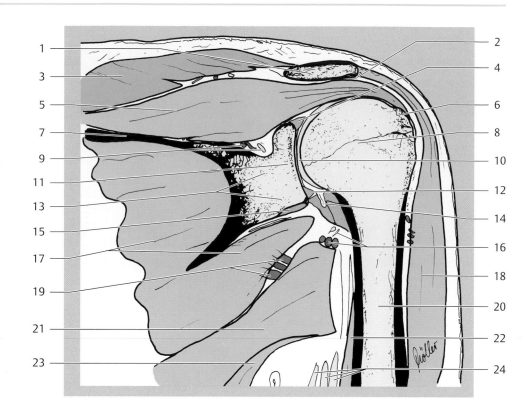

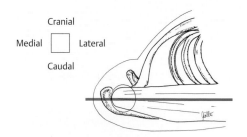

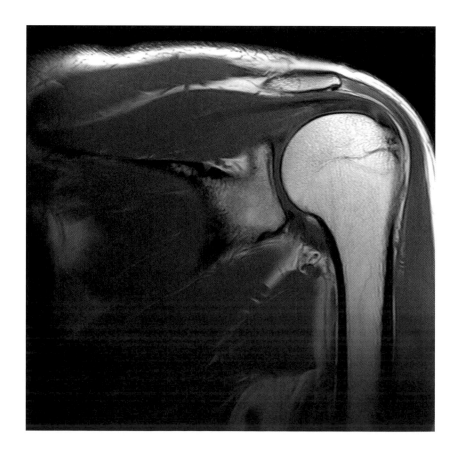

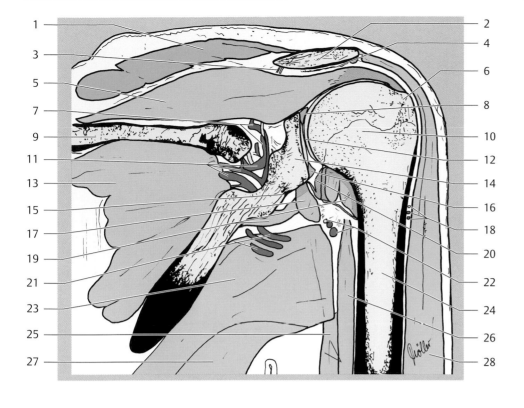

1 Trapezius muscle
2 Acromion
3 Suprascapular artery and vein (acromial branch)
4 Subacromial bursa
5 Supraspinatus muscle
6 Lesser tubercle
7 Suprascapular artery, vein, and nerve
8 Glenoid labrum (superior)
9 Scapula
10 Humerus (head)
11 Circumflex scapular artery and vein
12 Glenohumeral joint
13 Infraspinatus muscle
14 Glenoid
15 Neck of scapula
16 Glenoid labrum (inferior)
17 Triceps brachii muscle (long head, tendon attachment)
18 Posterior circumflex humeral artery and vein and axillary nerve (muscular branches)
19 Teres minor muscle
20 Axillary recess
21 Subscapular artery and vein
22 Posterior circumflex humeral artery and vein and axillary nerve
23 Teres major muscle
24 Humerus (shaft)
25 Triceps brachii muscle (long head)
26 Triceps brachii muscle (lateral head)
27 Latissimus dorsi muscle
28 Deltoid muscle

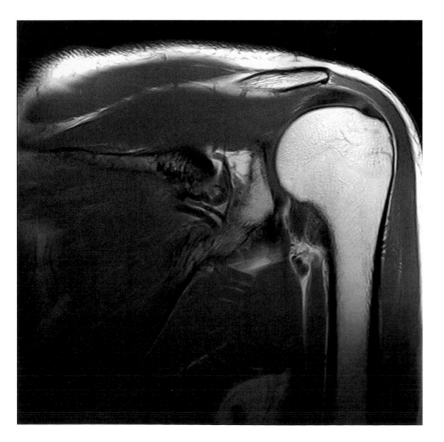

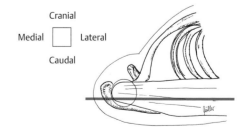

Cranial
Medial Lateral
Caudal

1 Trapezius muscle
2 Acromion
3 Subscapular artery, vein, and nerve (acromial branch)
4 Supraspinatus muscle
5 Scapula (spine)
6 Humerus (head)
7 Scapular artery, vein, and nerve
8 Glenohumeral joint
9 Infraspinatus muscle
10 Glenoid
11 Circumflex scapular artery and vein
12 Joint capsule
13 Teres minor muscle
14 Posterior circumflex humeral artery and vein and axillary nerve (muscular branches)
15 Subscapular artery and vein
16 Posterior circumflex humeral artery and vein and axillary nerve
17 Triceps brachii muscle (long head)
18 Deltoid muscle
19 Teres major muscle
20 Humerus (shaft)
21 Scapula
22 Triceps brachii muscle (lateral head)
23 Latissimus dorsi muscle

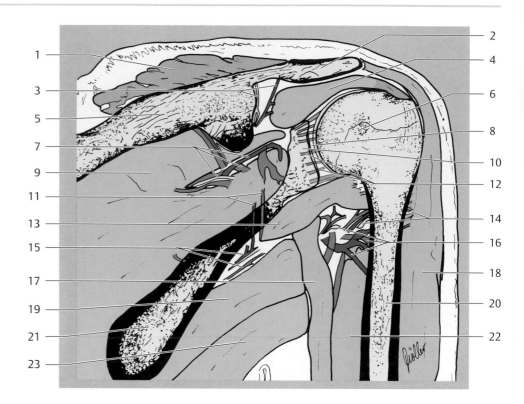

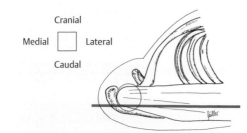

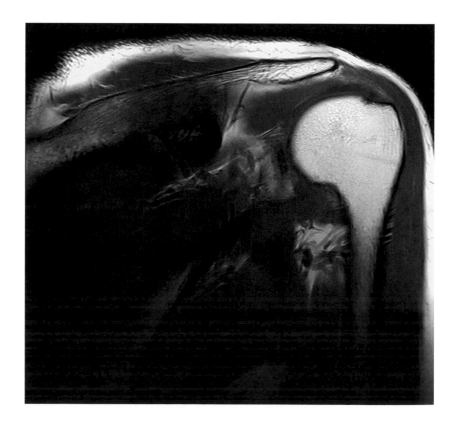

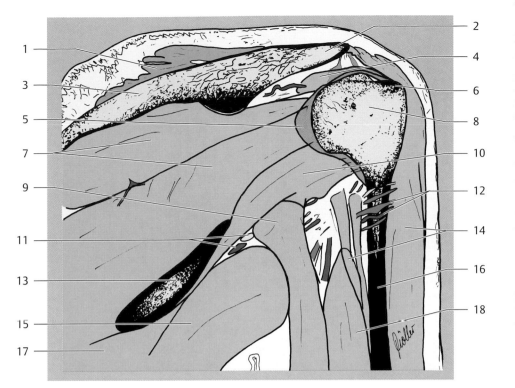

1 Trapezius muscle
2 Acromion
3 Scapula (spine)
4 Supraspinatus muscle
5 Joint capsule
6 Lesser tubercle
7 Infraspinatus muscle
8 Humerus (head)
9 Triceps brachii muscle (long head)
10 Teres minor muscle
11 Subscapular artery and nerve
12 Posterior circumflex humeral artery and vein and axillary nerve
13 Scapula
14 Deltoid muscle
15 Teres major muscle
16 Humerus (shaft)
17 Latissimus dorsi muscle
18 Triceps brachii muscle (lateral head)

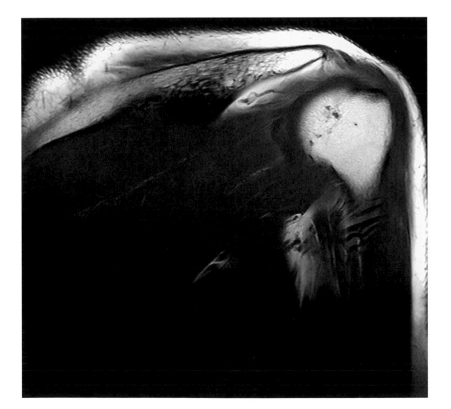

Cranial

Medial   Lateral

Caudal

1 Acromion
2 Joint capsule
3 Scapula (spine)
4 Deltoid muscle (acromial part)
5 Infraspinatus muscle
6 Humerus (head)
7 Teres minor muscle
8 Axillary nerve
9 Thoracodorsal artery and vein
10 Posterior circumflex humeral artery and vein
11 Teres major muscle
12 Deltoid muscle (spinal part)
13 Latissimus dorsi muscle
14 Triceps brachii muscle (long head)

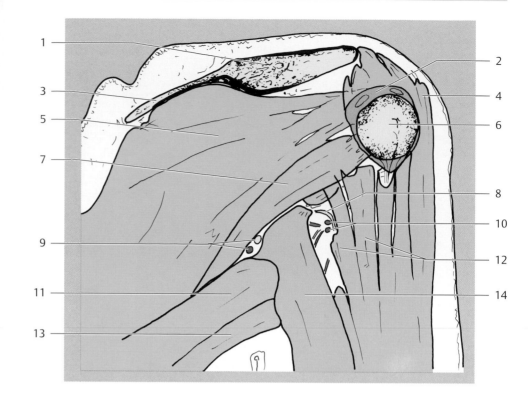

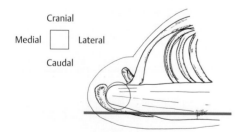

Cranial

Medial   Lateral

Caudal

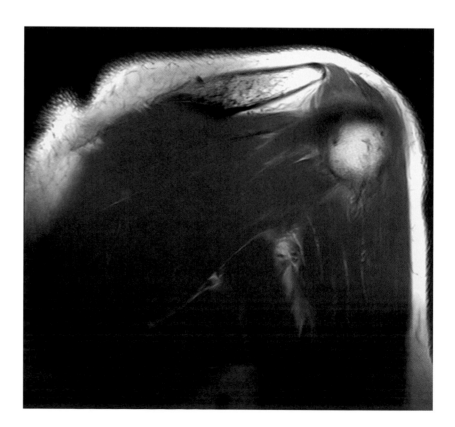

1 Deltoid muscle (spinal part)
2 Acromion
3 Infraspinatus muscle
4 Deltoid muscle (acromial part)
5 Thoracodorsal artery and vein
6 Joint capsule
7 Teres major muscle
8 Posterior circumflex humeral artery and vein
9 Latissimus dorsi muscle
10 Triceps brachii muscle (long head)

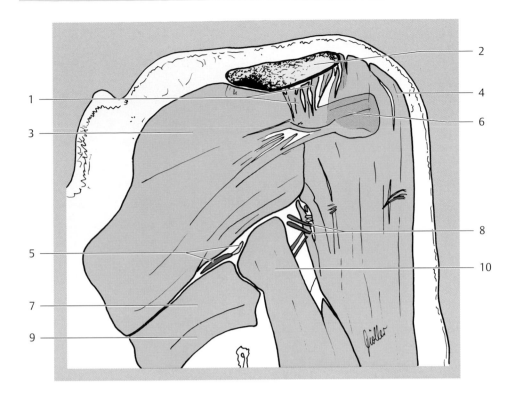

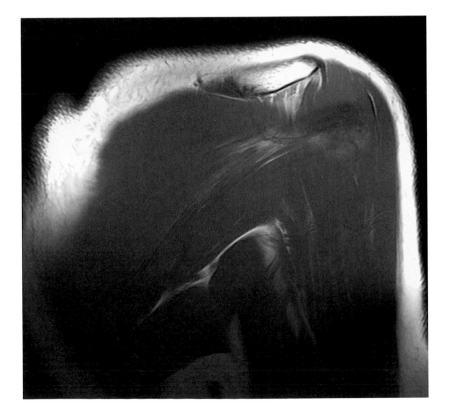

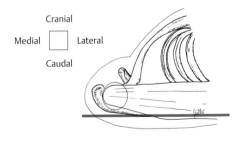

Cranial

Medial Lateral

Caudal

Shoulder, Sagittal

1 Deltoid muscle (acromial part)
2 Supraspinatus muscle (tendon)
3 Glenohumeral ligament (superior)
4 Infraspinatus muscle (tendon)
5 Intertubercular sulcus (bicipital groove)
6 Greater tubercle
7 Glenohumeral ligament (middle)
8 Biceps brachii muscle
   (long head, tendon)
9 Lesser tubercle
10 Crest of greater tubercle
11 Anterior circumflex humeral artery
   and vein
12 Posterior circumflex humeral artery
   and vein
13 Cephalic vein
14 Humerus (shaft)
15 Biceps brachii muscle (long head)

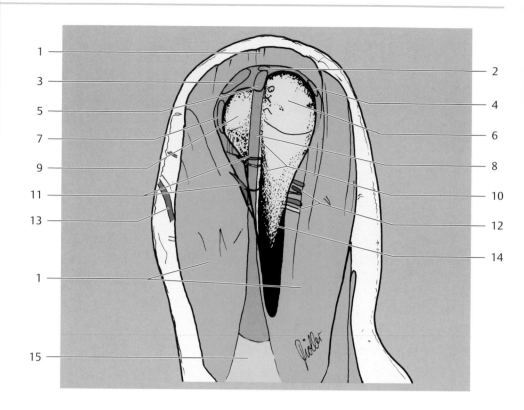

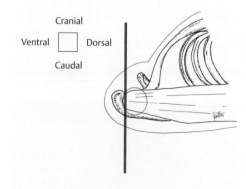

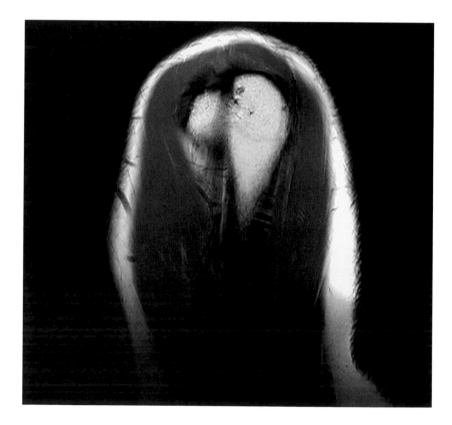

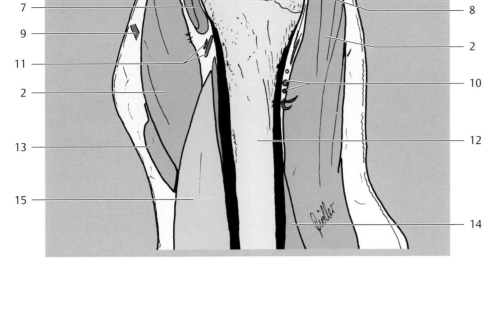

1 Biceps brachii muscle
  (long head, tendon)
2 Deltoid muscle (acromial part)
3 Glenohumeral ligament (superior)
4 Supraspinatus muscle (tendon)
5 Glenohumeral ligament (middle)
6 Infraspinatus muscle (tendon)
7 Joint capsule
8 Humerus (head)
9 Cephalic vein
10 Posterior circumflex humeral artery
   and vein
11 Anterior circumflex humeral artery
   and vein
12 Humerus (shaft)
13 Pectoralis major muscle
14 Triceps brachii muscle (medial head)
15 Biceps brachii muscle (long head)

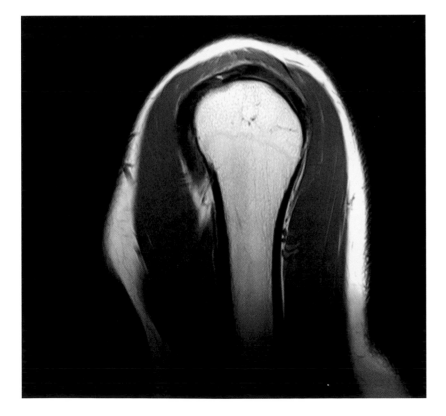

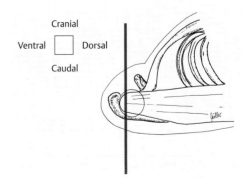

Cranial
Ventral Dorsal
Caudal

1 Transverse humeral ligament
2 Acromion
3 Biceps brachii muscle
   (long head, tendon)
4 Subdeltoid bursa
5 Glenohumeral ligament (superior)
6 Supraspinatus muscle (tendon)
7 Subscapularis muscle
8 Infraspinatus muscle (tendon)
9 Cephalic vein
10 Humerus (head)
11 Glenohumeral ligament (middle)
12 Teres minor muscle
   (and tendon attachment)
13 Glenohumeral ligament (inferior)
14 Deltoid muscle (acromial part)
15 Anterior circumflex humeral artery
   and vein
16 Posterior circumflex humeral artery
   and vein
17 Pectoralis major muscle
18 Latissimus dorsi muscle
19 Teres major muscle
20 Humerus (shaft)
21 Biceps brachii muscle (long head)
22 Triceps brachii muscle (medial head)
23 Coracobrachialis muscle

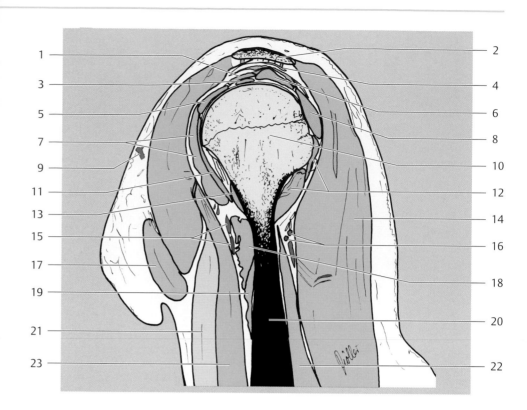

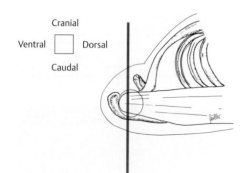

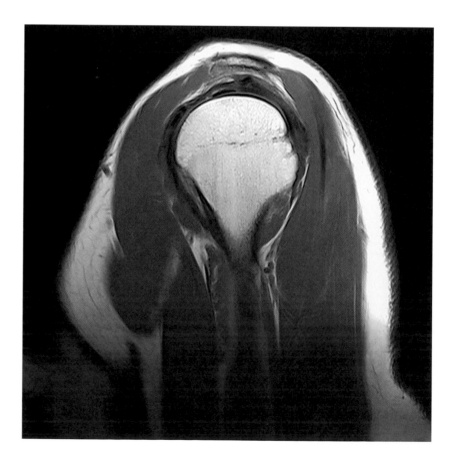

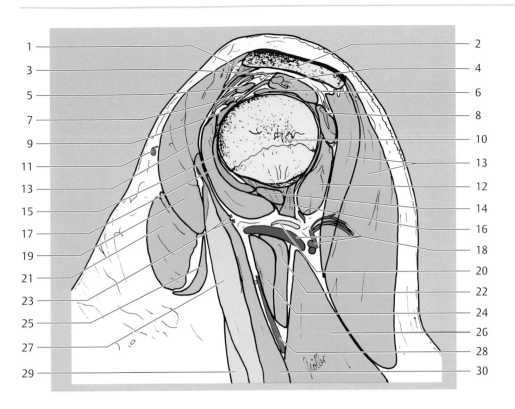

1 Coraco-acromial ligament
2 Acromion
3 Subacromial bursa
4 Supraspinatus muscle (and tendon)
5 Coracohumeral ligament
6 Biceps brachii muscle
   (long head, tendon)
7 Transverse humeral ligament
8 Infraspinatus muscle (and tendon)
9 Superior glenohumeral ligament
10 Humerus (head)
11 Cephalic vein
12 Teres minor muscle
13 Deltoid muscle (acromial part)
14 Inferior glenohumeral ligament
15 Medial glenohumeral ligament
16 Teres major muscle (tendon)
17 Subscapularis muscle
18 Posterior circumflex humeral artery
   and vein and muscular branches
19 Deltoid muscle (clavicular part)
20 Axillary nerve
21 Pectoralis major muscle
22 Teres major muscle
23 Anterior circumflex humeral artery
   and vein
24 Latissimus dorsi muscle
25 Pectoralis minor muscle
26 Triceps brachii muscle (long head)
27 Biceps brachii muscle
   (short head and tendon)
28 Basilic vein
29 Biceps brachii muscle (long head)
30 Coracobrachialis muscle

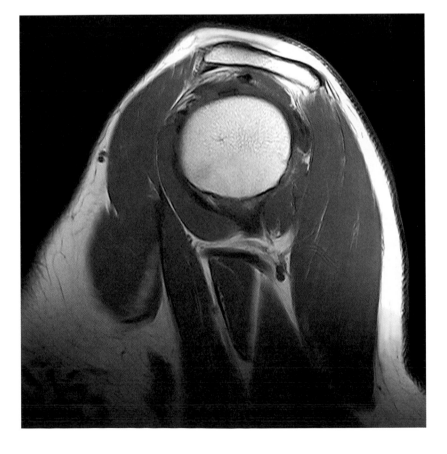

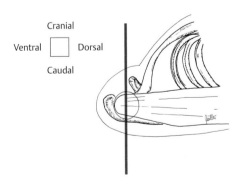

1 Acromioclavicular joint
2 Acromioclavicular ligament
3 Thoraco-acromial artery
(acromial branch)
4 Acromion
5 Deltoid muscle (clavicular part)
6 Subacromial bursa
7 Coraco-acromial ligament
8 Supraspinatus muscle (and tendon)
9 Coracohumeral ligament
10 Biceps brachii muscle
(long head, tendon)
11 Coracoid process
12 Infraspinatus muscle (and tendon)
13 Thoraco-acromial artery (deltoid
branch) and cephalic vein
14 Joint capsule
15 Glenohumeral ligament (superior)
16 Humerus (head)
17 Glenohumeral ligament (medial)
18 Teres minor muscle
19 Coracobrachialis muscle
20 Glenohumeral ligament (inferior)
21 Subscapularis muscle
22 Deltoid muscle (acromial part)
23 Axillary nerve
24 Posterior circumflex humeral artery
and vein (muscular branches)
25 Anterior circumflex humeral artery
and vein
26 Deltoid muscle (spinal part)
27 Pectoralis major muscle
28 Teres major muscle
29 Biceps brachii muscle
(short head, tendon)
30 Radial nerve
31 Pectoralis minor muscle
32 Latissimus dorsi muscle
33 Posterior circumflex humeral artery
and vein
34 Brachial artery and vein
35 Ulnar nerve
36 Triceps brachii muscle (long head)
37 Median nerve

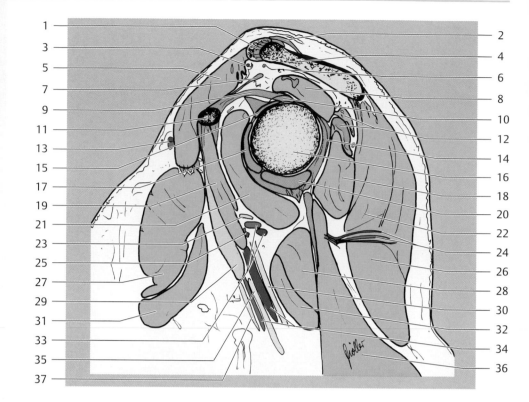

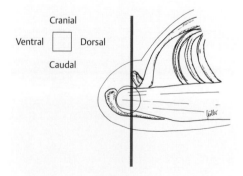

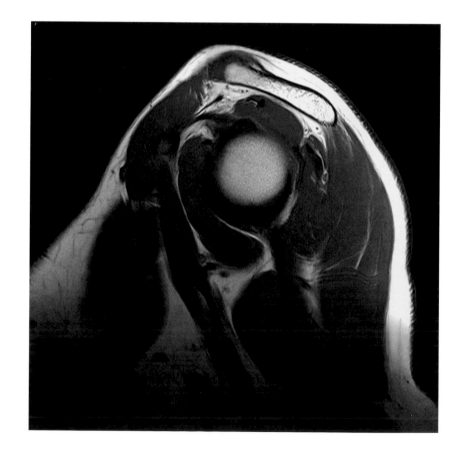

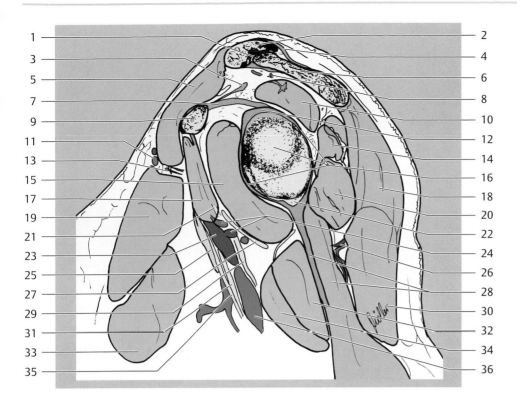

1 —
3 —
5 —
7 —
9 —
11 —
13 —
15 —
17 —
19 —
21 —
23 —
25 —
27 —
29 —
31 —
33 —
35 —

— 2
— 4
— 6
— 8
— 10
— 12
— 14
— 16
— 18
— 20
— 22
— 24
— 26
— 28
— 30
— 32
— 34
— 36

1 Acromioclavicular joint
2 Clavicle
3 Coraco-acromial ligament
4 Acromioclavicular ligament
5 Deltoid muscle (clavicular part)
6 Acromion
7 Coracohumeral ligament
8 Thoraco-acromial artery
  (acromial branch)
9 Coracoid process
10 Supraspinatus muscle (and tendon)
11 Cephalic vein
12 Biceps brachii muscle
  (long head, tendon attachment)
13 Thoraco-acromial artery (deltoid
  branch)
14 Infraspinatus muscle (and tendon)
15 Subscapularis muscle
16 Glenohumeral joint and joint capsule
17 Coracobrachialis muscle
18 Deltoid muscle (acromial part)
19 Pectoralis major muscle
20 Teres major muscle
21 Musculocutaneous nerve
22 Infraglenoid tubercle
23 Brachial artery
24 Posterior circumflex humeral artery
  and vein
25 Biceps brachii muscle (short head)
26 Posterior circumflex humeral artery
  and vein (muscular branches)
27 Axillary nerve
28 Triceps brachii muscle
  (long head and tendon)
29 Radial nerve
30 Deltoid muscle (spinal part)
31 Ulnar nerve
32 Teres major muscle
33 Pectoralis minor muscle
34 Latissimus dorsi muscle
35 Median nerve
36 Brachial vein

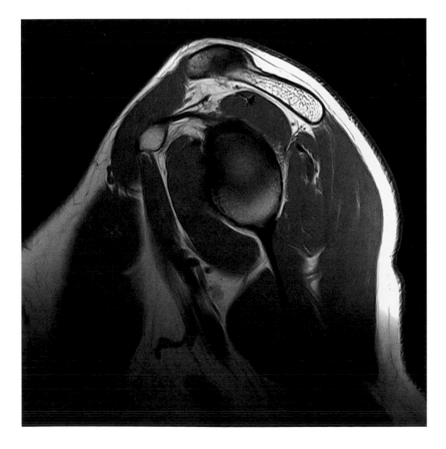

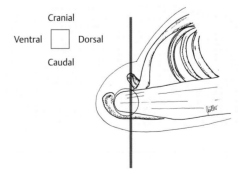

Cranial

Ventral ☐ Dorsal

Caudal

1 Clavicle
2 Trapezius muscle (tendon attachment)
3 Deltoid muscle (clavicular part)
4 Acromion
5 Coracoclavicular ligament
6 Supraspinatus muscle
7 Coracoid process
8 Deltoid muscle (acromial part)
9 Cephalic vein
10 Scapula (neck)
11 Thoraco-acromial artery (pectoral part)
12 Infraspinatus muscle (and tendon)
13 Subscapularis muscle
14 Circumflex scapular artery and vein
15 Axillary artery and vein
16 Teres minor muscle
17 Brachial plexus
18 Axillary nerve
19 Pectoralis major muscle
20 Deltoid muscle (spinal part)
21 Pectoralis minor muscle
22 Triceps brachii muscle
    (long head and tendon)
23 Circumflex scapular artery and vein
24 Teres major muscle
25 Axillary lymph nodes
26 Latissimus dorsi muscle

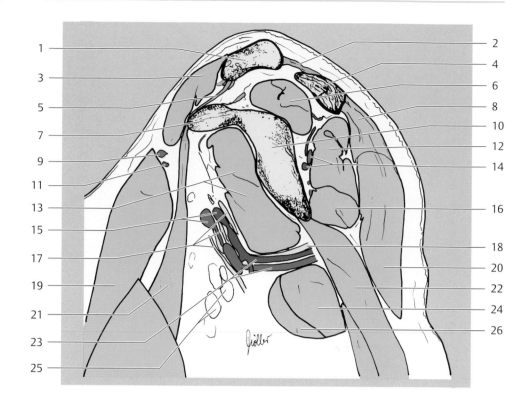

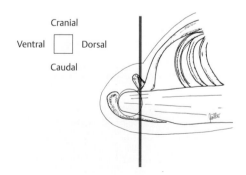

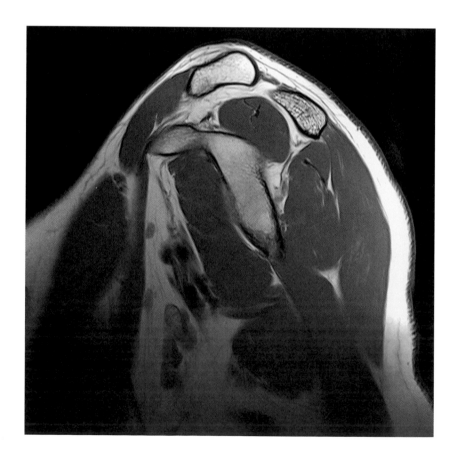

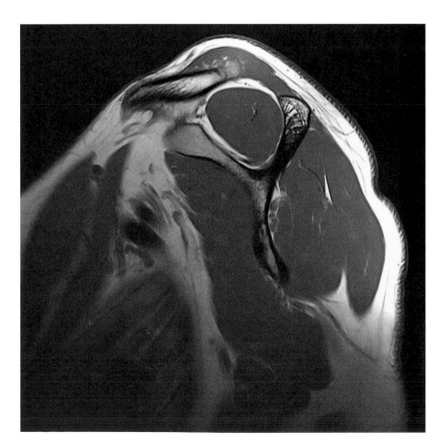

1 Clavicle
2 Trapezius muscle
3 Coracoclavicular ligament
4 Acromion
5 Deltoid muscle (clavicular part)
6 Supraspinatus muscle
7 Scapula (spine)
8 Suprascapular artery and vein
9 Cephalic vein
10 Infraspinatus muscle
11 Thoraco-acromial artery
   (pectoral branch)
12 Circumflex scapular artery and vein
13 Brachial plexus
14 Deltoid muscle (spinal part)
15 Axillary artery and vein
16 Subscapularis muscle
17 Pectoralis major muscle
18 Scapula (body)
19 Pectoralis minor muscle
20 Teres minor muscle
21 Serratus anterior muscle
22 Teres major muscle
23 Ribs
24 Latissimus dorsi muscle

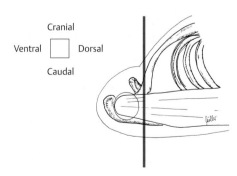

Cranial

Ventral ☐ Dorsal

Caudal

1 Median nerve
2 Brachialis muscle
3 Brachial artery and vein
4 Lateral cutaneous nerve of forearm
5 Basilic vein
6 Radial artery (recurrent branch)
7 Median cubital vein
8 Biceps brachii muscle (tendon)
9 Pronator teres muscle
10 Median cephalic vein
11 Ulnar artery
12 Cephalic vein
13 Median nerve
14 Brachioradialis muscle
15 Flexor carpi radialis muscle
16 Radial artery
17 Median vein of forearm

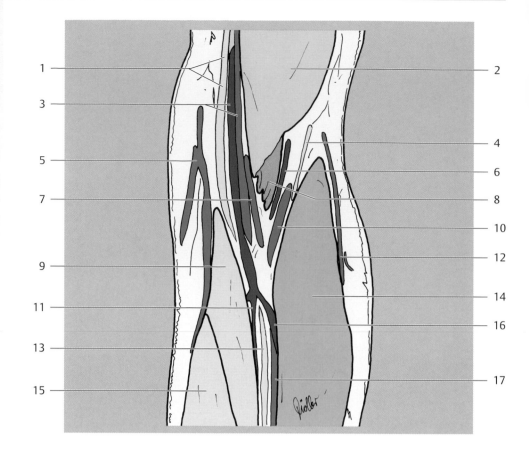

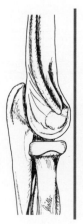

Proximal

Ulnar   Radial
Medial   Lateral

Distal

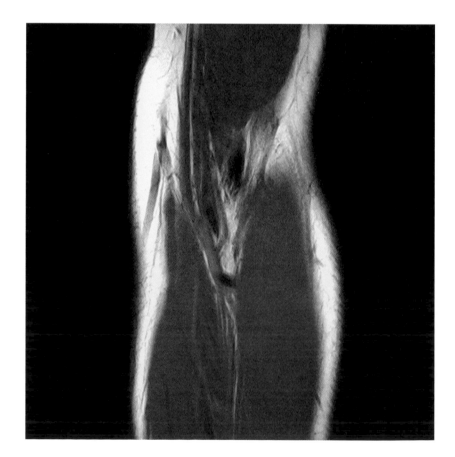

1 Brachialis muscle
2 Radial nerve
3 Humerus (trochlea)
4 Brachioradialis muscle
5 Pronator teres muscle
6 Humerus (capitulum)
7 Brachialis muscle (tendon)
8 Anular and radial collateral ligaments of wrist joint
9 Biceps brachii muscle (tendon)
10 Radius (head)
11 Median nerve
12 Radial nerve (deep branch)
13 Flexor carpi radialis muscle
14 Extensor carpi radialis longus and brevis muscles
15 Palmaris longus muscle
16 Supinator muscle
17 Flexor carpi ulnaris muscle
18 Anterior interosseous artery and vein
19 Flexor digitorum profundus muscle
20 Radius (shaft)

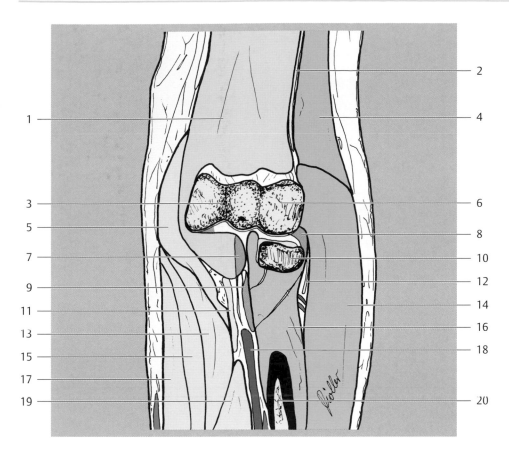

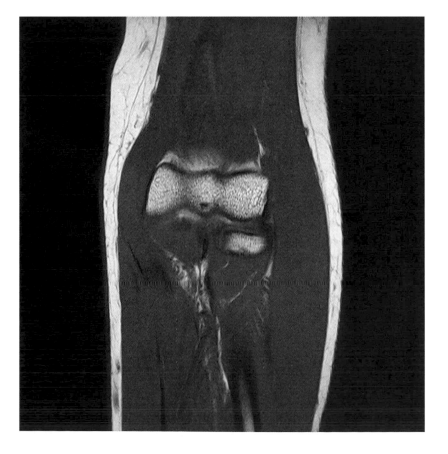

Proximal

Ulnar   Radial
Medial   Lateral

Distal

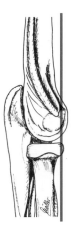

1 Triceps brachii muscle
2 Brachioradialis muscle
3 Brachialis muscle
4 Humerus (shaft)
5 Coronoid fossa
6 Extensor carpi radialis longus muscle
7 Medial epicondyle
8 Lateral epicondyle
9 Pronator teres muscle
10 Common extensor tendons
      (attachment)
11 Medial collateral ligament
12 Radial collateral ligament
13 Humerus (trochlea)
14 Humerus (capitulum)
15 Humero-ulnar joint
16 Humeroradial joint
17 Ulna (coronoid process)
18 Radius (head)
19 Flexor carpi radialis muscle
20 Supinator muscle
21 Biceps brachii muscle (tendon)
22 Radial tuberosity
23 Palmaris longus muscle
24 Extensor digitorum muscle
25 Flexor digitorum superficialis muscle
26 Radius (shaft)
27 Flexor digitorum profundus muscle

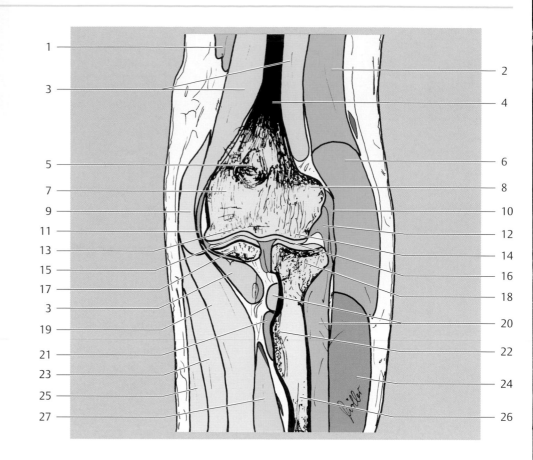

Proximal
Ulnar   Radial
Medial   Lateral
Distal

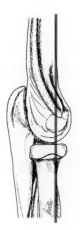

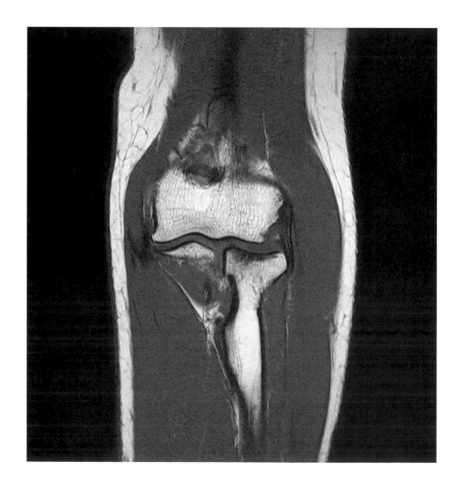

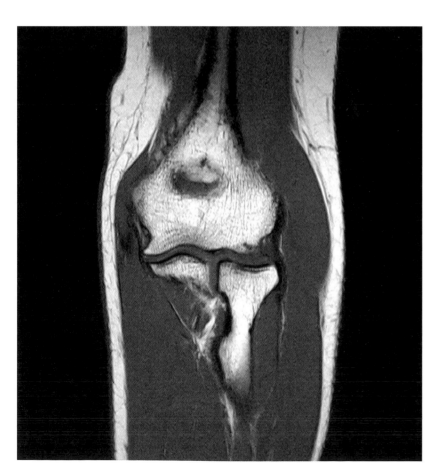

1 Triceps brachii muscle
2 Brachioradialis muscle
3 Brachialis muscle
4 Humerus (shaft)
5 Coronoid fossa
6 Extensor carpi radialis longus muscle
7 Pronator teres muscle
8 Common extensor tendons (attachment)
9 Medial epicondyle
10 Lateral epicondyle
11 Medial collateral ligament
12 Radial collateral ligament
13 Humerus (trochlea)
14 Humerus (capitulum)
15 Humero-ulnar joint
16 Anular ligament
17 Ulna (coronoid process)
18 Humeroradial joint
19 Flexor digitorum superficialis muscle
20 Radius (head)
21 Radius (shaft) and radial tuberosity
22 Radio-ulnar joint
23 Median nerve
24 Biceps brachii muscle (tendon)
25 Posterior interosseous artery and vein
26 Supinator muscle
27 Flexor digitorum profundus muscle
28 Extensor digitorum muscle
29 Abductor pollicis longus muscle

Proximal

Ulnar   Radial
Medial   Lateral

Distal

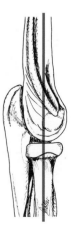

1 Triceps brachii muscle
2 Brachioradialis muscle
3 Humerus (shaft)
4 Brachialis muscle
5 Olecranon fossa (posterior fat pad)
6 Extensor carpi radialis longus muscle
7 Medial epicondyle
8 Olecranon
9 Common flexor tendons (attachment)
10 Lateral epicondyle
11 Humerus (trochlea)
12 Anular ligament
13 Ulna (coronoid process)
14 Radial nerve (deep branch)
15 Brachialis muscle (tendon attachment)
16 Radius (head)
17 Ulnar nerve
18 Common extensor tendons
19 Flexor carpi ulnaris muscle
20 Supinator muscle
21 Flexor digitorum superficialis muscle
22 Posterior interosseous artery and vein
23 Flexor digitorum profundus muscle
24 Extensor digitorum muscle

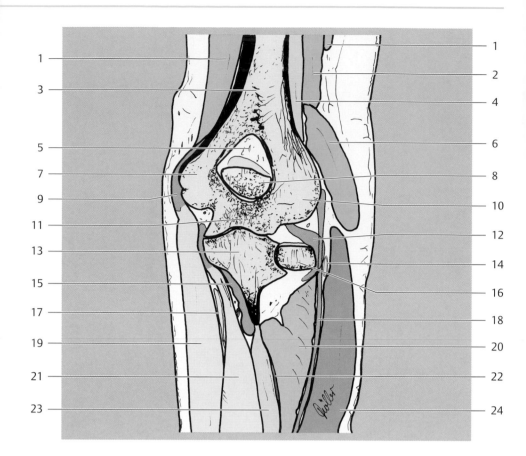

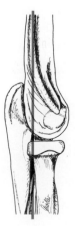

Proximal

Ulnar   Radial
Medial   Lateral

Distal

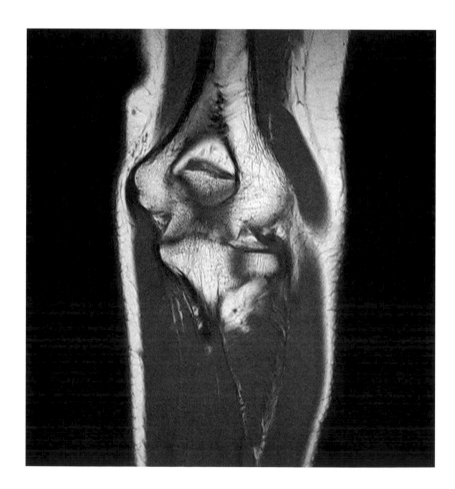

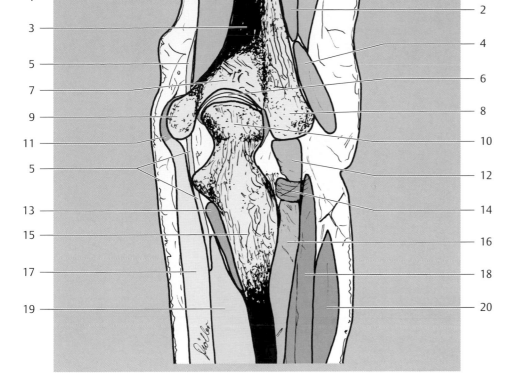

1 Triceps brachii muscle
2 Brachioradialis muscle
3 Humerus (shaft)
4 Extensor carpi radialis longus muscle
5 Ulnar nerve
6 Humero-ulnar joint
7 Olecranon fossa
8 Lateral epicondyle
9 Medial epicondyle
10 Olecranon
11 Common flexor tendons (attachment)
12 Anconeus muscle
13 Brachialis muscle (tendon attachment)
14 Anular ligament
15 Ulna (shaft)
16 Supinator muscle
17 Flexor carpi ulnaris muscle
18 Extensor carpi ulnaris muscle
19 Flexor digitorum profundus muscle
20 Extensor digitorum muscle

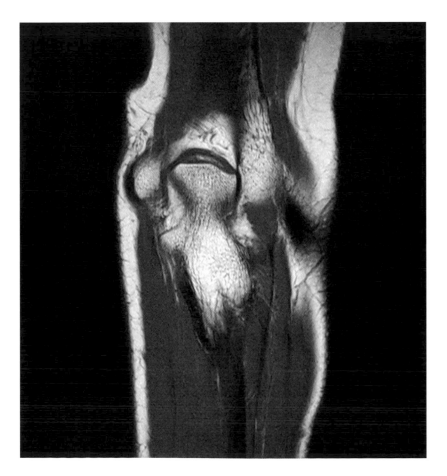

Proximal

Ulnar ☐ Radial
Medial ☐ Lateral

Distal

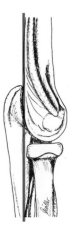

1 Brachial artery
2 Biceps brachii muscle
3 Brachialis muscle
4 Brachial vein
5 Median nerve
6 Humerus (trochlea)
7 Humerus (medial epicondyle)
8 Pronator teres muscle
9 Flexor carpi ulnaris muscle
10 Palmaris longus muscle
11 Flexor digitorum superficialis muscle
12 Flexor carpi radialis muscle
13 Flexor digitorum profundus muscle
14 Basilic vein

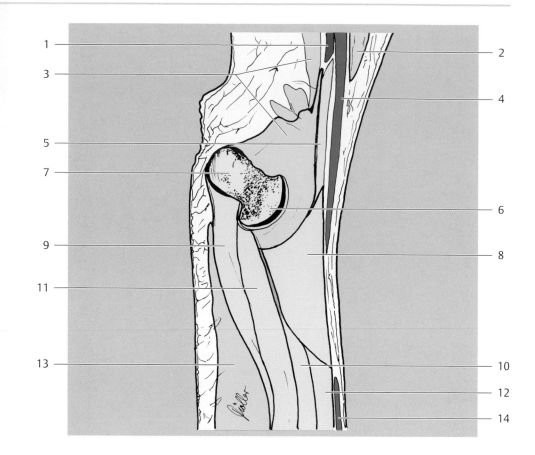

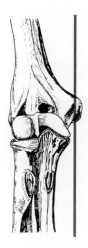

Proximal

Dorsal ☐ Ventral

Distal

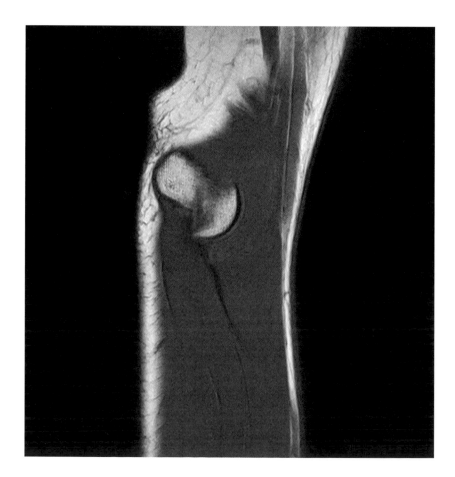

1 Triceps brachii muscle
2 Biceps brachii muscle
3 Ulnar nerve
4 Brachial artery and nerve
5 Brachialis muscle
6 Median nerve
7 Collateral ulnar ligament, posterior part
   (and posterior capsule of elbow joint)
8 Humerus (trochlea)
9 Humero-ulnar joint
10 Median cubital vein
11 Olecranon
12 Pronator teres muscle
13 Ulnar recurrent artery
14 Flexor digitorum superficialis muscle
15 Flexor digitorum profundus muscle
16 Flexor carpi radialis muscle

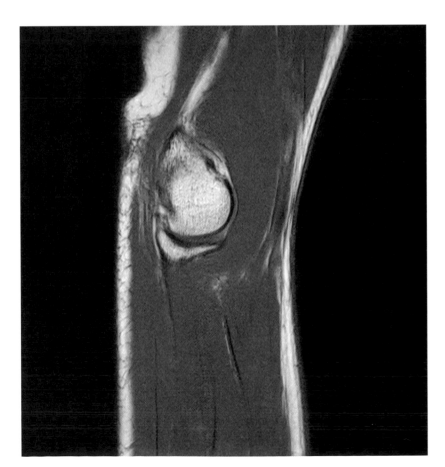

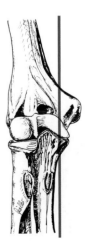

Proximal

Dorsal ☐ Ventral

Distal

1 Triceps brachii muscle
2 Biceps brachii muscle
3 Humerus (shaft)
4 Brachialis muscle
5 Joint capsule
6 Radial nerve
7 Humeroradial joint
8 Humerus (capitulum)
9 Radius (head)
10 Anular ligament of radius
11 Radial collateral ligament
12 Cephalic vein
13 Anconeus muscle
14 Supinator muscle
15 Interosseous artery and vein
16 Brachioradialis muscle
17 Ulna (shaft)
18 Radial nerve (deep branch)
19 Extensor carpi ulnaris muscle
20 Extensor carpi radialis longus muscle
21 Pronator teres muscle (ulnar head)
22 Flexor digitorum superficialis muscle
   (radial head)
23 Radius (shaft)

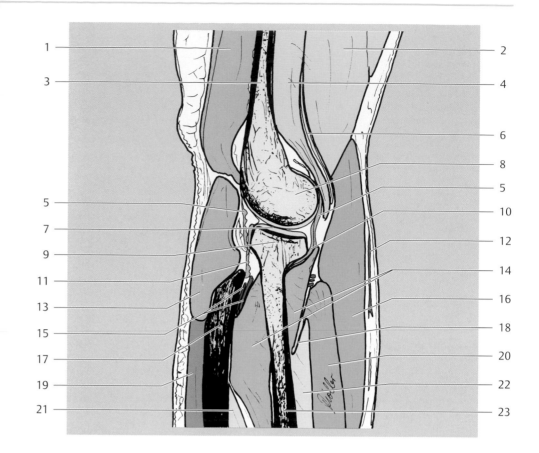

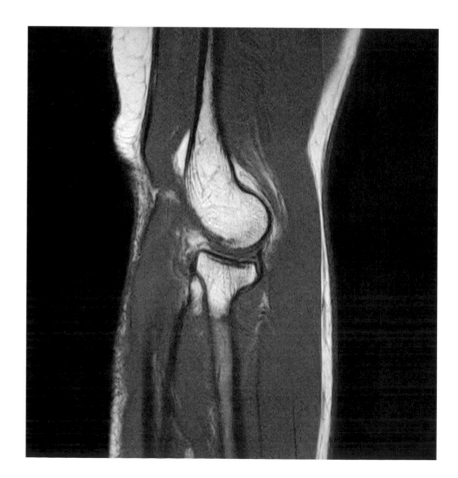

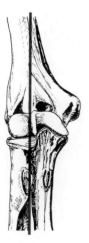

Proximal

Dorsal   ☐   Ventral

Distal

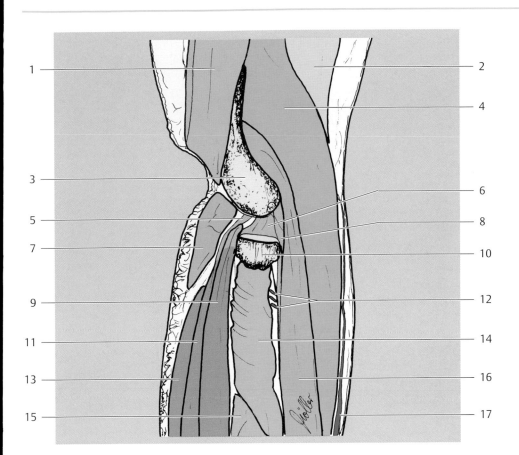

1 Triceps brachii muscle
2 Brachialis muscle
3 Humerus (capitulum)
4 Brachioradialis muscle
5 Joint capsule
6 Radial collateral ligament
7 Anconeus muscle
8 Anular ligament of radius
9 Extensor digitorum muscle
10 Radius (head)
11 Extensor digiti minimi muscle
12 Anterior interosseous artery and veins
13 Extensor carpi ulnaris muscle
14 Supinator muscle
15 Abductor pollicis longus muscle
16 Extensor carpi radialis longus muscle
17 Cephalic vein

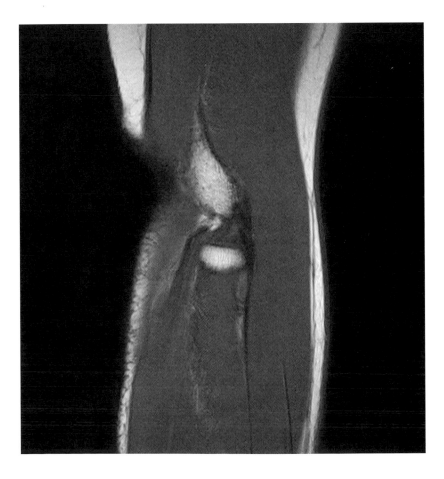

Proximal

Dorsal ☐ Ventral

Distal

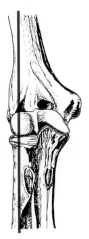

1 Proper palmar digital arteries
2 Proper palmar digital nerves
   (median nerve)
3 Adductor pollicis muscle
4 Palmar aponeurosis
5 Metacarpal I (head)
6 Abductor digiti minimi muscle
7 Palmar digital nerve of thumb
8 Proper palmar digital nerves
   (ulnar nerve)
9 Flexor pollicis brevis muscle
   (superficial head)
10 Ulnar nerve
11 Abductor pollicis muscle
12 Flexor digiti minimi muscle
13 Median nerve
14 Palmar carpometacarpal ligaments and
   pisohamate ligament
15 Opponens pollicis muscle
16 Retinaculum of flexor muscles
   (transverse carpal ligament)
17 Metacarpal I (base)
18 Pisiform
19 Palmar carpometacarpal ligaments
20 Flexor digitorum superficialis muscle
   (tendons)
21 Trapezium
22 Ulnar artery
23 Scaphoid
24 Palmaris longus muscle
25 Radial artery (superficial palmar
   branch)
26 Flexor carpi ulnaris muscle (tendon)
27 Flexor carpi radialis muscle (tendon)

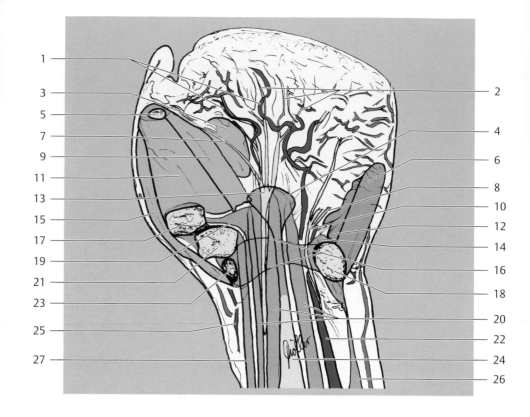

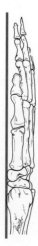

Distal

Radial   Ulnar

Proximal

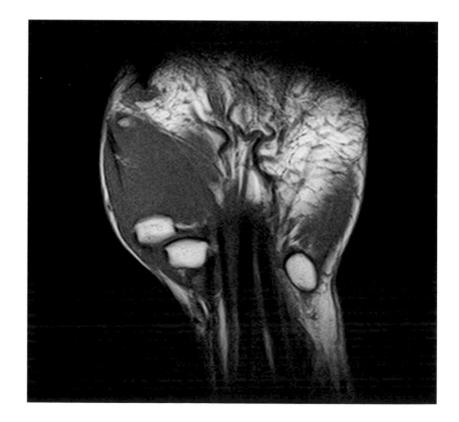

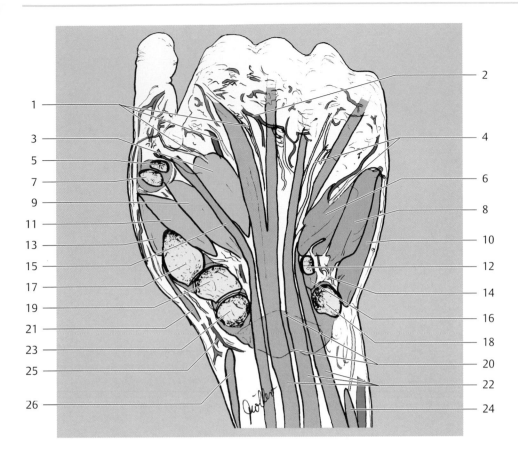

1 Proper palmar digital nerves
   (of median nerve)
2 Proper palmar digital arteries
3 Adductor pollicis muscle
   (transverse head)
4 Proper palmar digital nerves
   (of ulnar nerve)
5 Proximal phalanx I (base)
6 Opponens digiti minimi muscle
7 Metacarpal I (head)
8 Flexor digiti minimi muscle
9 Flexor pollicis brevis muscle
   (deep head)
10 Abductor digiti minimi muscle
11 Abductor pollicis muscle
12 Hamate (hook)
13 Opponens pollicis muscle
14 Ulnar nerve (deep branch)
15 Flexor pollicis longus muscle (tendon)
16 Pisohamate ligament
17 Metacarpal I (base)
18 Pisiform
19 Trapezium
20 Palmar radiocarpal ligament
21 Abductor pollicis longus muscle
   (tendon attachment)
22 Flexor digitorum profundus muscle
   (tendons)
23 Scaphoid
24 Flexor carpi ulnaris muscle
25 Radial artery (superficial palmar branch)
26 Brachioradialis muscle (tendon)

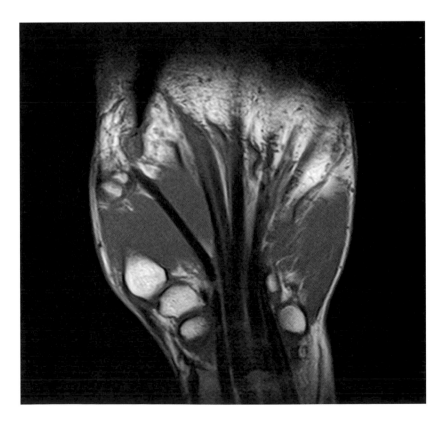

Distal

Radial ☐ Ulnar

Proximal

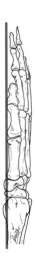

1 Distal phalanx I
2 Proper palmar digital arteries and nerves
3 Proximal phalanx I (head)
4 Lumbrical muscles
5 Flexor pollicis longus muscle (tendon)
6 Proximal phalanx V (base)
7 Adductor pollicis muscle (transverse head)
8 Metacarpal V (head)
9 Proximal phalanx I (base)
10 Flexor digitorum profundus muscle (tendons)
11 Sesamoid bone
12 Opponens digiti minimi muscle
13 Metacarpophalangeal joint I
14 Flexor digiti minimi muscle
15 Joint capsule
16 Abductor digiti minimi muscle
17 Adductor pollicis muscle (oblique head)
18 Hamate (hook)
19 Abductor pollicis muscle
20 Pisohamate ligament
21 Flexor pollicis brevis muscle
22 Radiate carpal ligament
23 Opponens pollicis muscle
24 Pisiform
25 Metacarpal I
26 Ulnar collateral ligament of wrist joint
27 Carpometacarpal joint I
28 Lunate
29 Trapezium
30 Palmar ulnocarpal ligament
31 Scaphoid
32 Radius
33 Extensor pollicis brevis muscle
34 Pronator quadratus muscle
35 Palmar radiocarpal ligament
36 Radial artery

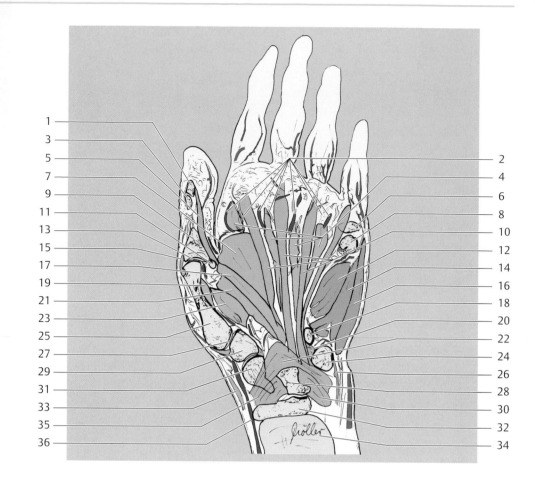

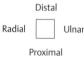

Distal
Radial | | Ulnar
Proximal

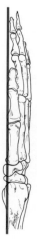

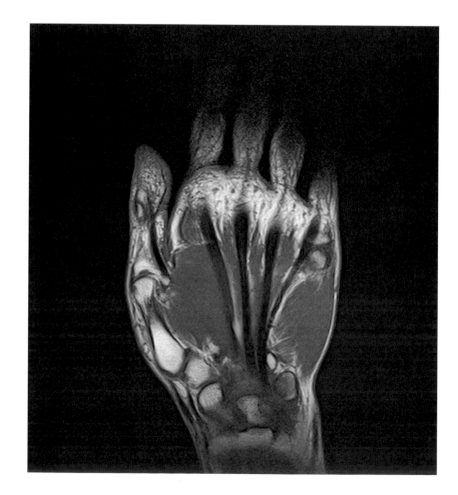

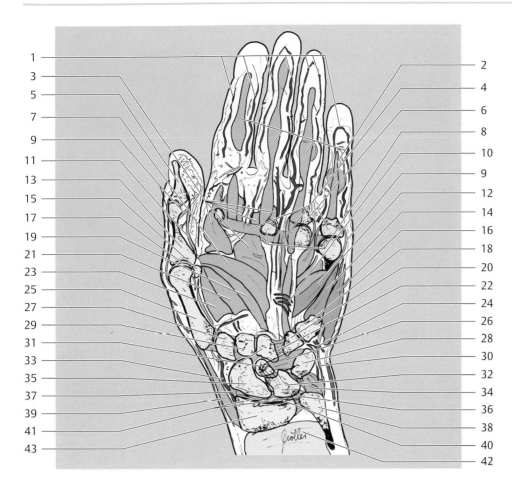

1 Proper palmar digital arteries
2 Flexor digitorum muscle (tendon)
3 Lumbrical muscles
4 Metacarpal ligaments
5 Distal phalanx I (thumb)
6 Proximal phalanges (bases)
7 Adductor pollicis muscle
  (transverse head)
8 Metacarpal (head)
9 Joint capsule
10 Deep palmar arch (of radial artery)
11 Flexor pollicis muscle
12 Opponens digiti minimi muscle
13 Proximal phalanx I (thumb)
14 Flexor digiti minimi muscle
15 Sesamoid bone
16 Abductor digiti minimi muscle
17 Metacarpophalangeal joint (proximal
  thumb joint)
18 Metacarpal V (base)
19 Adductor pollicis muscle (oblique head)
20 Hamate
21 Flexor pollicis brevis muscle
22 Interosseous (capitohamate) ligament
23 Opponens pollicis muscle
24 Ulnar artery (deep branch)
25 Metacarpal I
26 Radial carpal ligament
27 Trapezium
28 Triquetrum
29 Trapezoid
30 Ulnar collateral ligament of wrist
31 Capitate
32 Lunate
33 Radial artery
34 Palmar ulnocarpal ligament
35 Scaphoid
36 Ulnolunate ligament
37 Radial collateral ligament
38 Ulna (head)
39 Abductor pollicis longus muscle
  (tendon)
40 Interosseous (scapholunate) ligament
41 Radiocarpal joint
42 Pronator quadratus muscle
43 Radius

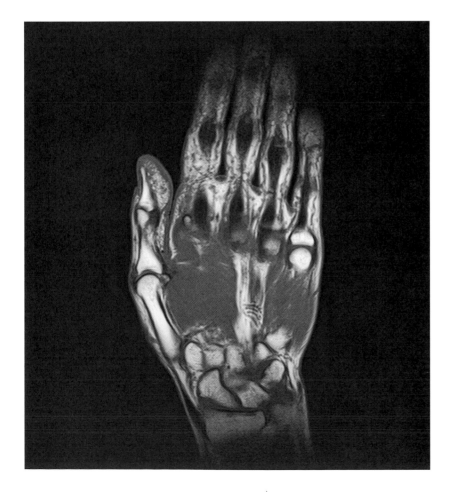

Distal

Radial ☐ Ulnar

Proximal

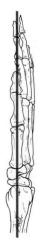

1 Distal phalanx II
2 Distal interphalangeal joint
3 Middle phalanx (base)
4 Proper palmar digital nerve and artery
5 Proximal phalanx (head)
6 Flexor digitorum muscle (tendon)
7 Distal phalanx I
8 Proximal interphalangeal joint
9 Metacarpal II (head)
10 Collateral ligament
11 Interphalangeal joint I
12 Metacarpophalangeal joint
13 Extensor pollicis longus muscle (tendon)
14 Interosseous muscles
15 Proximal phalanx I
16 Adductor pollicis muscle (transverse head)
17 Sesamoid bone
18 Abductor digiti minimi muscle
19 Adductor pollicis muscle (oblique head)
20 Deep palmar arch and palmar carpal branch
21 Metacarpal I (head)
22 Metacarpals (bases)
23 Flexor pollicis brevis muscle
24 Carpometacarpal joint
25 Trapezium
26 Hamate
27 Trapezoid
28 Capitate
29 Radial artery
30 Ulnar collateral ligament of wrist joint
31 Scaphoid
32 Triquetrum
33 Lunate
34 Ulnar styloid process
35 Interosseous (scapholunate) ligament
36 Triangular fibrocartilage complex
37 Wrist joint
38 Ulna
39 Brachioradialis muscle (tendon)
40 Pronator quadratus muscle
41 Radius

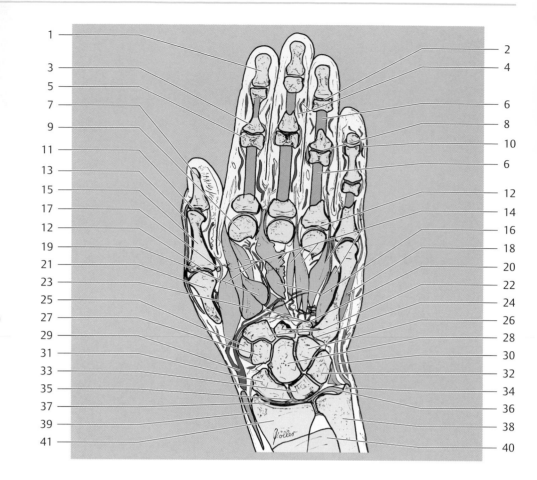

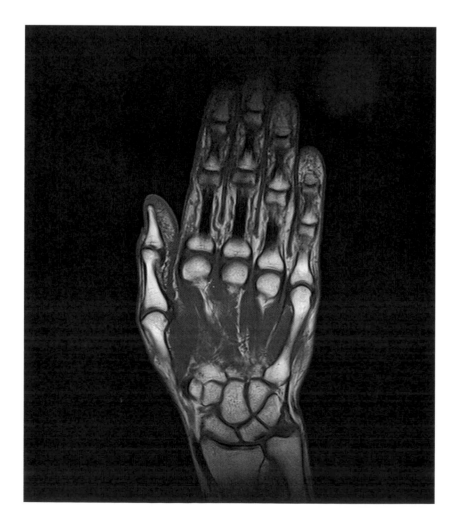

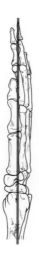

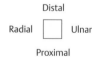

Distal

Radial | | Ulnar

Proximal

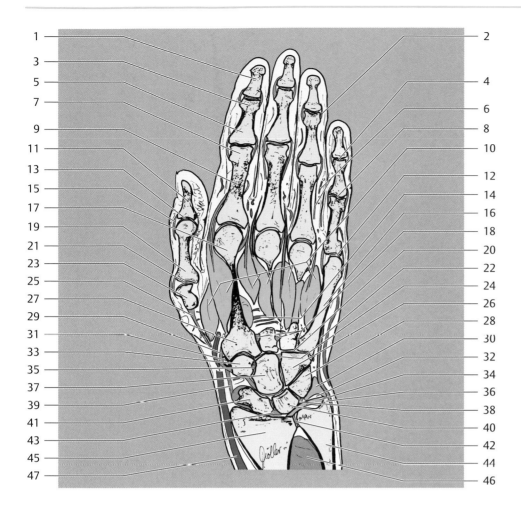

1 Distal phalanx II
2 Collateral ligament
3 Middle phalanx II (head)
4 Distal interphalangeal joint V
5 Middle phalanx II (base)
6 Proper palmar digital artery and nerves
7 Proximal phalanx II (head)
8 Proximal interphalangeal joint V
9 Proximal phalanx II (shaft)
10 Dorsal interossei muscles
11 Distal phalanx I
12 Metacarpophalangeal joint V
13 Interphalangeal joint I
14 Deep palmar arch
15 Extensor pollicis longus muscle (tendon)
16 Metacarpal V (shaft)
17 Metacarpal II (head)
18 Interosseous metacarpal ligaments
19 Proximal phalanx I (base)
20 Carpometacarpal joint
21 Metacarpophalangeal joint I
22 Ulnar ligament of wrist
23 Metacarpal I (head)
24 Dorsal intercarpal (capitohamate) ligament
25 Extensor pollicis longus muscle (tendon)
26 Hamate
27 Metacarpal II (base)
28 Triquetrum
29 Dorsal carpometacarpal ligament
30 Meniscal homologen
31 Trapezium
32 Prestyloid recess
33 Trapezoid
34 Ulnar triangular fibrocartilage
35 Dorsal intercarpal (trapeziocapitate) ligament
36 Ulnar styloid process
37 Capitate
38 Dorsal intercarpal (lunotriquetral) ligament
39 Radial collateral ligament
40 Lunate
41 Scaphoid
42 Distal radio-ulnar joint
43 Interosseous (scapholunate) ligament
44 Ulna
45 Radius
46 Interosseous membrane
47 Radial artery

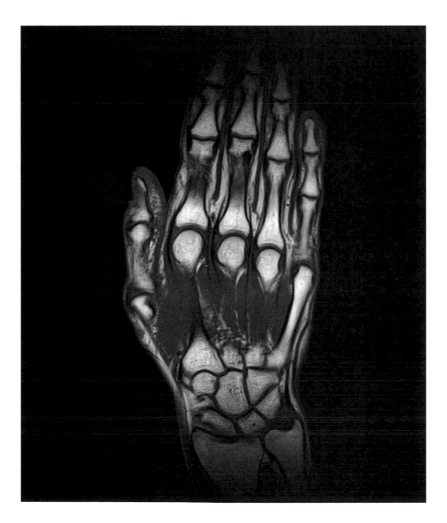

Distal

Radial ☐ Ulnar

Proximal

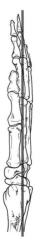

1 Middle phalanx (base)
2 Dorsal digital arteries and nerves
3 Collateral ligament
4 Proximal interphalangeal joint
5 Proximal phalanx (head)
6 Metacarpophalangeal joint
7 Proximal phalanx (shaft)
8 Interosseous muscles
9 Proximal phalanx (base)
10 Dorsal metacarpal vein
11 Metacarpal (head)
12 Joint capsule
13 Metacarpal (shaft)
14 Dorsal metacarpal arteries
15 Dorsal metacarpal artery and nerve of thumb
16 Extensor digitorum muscle (tendon)
17 Metacarpal I (head)
18 Dorsal metacarpal arteries (perforating branches)
19 Interosseous metacarpal ligament
20 Carpometacarpal joint
21 Extensor pollicis longus muscle (tendon)
22 Hamate
23 Radial artery (dorsal carpal branch)
24 Triquetrum
25 Metacarpal II (base)
26 Lunate
27 Trapezoid
28 Dorsal radiocarpal ligament
29 Interosseous intercarpal (trapeziocapitate and capitohamate) ligaments
30 Ulnar collateral ligament of wrist joint
31 Capitate
32 Ulnar articular disk
33 Extensor carpi radialis longus muscle (tendon)
34 Styloid process of ulna
35 Radial collateral ligament of wrist joint
36 Extensor carpi ulnaris muscle (tendon)
37 Scaphoid
38 Ulna
39 Radius
40 Interosseous membrane
41 Brachioradialis muscle (tendon)

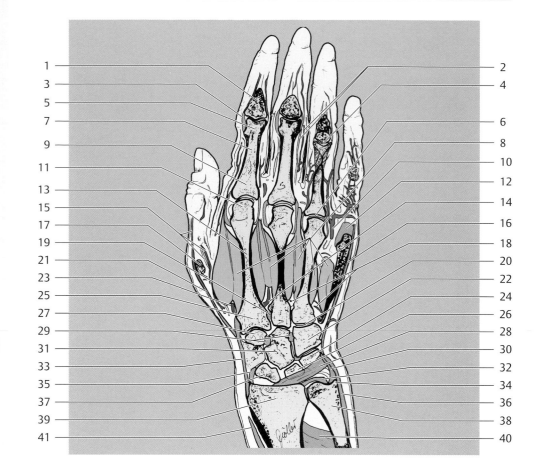

Distal

Radial ☐ Ulnar

Proximal

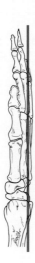

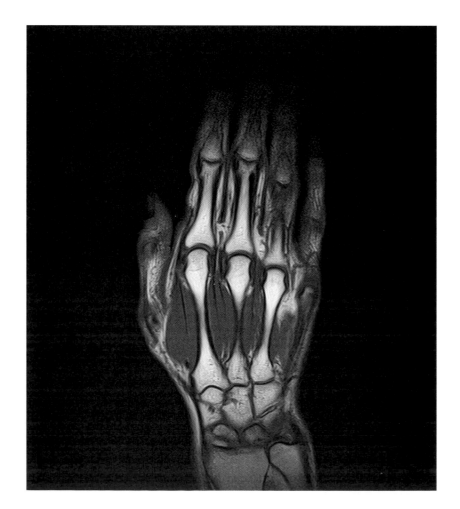

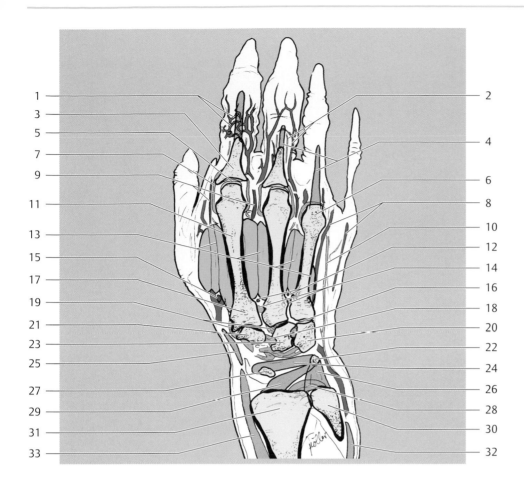

1 Dorsal digital veins
2 Dorsal digital arteries and nerves
3 Proximal phalanx II (base)
4 Extensor digitorum muscles (tendons)
5 Metacarpophalangeal joint II
6 Metacarpal IV (head)
7 Collateral ligament
8 Dorsal metacarpal veins
9 Dorsal metacarpal arteries
10 Ulnar nerve (dorsal branch of the hand)
11 Metacarpal II (shaft)
12 Dorsal metacarpal arteries
13 Dorsal interossei muscles
14 Dorsal metacarpal ligaments
15 Radial artery
16 Carpometacarpal joint IV
17 Metacarpal II (base)
18 Dorsal intercarpal (trapeziocapitate) ligament
19 Dorsal carpometacarpal ligaments
20 Hamate
21 Trapezoid
22 Triquetrum
23 Capitate
24 Dorsal intercarpal (scaphotriquetral) ligament
25 Extensor pollicis longus muscle (tendon)
26 Dorsal ulnocarpal (ulnotriquetral) ligament
27 Scaphoid
28 Dorsal radio-ulnar ligament and joint capsule
29 Dorsal radiocarpal ligament
30 Ulna
31 Radius
32 Extensor carpi ulnaris muscle (tendon)
33 Extensor carpi radialis longus muscle (tendon)

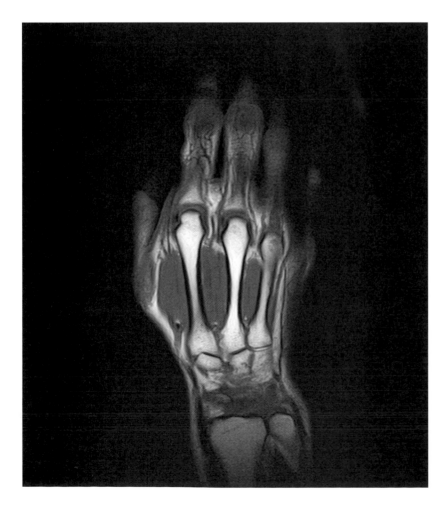

Distal

Radial | | Ulnar

Proximal

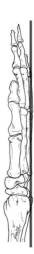

1 Distal phalanx
2 Distal interphalangeal joint
3 Joint capsule
4 Middle phalanx (head)
5 Middle phalanx (base)
6 Palmar collateral ligament
7 Proximal interphalangeal joint
8 Flexor digitorum muscle (tendon)
9 Proximal phalanx (head)
10 Metacarpophalangeal joint
11 Extensor digitorum muscle (tendon)
12 Lumbrical muscle
13 Proximal phalanx (base)
14 Palmar metacarpal artery
15 Metacarpal (head)
16 Flexor digiti minimi muscle (tendon)
17 Collateral ligament and attachment of dorsal interosseous muscle
18 Opponens digiti minimi muscle
19 Dorsal interosseous muscle
20 Flexor digiti minimi brevis muscle
21 Palmar interosseous muscle
22 Deep palmar arch
23 Metacarpal V (base)
24 Abductor digiti minimi muscle
25 Dorsal carpometacarpal ligament
26 Ulnar nerve (deep branch)
27 Triquetrum
28 Palmaris brevis muscle
29 Lunate
30 Pisiform
31 Dorsal radiocarpal ligament
32 Palmar ulnocarpal ligament
33 Triangular fibrocartilage complex
34 Ulnar artery and nerve
35 Ulna
36 Palmar radio-ulnar ligament
37 Dorsal radio-ulnar ligament
38 Flexor digitorum profundus muscle (tendon)
39 Extensor carpi ulnaris muscle
40 Extensor digitorum superficialis muscle (tendon)
41 Pronator quadratus muscle

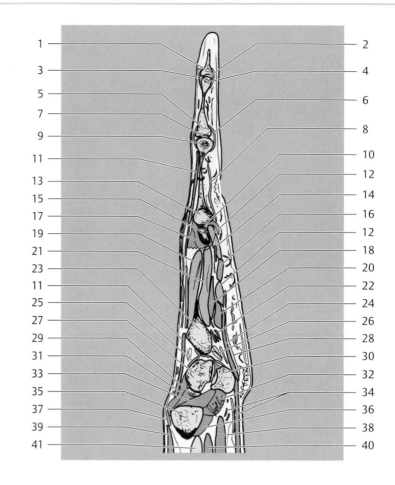

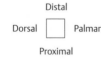

Distal

Dorsal ☐ Palmar

Proximal

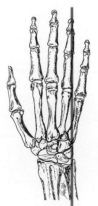

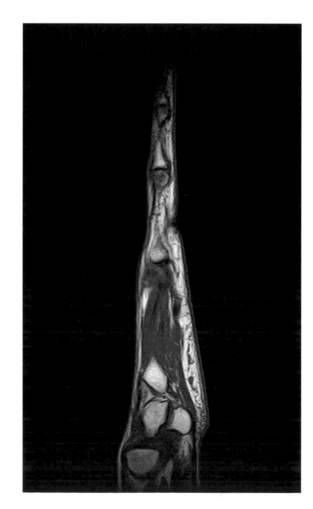

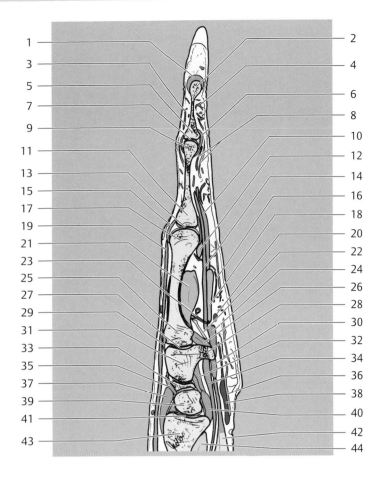

1 Collateral ligament
2 Middle phalanx (head)
3 Dorsal digital vein
4 Palmar digital vein
5 Middle phalanx (base)
6 Palmar (collateral) ligament
7 Proximal interphalangeal joint
8 Palmar digital artery and nerve
9 Proximal phalanx (head)
10 Flexor digitorum superficialis muscle (tendon)
11 Proximal phalanx (base)
12 Palmar interosseous muscle
13 Metacarpophalangeal joint
14 Flexor digitorum profundus muscle (tendon)
15 Joint capsule
16 Palmar digital artery
17 Metacarpal (head)
18 Lumbrical muscle
19 Extensor digitorum muscle (tendon)
20 Superficial palmar arch
21 Palmar interosseous muscle
22 Ulnar nerve (deep branch)
23 Deep palmar arch
24 Flexor digiti minimi brevis muscle
25 Metacarpal (base)
26 Palmar carpometacarpal ligament
27 Carpometacarpal joint
28 Hamate (hook)
29 Dorsal carpometacarpal ligament
30 Flexor retinaculum
31 Hamate
32 Palmar intercarpal ligament
33 Triquetrum
34 Flexor digitorum muscle (tendon)
35 Dorsal intercarpal ligament
36 Palmar carpal ligament
37 Dorsal radiocarpal ligament
38 Ulnar artery
39 Lunate
40 Palmar ulnocarpal ligament
41 Radiocarpal joint
42 Flexor carpi ulnaris muscle
43 Radius
44 Pronator quadratus muscle

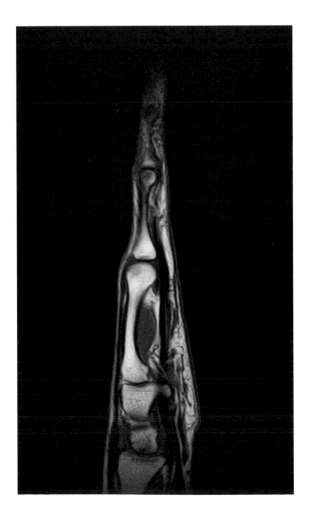

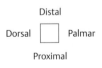

Distal

Dorsal ☐ Palmar

Proximal

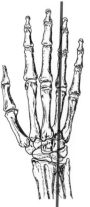

1 Distal phalanx
2 Middle phalanx (head)
3 Distal interphalangeal joint
4 Palmar ligament
5 Joint capsule
6 Palmar digital artery
7 Middle phalanx (base)
8 Flexor digitorum muscle (tendon)
9 Proximal interphalangeal joint
10 Proximal phalanx (shaft)
11 Proximal phalanx (head)
12 Flexor digitorum superficialis muscle
   (tendon)
13 Proximal phalanx (base)
14 Flexor digitorum profundus muscle
   (tendon)
15 Metacarpophalangeal joint
16 Adductor pollicis muscle
   (transverse head)
17 Metacarpal (head)
18 Lumbrical muscles
19 Extensor digitorum muscle (tendon)
20 Superficial palmar arch
21 Palmar digital vein
22 Ulnar nerve (deep branch)
23 Deep palmar arch
24 Adductor pollicis muscle (deep head)
25 Metacarpal (base)
26 Palmar aponeurosis
27 Carpometacarpal joint
28 Palmar carpometacarpal ligament
29 Dorsal carpometacarpal ligament
30 Flexor retinaculum
31 Capitate
32 Median nerve
33 Dorsal intercarpal ligament
34 Palmar intercarpal ligament
35 Intercarpal (scaphocapitate) joint
36 Lunate
37 Scaphoid
38 Palmar radiocarpal ligament
39 Dorsal radiocarpal ligament
40 Wrist joint
41 Radius
42 Pronator quadratus muscle

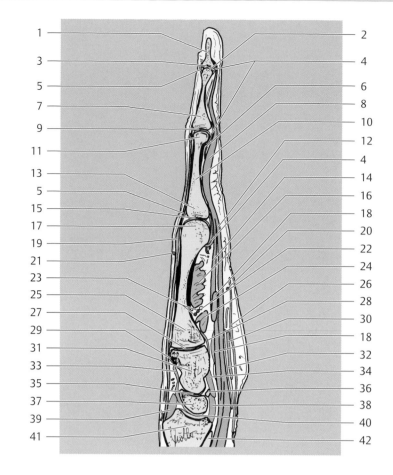

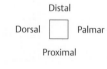

Distal

Dorsal [ ] Palmar

Proximal

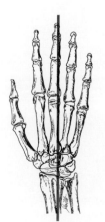

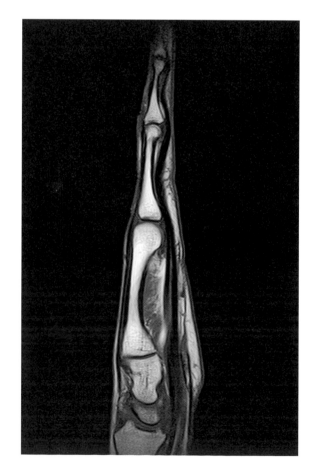

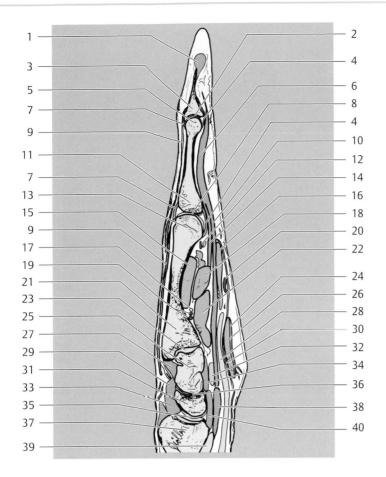

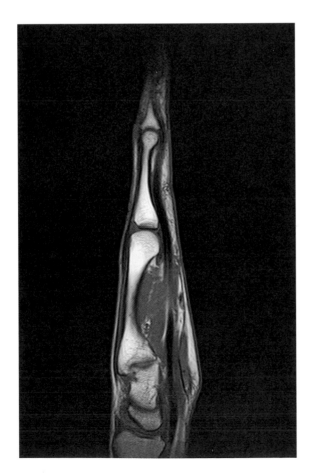

1 Collateral ligament
 (distal interphalangeal joint)
2 Proximal interphalangeal joint
3 Middle phalanx (base)
4 Palmar ligament
5 Proximal phalanx (head)
6 Flexor digitorum muscle (tendon)
7 Joint capsule
8 Metacarpophalangeal joint
9 Extensor digitorum muscle (tendon)
10 Flexor digitorum superficialis muscle
 (tendon)
11 Proximal phalanx (base)
12 Common palmar arteries
13 Metacarpal (head)
14 Flexor digitorum profundus muscle
 (tendon)
15 Palmar interosseous muscle
16 Lumbrical muscle
17 Ulnar nerve (deep branch)
18 Adductor pollicis muscle
 (transverse head)
19 Deep palmar arch
20 Superficial palmar arch
21 Metacarpal (base)
22 Adductor pollicis muscle (oblique head)
23 Carpometacarpal joint
24 Palmar aponeurosis
25 Capitate
26 Abductor pollicis brevis muscle
27 Dorsal carpometacarpal ligament
28 Median nerve
29 Dorsal intercarpal ligament
30 Flexor retinaculum
31 Scaphoid
32 Flexor pollicis muscle (deep head)
33 Dorsal radiocarpal ligament
34 Palmar intercarpal ligament
35 Radiocarpal joint
36 Intercarpal (scaphocapitate) joint
37 Radius
38 Flexor pollicis longus muscle
39 Pronator quadratus muscle
40 Palmar radiocarpal ligament

Distal

Dorsal ☐ Palmar

Proximal

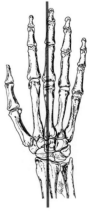

1 Dorsal digital vein
2 Common palmar digital artery
3 Proximal phalanx (base)
4 Lumbrical muscle
5 Collateral ligament
  (metacarpophalangeal joint)
6 Adductor pollicis muscle
  (transverse head)
7 Metacarpal (head)
8 Palmar aponeurosis
9 Dorsal interosseous muscle
10 Flexor digitorum muscle (tendon)
11 Dorsal digital artery
12 Superficial palmar arch
13 Extensor digitorum muscle (tendon)
14 Adductor pollicis muscle
  (oblique head)
15 Ulnar nerve (deep branch)
16 Common palmar digital nerve
  (of median nerve)
17 Dorsal digital artery and nerve
18 Deep palmar arch
19 Metacarpal II (base)
20 Flexor pollicis brevis muscle
  (superficial head)
21 Metacarpal III (base)
22 Flexor pollicis longus muscle (tendon)
23 Carpometacarpal joint
24 Flexor pollicis brevis muscle (deep head)
25 Trapezoid
26 Opponens pollicis muscle
27 Extensor carpi radialis brevis muscle
28 Abductor pollicis brevis muscle
29 Scaphoid
30 Hamate (hook)
31 Palmar radiocarpal ligament
32 Flexor retinaculum
33 Radial collateral ligament of wrist joint
34 Flexor carpi radialis muscle
35 Radius
36 Radial artery
37 Pronator quadratus muscle

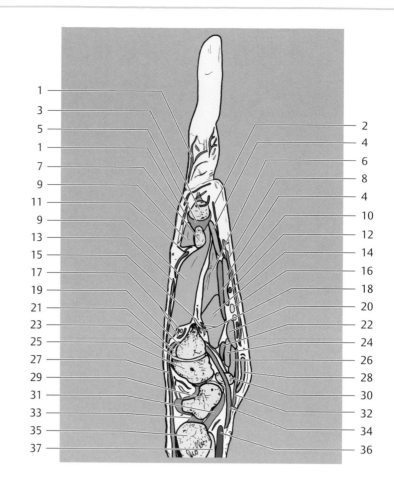

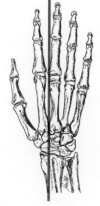

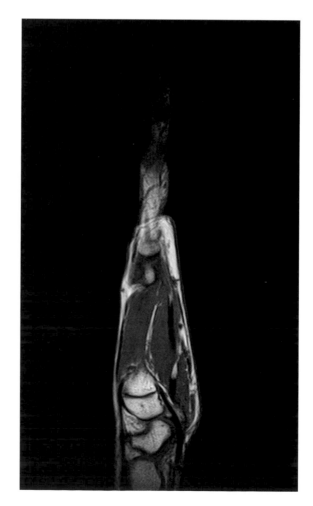

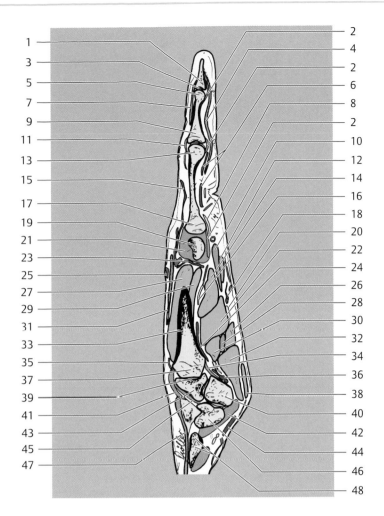

1 Distal phalanx
2 Palmar (collateral) ligament
3 Distal interphalangeal joint
4 Flexor digitorum muscle (tendon)
5 Middle phalanx (head)
6 Proper palmar digital artery
7 Extensor digitorum muscle (tendon)
8 Proper palmar digital nerve
9 Middle phalanx (base)
10 Flexor digitorum muscle (tendon)
11 Collateral ligament
12 Lumbrical muscle
13 Proximal phalanx (head)
14 Adductor pollicis muscle
   (transverse head)
15 Proper dorsal digital artery
16 Common palmar digital nerve
17 Proximal phalanx (base)
18 Superficial palmar arch
19 Metacarpal (head)
20 Median nerve
21 Collateral ligament
22 Adductor pollicis muscle (oblique head)
23 Digital artery (perforating branch)
24 Common metacarpal artery
25 Dorsal digital vein
26 Flexor pollicis brevis muscle
   (superficial head)
27 Dorsal interosseous muscle
28 Flexor pollicis longus muscle (tendon)
29 Palmar interosseous muscle
30 Flexor pollicis brevis muscle (deep head)
31 Extensor digitorum II muscle
32 Opponens pollicis muscle
33 Metacarpal II (shaft)
34 Palmar carpometacarpal ligament
35 Dorsal metacarpal artery
36 Deep palmar arch
37 Metacarpal II (base)
38 Abductor pollicis brevis muscle
39 Carpometacarpal joint
40 Trapezium (tubercle)
41 Dorsal carpometacarpal ligament
42 Radial collateral ligament of wrist
43 Trapezoid
44 Radial artery (superficial branch)
45 Dorsal intercarpal ligament
46 Scaphoid
47 Extensor carpi radialis longus muscle
48 Radius with styloid process

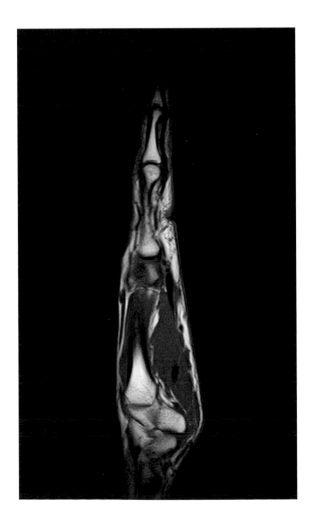

Distal

Dorsal [ ] Palmar

Proximal

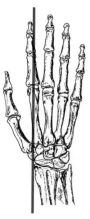

Anatomic Structures Color Code: Lower Extremity

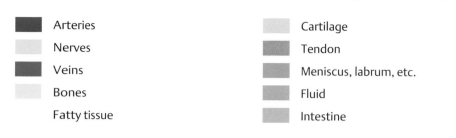

Arteries	Cartilage
Nerves	Tendon
Veins	Meniscus, labrum, etc.
Bones	Fluid
Fatty tissue	Intestine

Hip and Thigh Muscles

Sartorius
Tensor fasciae latae
Iliacus
Iliopsoas
Psoas
Gluteus maximus, medius, and minimus
Piriformis
Gemellus muscles
Quadratus femoris
Obturator internus
Semitendinosus
Semimembranosus
Biceps femoris

Abdominal Muscles
Rectus abdominis
Internal and
external oblique abdominal
Transversus abdominis

Adductors
Obturator externus
Pectineus
Adductor longus, brevis, and magnus
Gracilis

Quadriceps
Rectus femoris
Vastus lateralis, medialis,
and intermedius

Popliteus

Lower Leg Muscles

Extensor group
Tibialis anterior
Extensor digitorum longus
Extensor hallucis longus

Peroneus group
Peroneus brevis (fibularis brevis) and
peroneus longus (fibularis longus)

Flexor group
Tibialis posterior
Flexor digitorum longus
Flexor hallucis longus

Triceps surae
Gastrocnemius
Soleus
Plantaris

Muscles of Foot

Extensor digitorum brevis
Extensor hallucis brevis

Dorsal and plantar interossei
Flexor digitorum brevis
Quadratus plantae
Lumbricals

Muscles of Big Toe
Flexor hallucis brevis
Abductor hallucis
Adductor hallucis

Muscles of Little (Fifth) Toe
Abductor digiti minimi
Flexor digiti minimi
Opponens digiti minimi

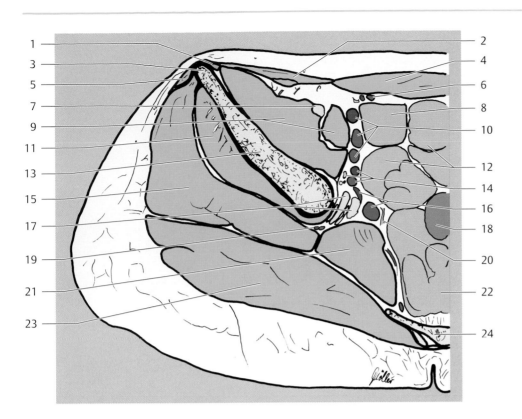

1 Inguinal ligament
2 Internal oblique abdominal muscle and transversus abdominis muscle
3 Anterior superior iliac spine
4 Rectus abdominis muscle
5 Tensor fasciae latae muscle
6 Inferior epigastric artery and vein
7 Femoral nerve
8 Urinary bladder
9 Iliopsoas muscle
10 External iliac artery and veins
11 Gluteus minimus muscle
12 Small intestine
13 Ilium
14 Obturator artery, vein, and nerve
15 Gluteus medius muscle
16 Internal iliac artery and vein
17 Sacral plexus
18 Uterus
19 Superior gluteal artery and vein
20 Ureter
21 Piriformis muscle
22 Sigmoid colon
23 Gluteus maximus muscle
24 Sacrum

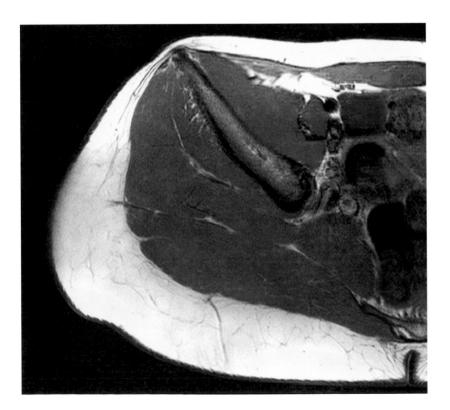

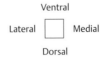

Ventral

Lateral ☐ Medial

Dorsal

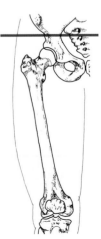

1 Inguinal ligament
2 Internal oblique abdominal muscle and transversus abdominis muscle
3 Sartorius muscle
4 Inferior epigastric artery and vein
5 Tensor fasciae latae muscle
6 Rectus abdominis muscle
7 Femoral nerve
8 Urinary bladder
9 Inferior anterior iliac spine
10 External iliac artery and veins
11 Iliopsoas muscle
12 Ovary and uterine tube
13 Gluteus minimus muscle
14 Obturator artery, vein, and nerve
15 Gluteus medius muscle
16 Uterus
17 Ilium
18 Small intestine
19 Obturator internus muscle
20 Ureter
21 Superior gluteal artery and vein
22 Lumbosacral plexus
23 Piriformis muscle
24 Internal iliac artery and vein
25 Gluteus maximus muscle
26 Rectum
27 Sacrotuberous ligament
28 Sacrum

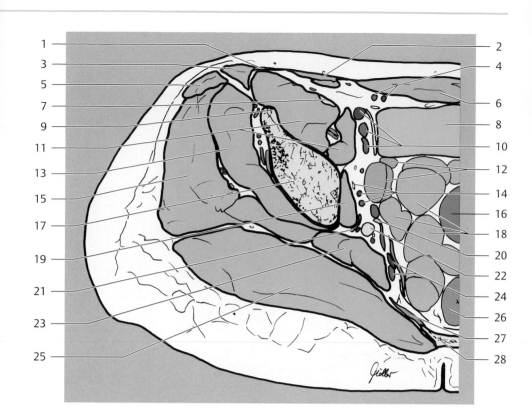

Ventral

Lateral | Medial

Dorsal

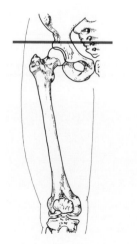

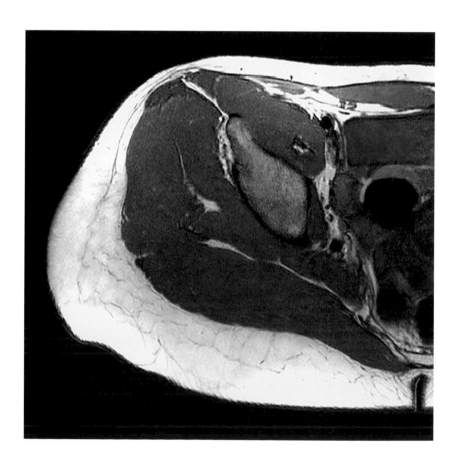

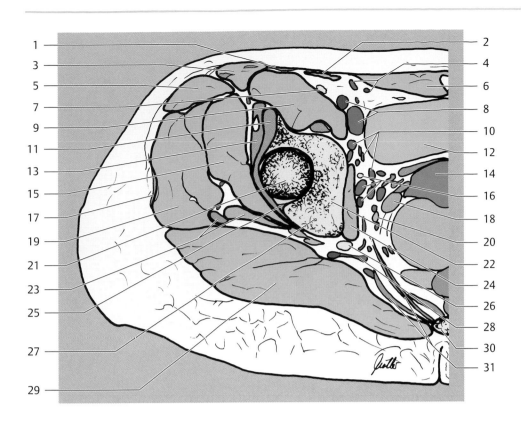

1 Inguinal ligament
2 Internal oblique abdominal muscle and transversus abdominis muscle
3 Sartorius muscle
4 Inferior epigastric artery and vein
5 Tensor fasciae latae muscle
6 Rectus abdominis muscle
7 Femoral nerve
8 External iliac artery and vein
9 Iliopsoas muscle
10 Venous plexus of urinary bladder
11 Iliofemoral ligament
12 Urinary bladder
13 Rectus femoris muscle (tendon)
14 Uterus
15 Gluteus minimus muscle
16 Obturator artery, vein, and nerve
17 Iliotibial tract
18 Ovary
19 Gluteus medius muscle
20 Ureter
21 Femur (head)
22 Pubis (superior ramus)
23 Piriformis muscle
24 Obturator internus muscle
25 Posterior acetabular labrum
26 Sciatic nerve
27 Ischium
28 Superior gluteal artery and vein
29 Gluteus maximus muscle
30 Coccyx
31 Sacrotuberous ligament

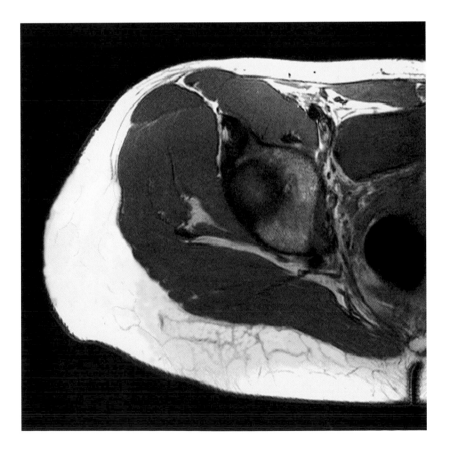

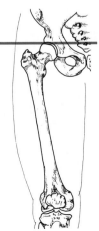

Ventral

Lateral ☐ Medial

Dorsal

1 Femoral nerve
2 Internal oblique abdominal muscle and
   transversus abdominis muscle
3 Sartorius muscle
4 Rectus abdominis muscle
5 Iliopsoas muscle
6 External iliac artery and vein
7 Tensor fasciae latae muscle
8 Urinary bladder
9 Rectus femoris muscle (tendon)
10 Pubis (superior ramus)
11 Anterior glenoid labrum
12 Ligament of head of femur
13 Iliofemoral ligament
14 Ureter
15 Gluteus minimus muscle
16 Uterus
17 Iliotibial tract
18 Obturator artery, vein, and nerve
19 Gluteus medius muscle (and tendon)
20 Uterine venous plexus
21 Femur (head)
22 Acetabular fossa
23 Posterior glenoid labrum
24 Rectum and levator ani muscle
25 Piriformis muscle
26 Obturator internus muscle
27 Sciatic nerve
28 Ischium
29 Superior gluteal artery and vein
30 Ischial spine
31 Gluteus maximus muscle
32 Sacrotuberous ligament

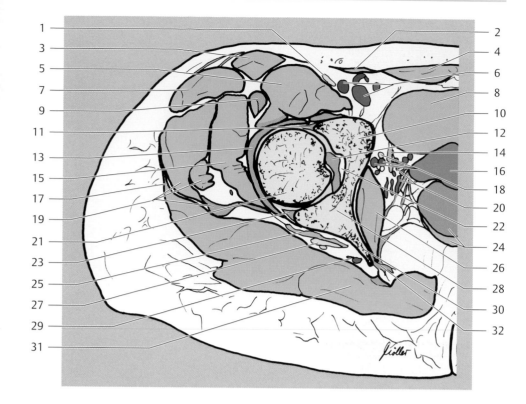

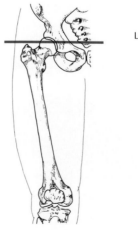

Ventral

Lateral   Medial

Dorsal

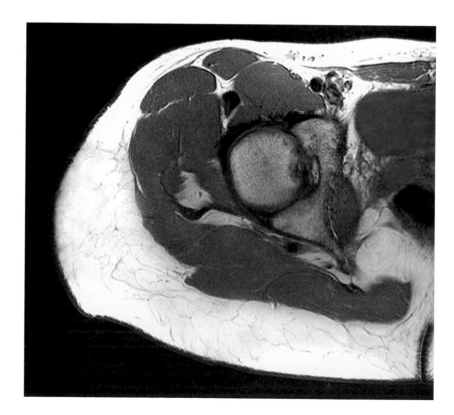

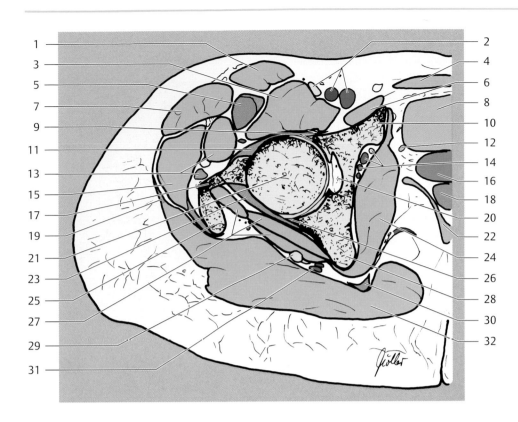

1 Sartorius muscle
2 Femoral artery, vein, and nerve
3 Iliopsoas muscle
4 Rectus abdominis muscle
5 Rectus femoris muscle (and tendon)
6 Pectineus muscle
7 Tensor fasciae latae muscle
8 Urinary bladder
9 Anterior glenoid labrum
10 Pubis (superior ramus)
11 Iliofemoral ligament
12 Ureter
13 Gluteus minimus muscle (and tendon)
14 Obturator artery, vein, and nerve
15 Gluteus medius muscle (and tendon)
16 Vagina
17 Femur (neck)
18 Rectum
19 Iliotibial tract
20 Acetabular fossa
21 Femur (head)
22 Levator ani muscle
23 Ischiofemoral ligament and
     ligamentous capsule
24 Obturator internus muscle
25 Greater trochanter
26 Posterior glenoid labrum
27 Gemellus inferior muscle
28 Ischium
29 Sciatic nerve
30 Sacrotuberous ligament
31 Superior gluteal artery and vein
32 Gluteus maximus muscle

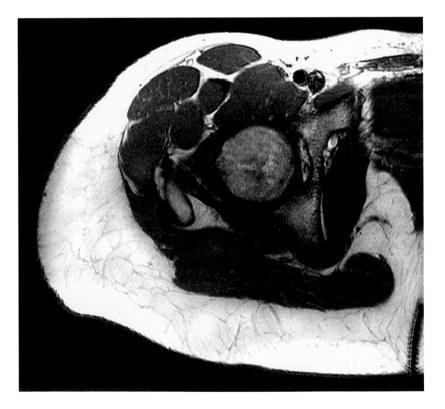

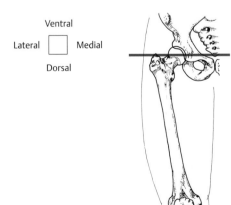

1 Sartorius muscle
2 Femoral artery, vein, and nerve
3 Rectus femoris muscle (and tendon)
4 Pectineus muscle
5 Iliopsoas muscle
6 Rectus abdominis muscle
7 Tensor fasciae latae muscle
8 Pubis (inferior ramus)
9 Vastus lateralis muscle
10 Obturator nerve (anterior branch)
11 Iliofemoral ligament
12 Adductor brevis muscle
13 Gluteus medius muscle (and tendon)
14 Vagina and urethra
15 Gluteus minimus muscle (and tendon)
16 Obturator externus muscle
17 Iliotibial tract
18 Rectum
19 Femur
20 Levator ani muscle
21 Ischiofemoral ligament
22 Ischiorectal fossa
23 Quadratus femoris muscle
24 Pubofemoral ligament
25 Sciatic nerve
26 Obturator internus muscle
27 Tendon attachment of dorsal thigh muscles
28 Ischial tuberosity
29 Gluteus maximus muscle
30 Sacrotuberous ligament

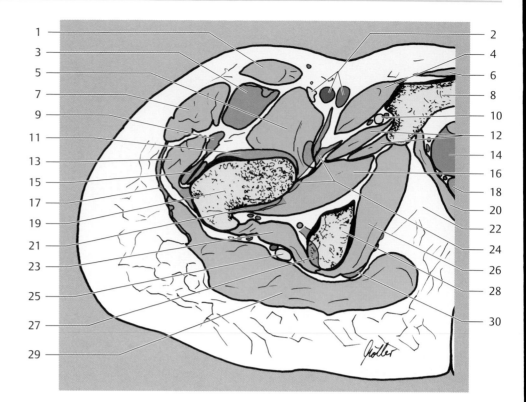

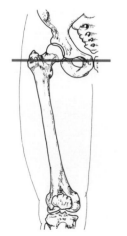

Ventral

Lateral ☐ Medial

Dorsal

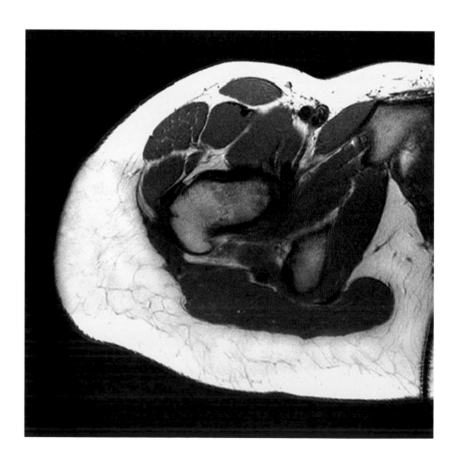

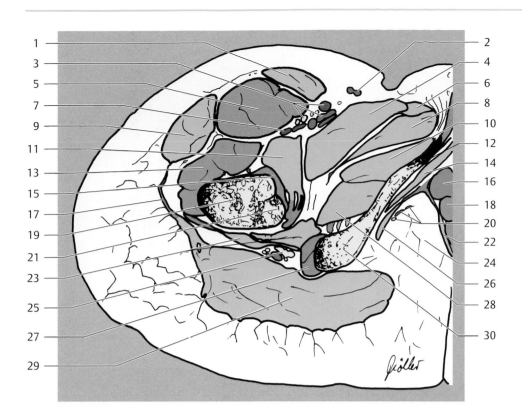

1 Sartorius muscle
2 Great saphenous vein
3 Femoral artery, vein, and nerve
4 Pectineus muscle
5 Rectus femoris muscle (and tendon)
6 Adductor longus muscle
7 Lateral circumflex femoral artery
  and vein
8 Adductor brevis muscle
9 Tensor fasciae latae muscle
10 Adductor magnus and adductor
   minimus muscles
11 Iliopsoas muscle
12 Pubis (inferior ramus)
13 Vastus lateralis muscle
14 Obturator internus muscle
15 Iliofemoral ligament
16 Vagina
17 Iliotibial tract
18 Rectum
19 Femur
20 Internal pudendal artery, vein, and nerve
21 Lesser trochanter
22 Levator ani muscle
23 Quadratus femoris muscle
24 Ischiorectal fossa
25 Sciatic nerve
26 Deep transverse perineal muscle
27 Ischiocrural muscles
   (tendon attachment)
28 External obturator muscle
29 Gluteus maximus muscle
30 Ischial tuberosity

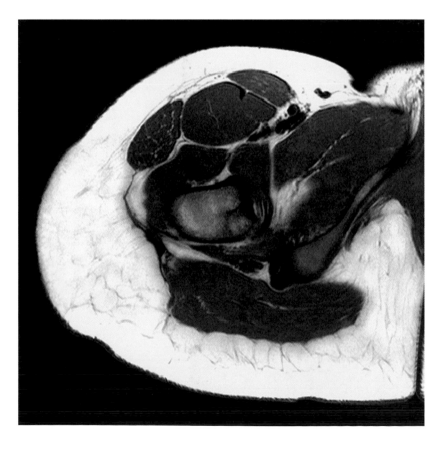

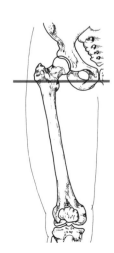

Ventral

Lateral ☐ Medial

Dorsal

1 Sartorius muscle
2 Femoral artery, vein, and nerve
3 Rectus femoris muscle
4 Great saphenous vein
5 Circumflex femoral artery and vein
6 Deep femoral artery and vein
7 Tensor fasciae latae muscle
8 Adductor longus muscle
9 Vastus medialis muscle
10 Pectineus muscle
11 Vastus intermedius muscle
12 Gracilis muscle
13 Vastus lateralis muscle
14 Adductor brevis muscle
15 Iliotibial tract
16 Iliopsoas muscle
17 Femur
18 Adductor magnus muscle
19 Lateral femoral intermuscular septum
20 Obturator internus muscle
21 Quadratus femoris muscle
22 Lesser trochanter
23 Sciatic nerve
24 Semimembranosus muscle (tendon)
25 Gluteus maximus muscle
26 Biceps femoris muscle (tendon)
27 Semitendinosus muscle (tendon)

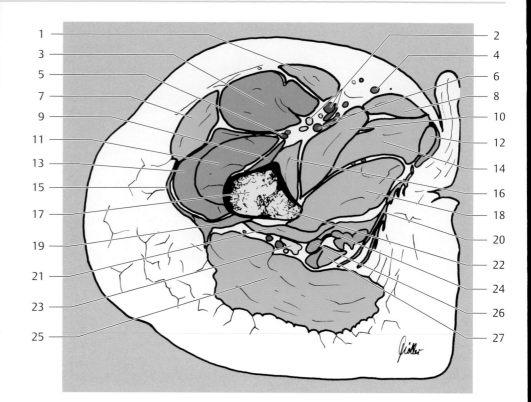

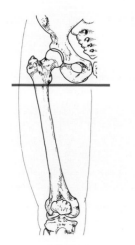

Ventral

Lateral ☐ Medial

Dorsal

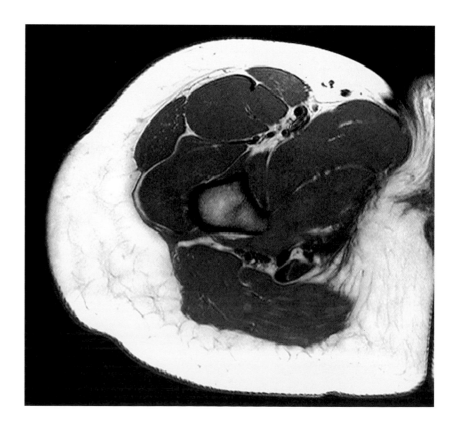

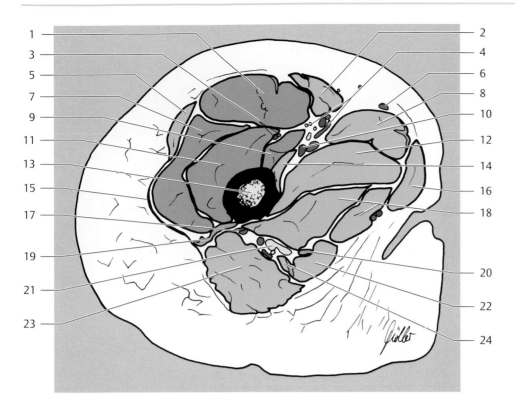

1 Rectus femoris muscle
2 Sartorius muscle
3 Circumflex femoral artery and vein
4 Femoral artery, vein, and nerve
5 Tensor fasciae latae muscle
6 Great saphenous vein
7 Vastus lateralis muscle
8 Adductor longus muscle
9 Vastus medialis muscle
10 Deep artery and vein of thigh
11 Vastus intermedius muscle
12 Adductor brevis muscle
13 Femur
14 Iliopsoas muscle
15 Iliotibial tract
16 Gracilis muscle
17 Perforating artery
18 Adductor magnus muscle
19 Lateral femoral intermuscular septum
20 Semimembranosus muscle (tendon)
21 Sciatic nerve
22 Semitendinosus muscle
23 Gluteus maximus muscle
24 Biceps femoris muscle (and tendon)

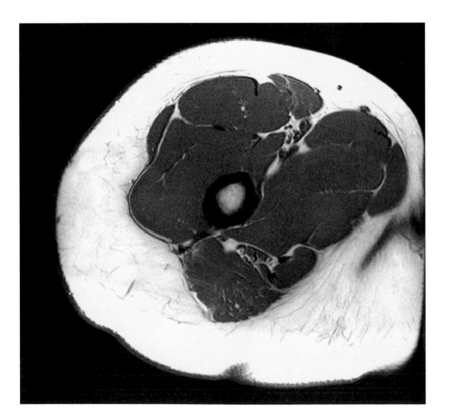

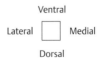

Ventral

Lateral Medial

Dorsal

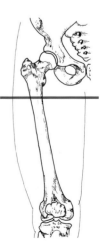

1 Rectus femoris muscle
2 Sartorius muscle
3 Vastus intermedius muscle
4 Femoral artery, veins, and nerve
5 Vastus lateralis muscle
6 Great saphenous vein
7 Iliotibial tract
8 Vastus medialis muscle
9 Femur
10 Adductor longus muscle
11 Perforating artery and vein
12 Deep artery and vein of thigh
13 Lateral femoral intermuscular septum
14 Gracilis muscle
15 Artery and vein to sciatic nerve
16 Adductor brevis muscle
17 Sciatic nerve
18 Adductor magnus muscle
19 Gluteus maximus muscle
20 Semimembranosus muscle (tendon)
21 Biceps femoris muscle
22 Semitendinosus muscle

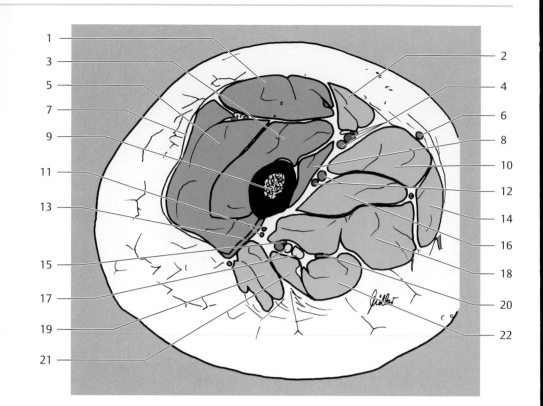

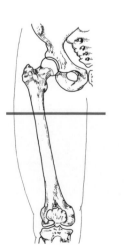

Ventral

Lateral ☐ Medial

Dorsal

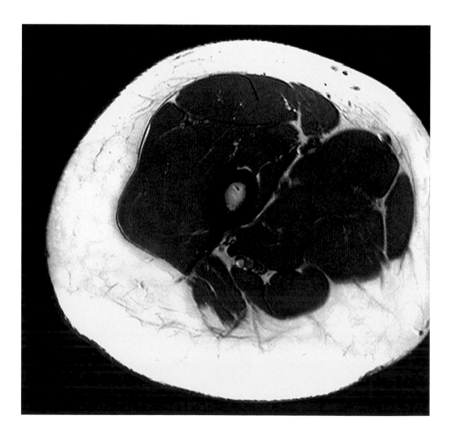

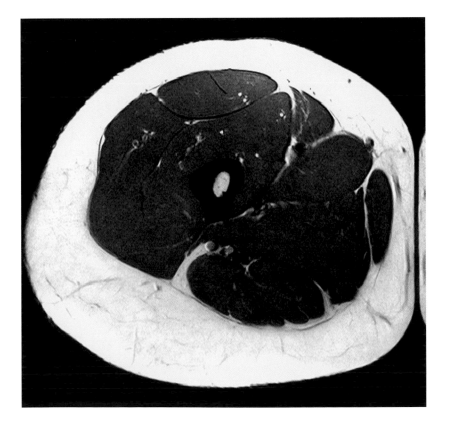

1 Rectus femoris muscle
2 Sartorius muscle
3 Vastus intermedius muscle
4 Saphenous nerve
5 Vastus lateralis muscle
6 Femoral artery and vein
7 Vastus medialis muscle
8 Great saphenous vein
9 Iliotibial tract
10 Adductor longus muscle
11 Femur
12 Gracilis muscle
13 Biceps femoris muscle (short head)
14 Adductor brevis muscle
15 Perforating artery
16 Deep artery and vein of thigh
17 Sciatic nerve
18 Adductor magnus muscle
19 Biceps femoris muscle (long head)
20 Semimembranosus muscle (tendon)
21 Semitendinosus muscle

Ventral

Lateral ☐ Medial

Dorsal

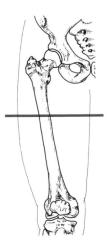

1 Rectus femoris muscle
2 Vastus medialis muscle
3 Vastus intermedius muscle
4 Sartorius muscle
5 Vastus lateralis muscle
6 Saphenous nerve
7 Femur
8 Great saphenous vein
9 Iliotibial tract
10 Femoral artery and vein
11 Deep artery and vein of thigh
12 Adductor longus muscle
13 Biceps femoris muscle (short head)
14 Adductor brevis muscle
15 Artery to sciatic nerve
16 Gracilis muscle
17 Sciatic nerve
18 Adductor magnus muscle
19 Biceps femoris muscle (long head)
20 Semimembranosus muscle
21 Semitendinosus muscle

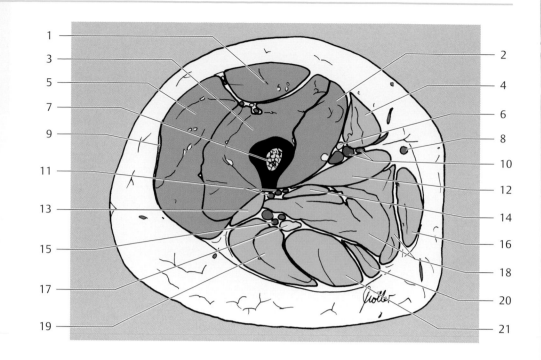

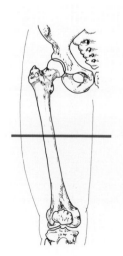

Ventral

Lateral ☐ Medial

Dorsal

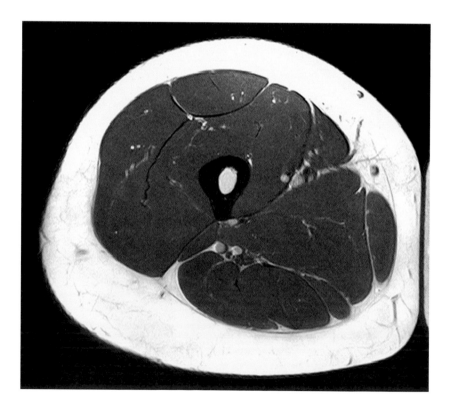

1 Rectus femoris muscle
2 Vastus medialis muscle
3 Vastus lateralis muscle
4 Sartorius muscle
5 Vastus intermedius muscle
6 Great saphenous vein
7 Iliotibial tract
8 Saphenous nerve
9 Femur
10 Femoral artery and vein
11 Perforating artery and vein
12 Adductor longus muscle
13 Biceps femoris muscle (short head)
14 Adductor magnus muscle
15 Sciatic nerve
16 Gracilis muscle
17 Biceps femoris muscle (long head)
18 Semimembranosus muscle
19 Semitendinosus muscle

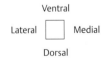

```
        Ventral
Lateral  □  Medial
        Dorsal
```

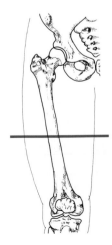

1 Rectus femoris muscle (and tendon)
2 Vastus medialis muscle
3 Vastus intermedius muscle
4 Sartorius muscle
5 Vastus lateralis muscle
6 Great saphenous vein
7 Femur
8 Saphenous nerve
9 Iliotibial tract
10 Femoral artery and vein
11 Linea aspera
12 Perforating artery and vein
13 Adductor magnus muscle
14 Gracilis muscle
15 Biceps femoris muscle (short head)
16 Semimembranosus muscle
17 Common fibular (peroneal) nerve
18 Semitendinosus muscle
19 Tibial nerve
20 Biceps femoris muscle (long head)
21 Posterior femoral cutaneous nerve

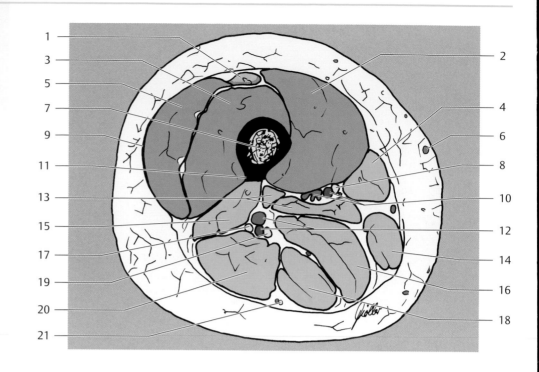

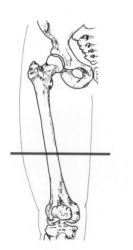

Ventral

Lateral ☐ Medial

Dorsal

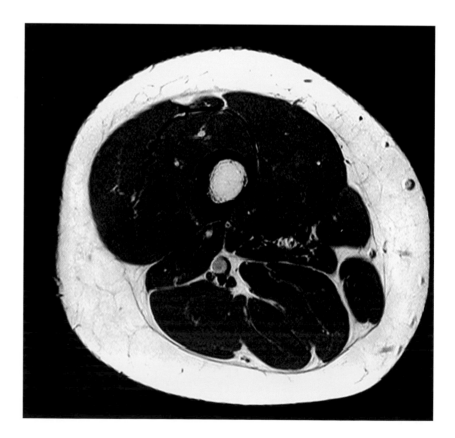

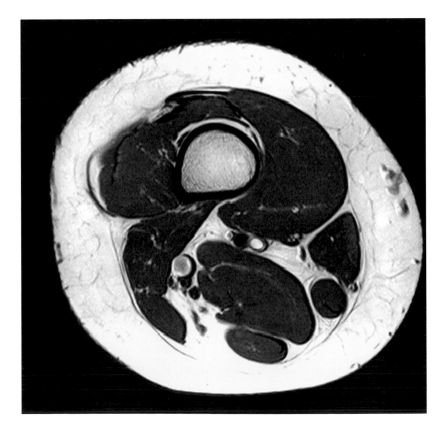

1 Rectus femoris muscle (tendon)
2 Vastus medialis muscle
3 Vastus intermedius muscle
4 Great saphenous vein
5 Femur
6 Muscular branch of femoral nerve
7 Iliotibial tract
8 Adductor magnus muscle (tendon)
9 Vastus lateralis muscle
10 Sartorius muscle
11 Biceps femoris muscle (short head)
12 Saphenous nerve
13 Femoral artery and vein
14 Gracilis muscle
15 Perforating artery and vein
16 Semimembranosus muscle
17 Common fibular (peroneal) nerve
18 Semitendinosus muscle
19 Tibial nerve
20 Biceps femoris muscle (long head)

Ventral

Lateral   Medial

Dorsal

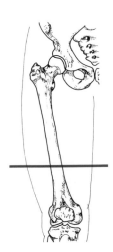

1 Rectus femoris muscle (tendon)
2 Vastus medialis muscle
3 Vastus intermedius muscle
4 Femur
5 Iliotibial tract
6 Sartorius muscle
7 Vastus lateralis muscle
8 Adductor magnus muscle (tendon)
9 Muscular branch of femoral nerve
10 Saphenous nerve
11 Femoral artery and vein
12 Great saphenous vein
13 Biceps femoris muscle (short head)
14 Gracilis muscle
15 Perforating artery and vein
16 Semimembranosus muscle
17 Common fibular (peroneal) nerve
18 Semitendinosus muscle
19 Tibial nerve
20 Biceps femoris muscle (long head)

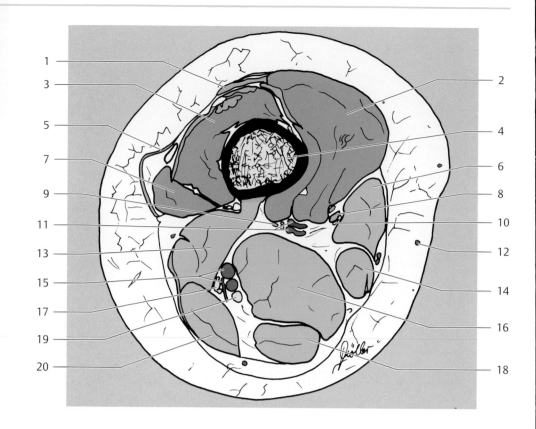

Ventral

Lateral [ ] Medial

Dorsal

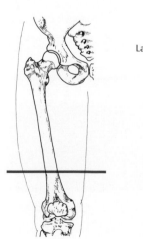

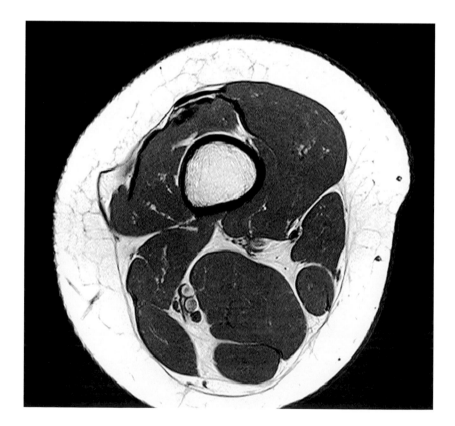

1 Rectus femoris muscle (tendon)
2 Vastus medialis muscle
3 Vastus intermedius muscle
4 Accessory saphenous vein
5 Femur
6 Sartorius muscle
7 Iliotibial tract
8 Femoral artery and vein
9 Vastus lateralis muscle
10 Adductor magnus muscle (tendon)
11 Muscular branch of femoral nerve
12 Great saphenous vein
13 Biceps femoris muscle (short head)
14 Saphenous nerve
15 Perforating artery and vein
16 Gracilis muscle
17 Common fibular (peroneal) nerve
18 Semimembranosus muscle
19 Tibial nerve
20 Semitendinosus muscle
21 Biceps femoris muscle (long head)

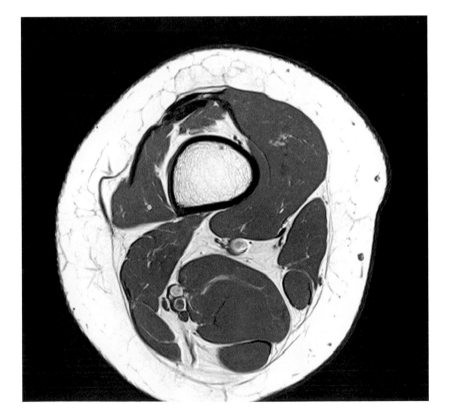

Ventral

Lateral ☐ Medial

Dorsal

1 Rectus femoris muscle (tendon)
2 Vastus medialis muscle
3 Vastus intermedius muscle
   (and tendon)
4 Femur
5 Vastus lateralis muscle
6 Adductor magnus muscle (tendon)
7 Iliotibial tract
8 Sartorius muscle
9 Femoral artery and vein
10 Great saphenous vein
11 Biceps femoris muscle (short head)
12 Saphenous nerve
13 Perforating vein
14 Gracilis muscle
15 Common fibular (peroneal) nerve
16 Semimembranosus muscle
17 Biceps femoris muscle (long head)
18 Semitendinosus muscle
19 Tibial nerve

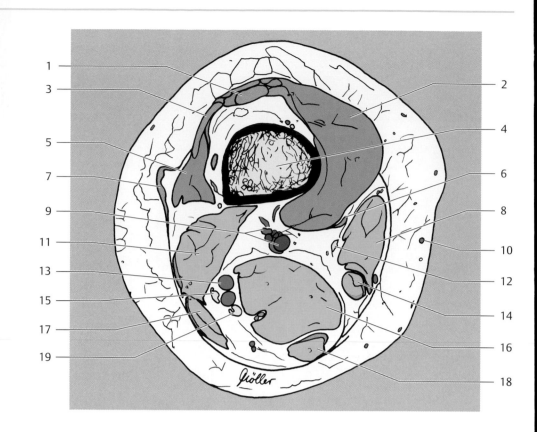

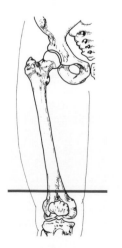

Ventral

Lateral ☐ Medial

Dorsal

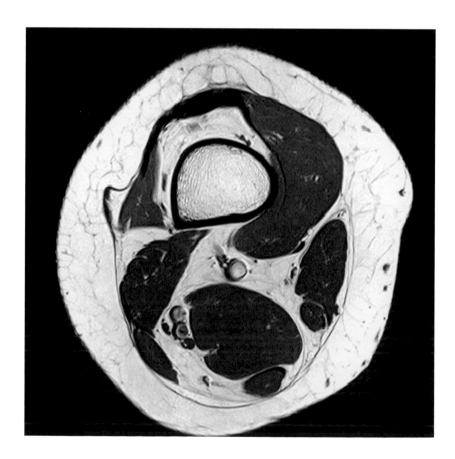

1 Rectus femoris muscle (tendon)
2 Patella
3 Suprapatellar recess
4 Medial patellar retinaculum
5 Lateral patellar retinaculum
6 Vastus medialis muscle
7 Femur
8 Superior medial genicular artery and vein
9 Iliotibial tract
10 Adductor magnus muscle (tendon)
11 Superior lateral genicular artery and vein
12 Great saphenous vein
13 Biceps femoris muscle (short head)
14 Sartorius muscle
15 Femoral artery and vein
16 Saphenous nerve
17 Common fibular (peroneal) nerve
18 Gracilis muscle (tendon)
19 Perforating vein
20 Semimembranosus muscle
21 Biceps femoris muscle (long head, tendon)
22 Semitendinosus muscle (tendon)
23 Tibial nerve

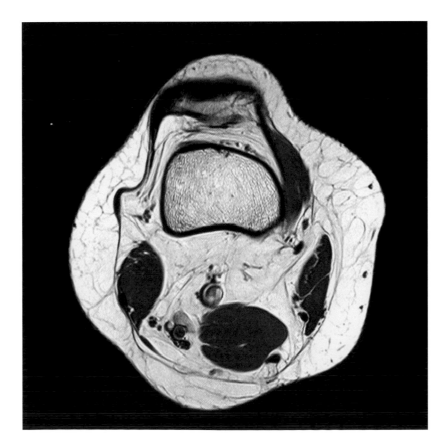

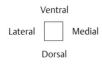

Ventral

Lateral ☐ Medial

Dorsal

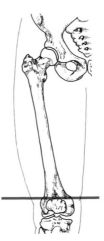

1 Patellar ligament
2 Patella
3 Retropatellar cartilage
4 Femoropatellar joint
5 Lateral patellar retinaculum
6 Medial patellar retinaculum
7 Vastus lateralis muscle (tendon)
8 Femur
9 Iliotibial tract
10 Gastrocnemius muscle (medial head, tendon)
11 Popliteus muscle (tendon)
12 Adductor magnus muscle (tendon)
13 Gastrocnemius muscle (lateral head)
14 Great saphenous vein
15 Superior lateral genicular artery and vein
16 Superior medial genicular artery and vein
17 Biceps femoris muscle (and tendon)
18 Sartorius muscle
19 Femoral artery and vein
20 Saphenous nerve
21 Common fibular (peroneal) nerve
22 Gracilis muscle (tendon)
23 Perforating artery
24 Semitendinosus muscle
25 Tibial nerve
26 Semimembranosus muscle

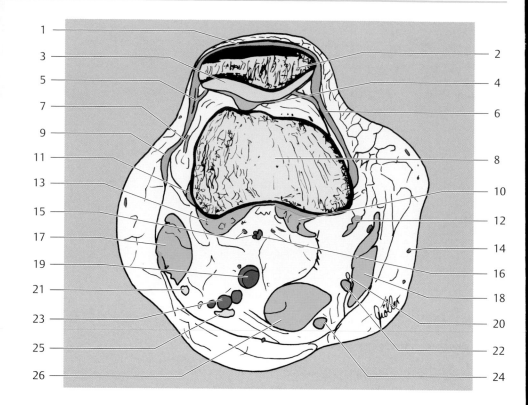

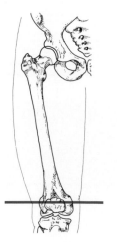

Ventral

Lateral ☐ Medial

Dorsal

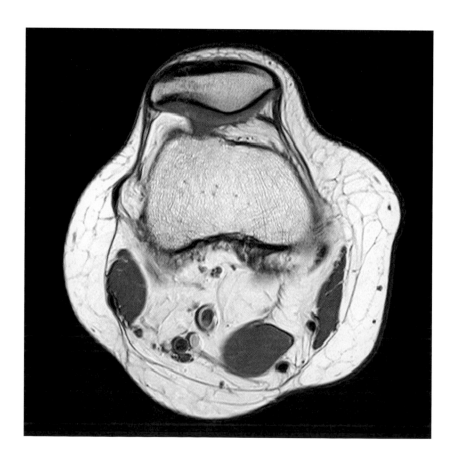

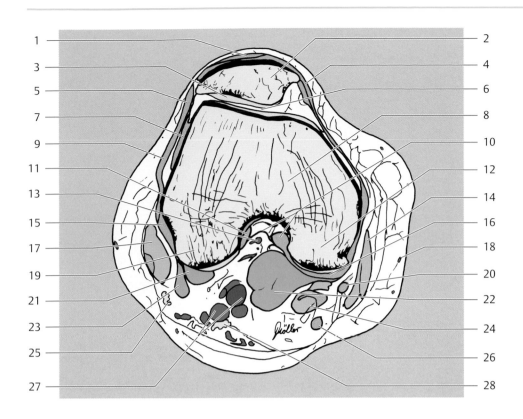

1 Patellar ligament
2 Patella
3 Retropatellar cartilage
4 Medial patellar retinaculum
5 Lateral patellar retinaculum
6 Femoropatellar joint
7 Lateral collateral ligament
8 Femur
9 Iliotibial tract
10 Joint capsule and posterior cruciate ligament (attachment)
11 Anterior cruciate ligament (attachment)
12 Medial femoral condyle
13 Middle genicular artery
14 Sartorius muscle
15 Popliteus muscle (tendon)
16 Joint capsule and oblique popliteal ligament
17 Biceps femoris muscle (and tendon)
18 Great saphenous vein
19 Lateral femoral condyle
20 Gracilis muscle (tendon)
21 Plantaris muscle
22 Gastrocnemius muscle (medial head)
23 Gastrocnemius muscle (lateral head)
24 Semimembranosus muscle (and tendon)
25 Common fibular (peroneal) nerve
26 Semitendinosus muscle (tendon)
27 Femoral artery and vein
28 Tibial nerve

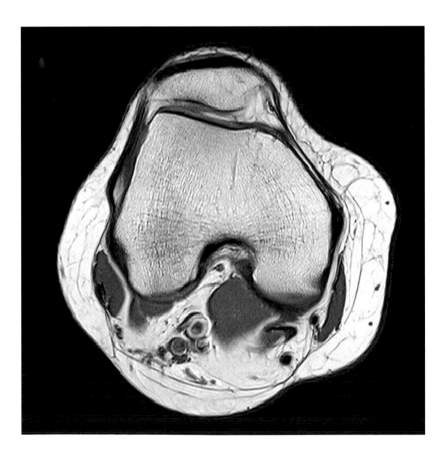

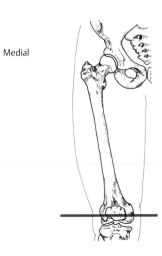

Ventral

Lateral   Medial

Dorsal

1 Patellar ligament
2 Infrapatellar (Hoffa) fat pad
3 Lateral patellar retinaculum
4 Medial patellar retinaculum
5 Lateral femoral condyle
6 Posterior cruciate ligament
7 Iliotibial tract
8 Medial collateral ligament
9 Lateral collateral ligament
10 Medial femoral condyle
11 Intercondylar fossa
12 Sartorius muscle
13 Anterior cruciate ligament
14 Gracilis muscle (tendon)
15 Popliteus muscle (tendon)
16 Great saphenous vein
17 Biceps femoris muscle (and tendon)
18 Semimembranosus muscle
   (and tendon)
19 Oblique popliteal ligament and joint
   capsule
20 Semitendinosus muscle (tendon)
21 Plantaris muscle
22 Gastrocnemius muscle (medial head)
23 Common fibular (peroneal) nerve
24 Popliteal vein
25 Femoral artery and vein
26 Gastrocnemius muscle (lateral head)
27 Tibial nerve

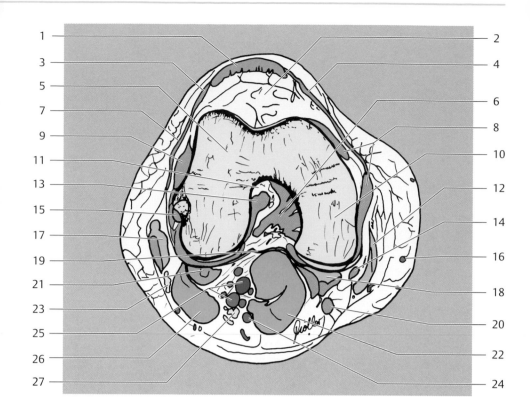

Ventral

Lateral ☐ Medial

Dorsal

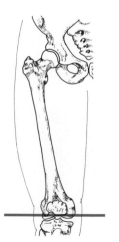

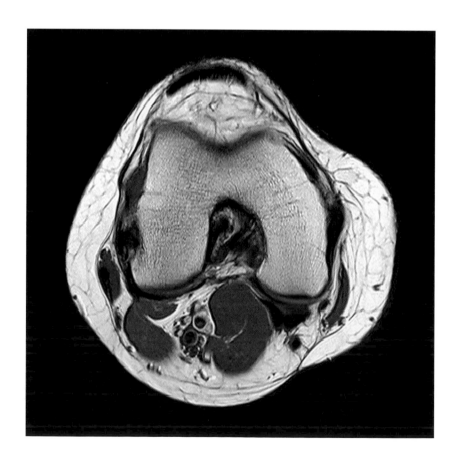

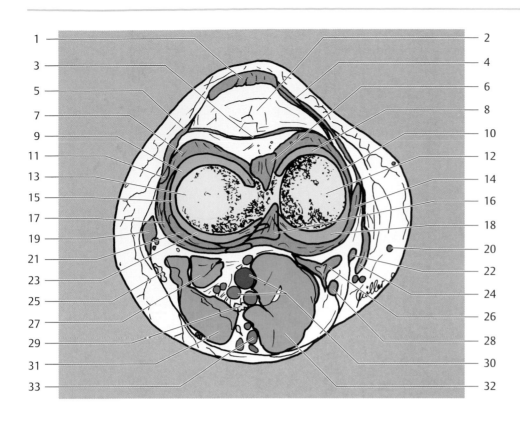

1 Patellar ligament
2 Infrapatellar (Hoffa) fat pad
3 Transverse patellar retinaculum
4 Medial patellar retinaculum
5 Lateral patellar retinaculum
6 Anterior cruciate ligament
7 Joint capsule
8 Medial meniscus (anterior horn)
9 Lateral meniscus (anterior horn)
10 Medial meniscus (intermediate portion)
11 Iliotibial tract
12 Medial femoral condyle with joint cartilage
13 Lateral femoral condyle with joint cartilage
14 Medial collateral ligament
15 Lateral meniscus (intermediate portion)
16 Posterior cruciate ligament
17 Lateral collateral ligament
18 Medial meniscus (posterior horn)
19 Biceps femoris muscle (tendon)
20 Great saphenous vein
21 Popliteus muscle (tendon)
22 Gracilis muscle (tendon)
23 Lateral meniscus (posterior horn)
24 Sartorius muscle (and tendon)
25 Common fibular (peroneal) nerve
26 Semimembranosus muscle (and tendon)
27 Plantaris muscle
28 Semitendinosus muscle (tendon)
29 Tibial nerve
30 Femoral artery and vein
31 Gastrocnemius muscle (lateral head, tendon)
32 Gastrocnemius muscle (medial head, tendon)
33 Popliteal vein

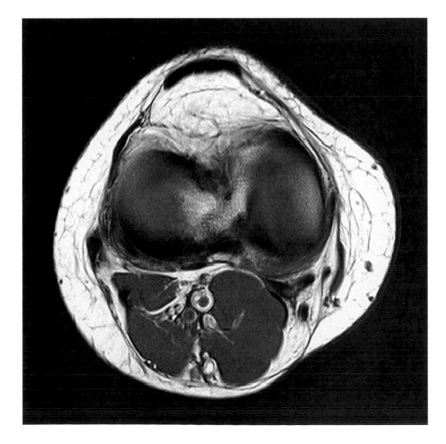

Ventral

Lateral ☐ Medial

Dorsal

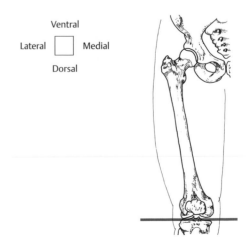

1 Patellar ligament
2 Infrapatellar (Hoffa) fat pad
3 Lateral patellar retinaculum
4 Medial patellar retinaculum
5 Iliotibial tract
6 Joint capsule
7 Lateral collateral ligament
8 Tibia (head)
9 Fibular collateral ligament
10 Medial collateral ligament
11 Posterior cruciate ligament
12 Sartorius muscle (tendon)
13 Biceps femoris muscle (tendon)
14 Great saphenous vein
15 Popliteus muscle (and tendon)
16 Gracilis muscle (tendon)
17 Common fibular (peroneal) nerve
18 Semimembranosus muscle
   (and tendon)
19 Plantaris muscle
20 Semitendinosus muscle (tendon)
21 Femoral artery and vein
22 Oblique popliteal ligament and joint
   capsule
23 Tibial nerve
24 Gastrocnemius muscle (medial head,
   tendon)
25 Gastrocnemius muscle (lateral head,
   tendon)
26 Popliteal vein

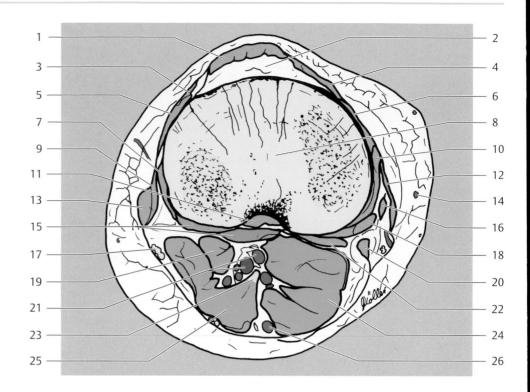

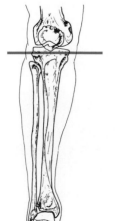

Anterior
Ventral

Lateral   □   Medial

Dorsal
Posterior

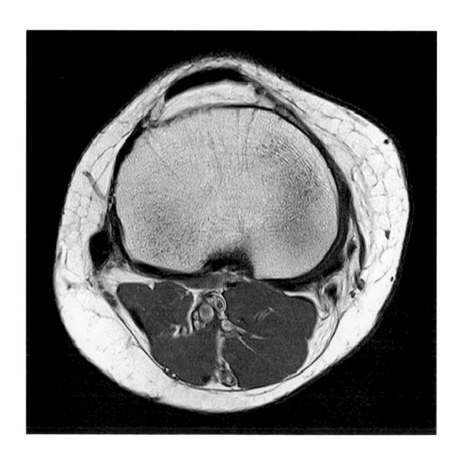

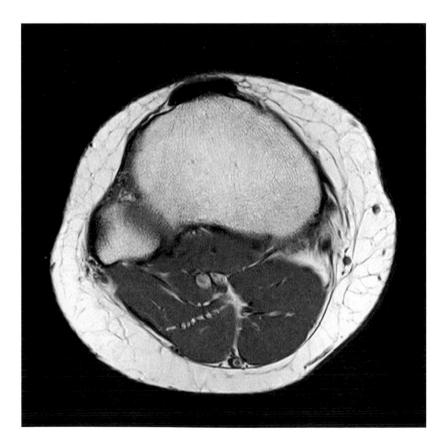

1 Patellar ligament
2 Medial patellar retinaculum
3 Lateral patellar retinaculum
4 Tibia (head)
5 Tibialis anterior muscle (tendon)
6 Sartorius muscle (tendon)
7 Anterior ligament of fibular head
8 Gracilis muscle (tendon)
9 Tibiofibular joint (proximal)
10 Great saphenous vein
11 Biceps femoris muscle
   (tendon attachment)
12 Semimembranosus muscle
   (and tendon)
13 Fibula (head)
14 Oblique popliteal ligament and joint
   capsule
15 Lateral collateral (fibular) ligament
16 Semitendinosus muscle (tendon)
17 Posterior ligament of fibular head
18 Popliteus muscle
19 Common fibular (peroneal) nerve
20 Femoral artery and vein
21 Soleus muscle
22 Tibial nerve
23 Plantaris muscle
24 Gastrocnemius muscle
   (medial head, tendon)
25 Gastrocnemius muscle
   (lateral head, tendon)
26 Popliteal vein
27 Medial sural cutaneous nerve

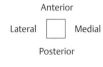

Anterior

Lateral ▢ Medial

Posterior

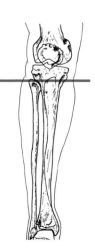

1 Patellar ligament
2 Tibial tuberosity
3 Tibia
4 Medial patellar retinaculum
5 Anterior tibial muscle
6 Sartorius muscle (tendon)
7 Extensor digitorum longus muscle
8 Gracilis muscle (tendon)
9 Interosseous membrane of leg
10 Great saphenous vein
11 Peroneus (fibularis) longus muscle
12 Semitendinosus muscle (tendon)
13 Fibula (head)
14 Popliteus muscle
15 Common fibular (peroneal) nerve
16 Femoral artery and vein
17 Soleus muscle
18 Tibial nerve
19 Plantaris muscle
20 Gastrocnemius muscle (medial head)
21 Gastrocnemius muscle (lateral head)
22 Popliteal vein
23 Medial sural cutaneous nerve

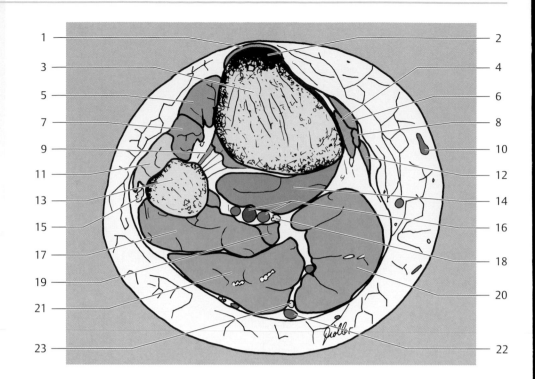

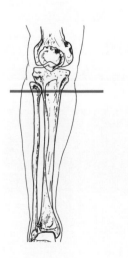

Anterior

Lateral | Medial

Posterior

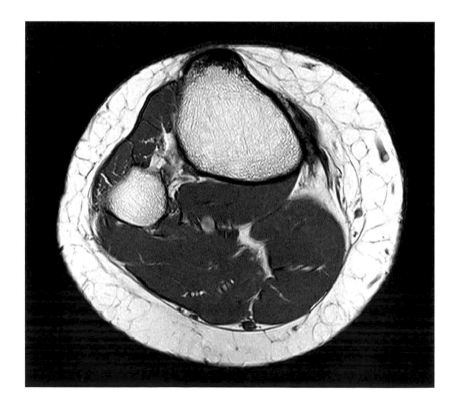

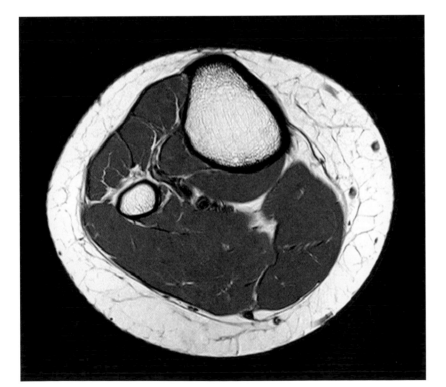

1 Patellar ligament
2 Tibial tuberosity
3 Tibialis anterior muscle
4 Tibia
5 Interosseous membrane of leg
6 Pes anserinus (tendinous expansions of sartorius, gracilis, and semitendinous muscles attaching to border of tibial tuberosity)
7 Extensor digitorum longus muscle
8 Great saphenous vein
9 Tibialis posterior muscle
10 Popliteus muscle
11 Peroneus longus muscle
12 Femoral artery and vein
13 Anterior tibial artery and vein
14 Tibial nerve
15 Common fibular (peroneal) nerve
16 Gastrocnemius muscle (medial head)
17 Fibula
18 Plantaris muscle
19 Soleus muscle
20 Medial sural cutaneous nerve
21 Gastrocnemius muscle (lateral head)
22 Popliteal vein

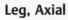

Anterior

Lateral ☐ Medial

Posterior

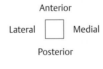

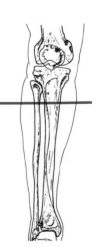

1 Tibialis anterior muscle
2 Tibial tuberosity
3 Interosseous membrane of leg
4 Tibia
5 Extensor digitorum longus muscle
6 Popliteus muscle
7 Tibialis posterior muscle
8 Great saphenous vein
9 Anterior tibial artery and vein
10 Tibial nerve
11 Deep fibular (peroneal) nerve
12 Plantaris muscle (tendon)
13 Peroneus (fibularis) longus muscle
14 Femoral artery and vein
15 Superficial fibular (peroneal) nerve
16 Gastrocnemius muscle (medial head)
17 Fibula
18 Soleus muscle
19 Gastrocnemius muscle (lateral head)
20 Medial sural cutaneous nerve
21 Popliteal vein

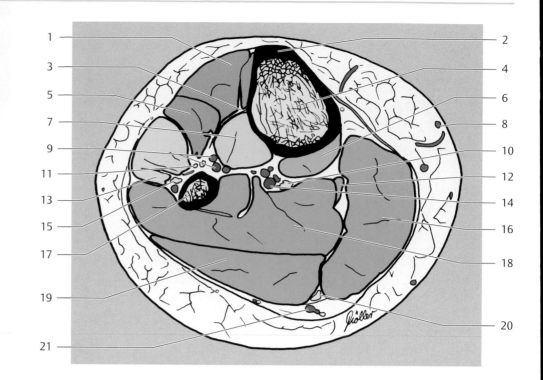

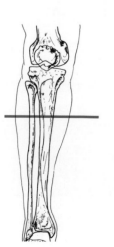

Anterior

Lateral   Medial

Posterior

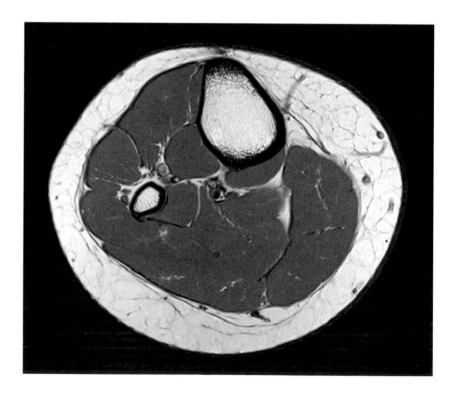

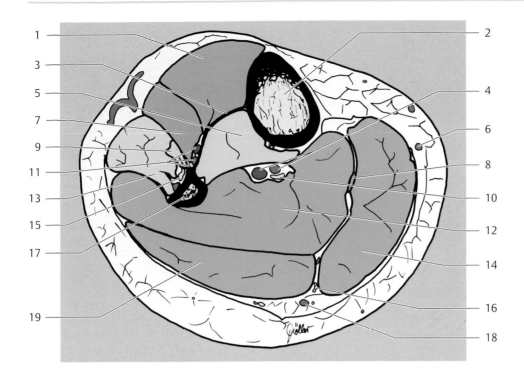

1 Tibialis anterior muscle
2 Tibia
3 Interosseous membrane of leg
4 Femoral artery and vein
5 Tibialis posterior muscle
6 Great saphenous vein
7 Extensor digitorum longus muscle
8 Plantaris muscle (tendon)
9 Peroneus (fibularis) brevis muscle
10 Tibial nerve
11 Anterior tibial artery and vein and deep fibular (peroneal) nerve
12 Soleus muscle
13 Peroneus (fibularis) longus muscle
14 Gastrocnemius muscle (medial head)
15 Superficial fibular (peroneal) nerve
16 Medial sural cutaneous nerve
17 Fibula
18 Small saphenous vein
19 Gastrocnemius muscle (lateral head)

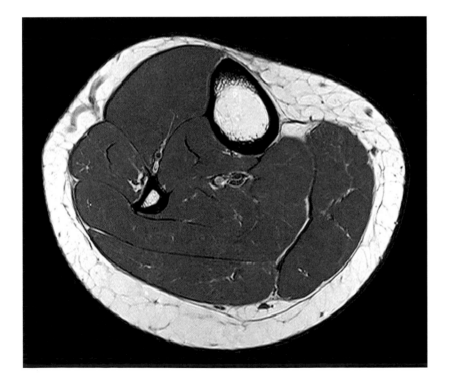

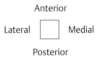

Anterior

Lateral ☐ Medial

Posterior

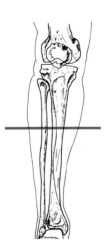

1 Tibialis anterior muscle
2 Tibia
3 Interosseous membrane of leg
4 Flexor digitorum longus muscle
5 Extensor digitorum longus muscle
6 Great saphenous vein
7 Anterior tibial artery and vein
8 Tibialis posterior muscle
9 Deep fibular (peroneal) nerve
10 Posterior tibial artery and vein
11 Peroneus brevis muscle
12 Plantaris muscle (tendon)
13 Peroneus longus muscle
14 Tibial nerve
15 Superficial fibular (peroneal) nerve
16 Gastrocnemius muscle (medial head)
17 Fibula
18 Fibular (peroneal) artery and vein
19 Soleus muscle
20 Flexor hallucis longus muscle
21 Gastrocnemius muscle (lateral head)
22 Medial sural cutaneous nerve
23 Small saphenous vein

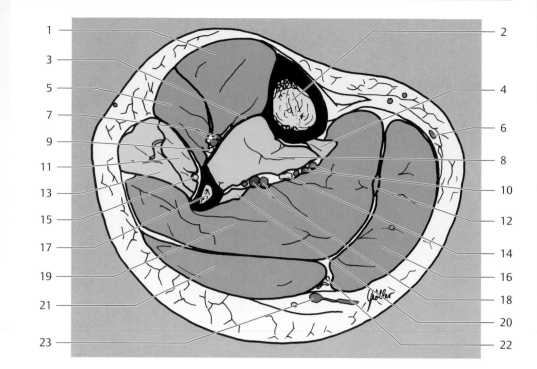

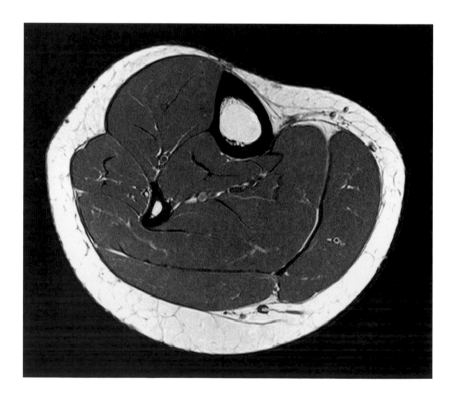

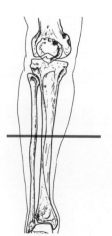

Anterior

Lateral ☐ Medial

Posterior

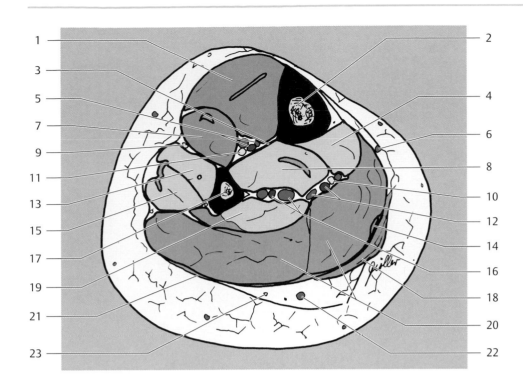

1 Tibialis anterior muscle (and tendon)
2 Tibia
3 Interosseous membrane of leg
4 Flexor digitorum longus muscle
5 Anterior tibial artery and vein
6 Great saphenous vein
7 Extensor digitorum longus muscle
(and tendon)
8 Tibialis posterior muscle
9 Superficial fibular (peroneal) nerve
10 Tibial nerve
11 Deep fibular (peroneal) nerve
12 Posterior tibial artery and vein
13 Peroneus (fibularis) brevis muscle
14 Plantaris muscle (tendon)
15 Peroneus longus muscle (and tendon)
16 Fibular (peroneal) artery and vein
17 Fibula
18 Gastrocnemius muscle (medial head
and tendon)
19 Flexor hallucis longus muscle
20 Soleus muscle
21 Gastrocnemius muscle (lateral head,
tendon)
22 Small saphenous vein
23 Medial sural cutaneous nerve

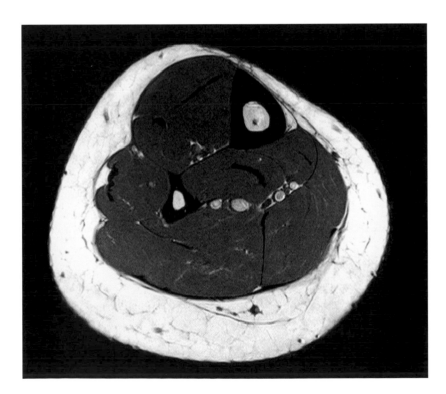

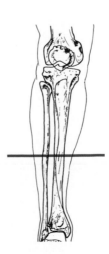

Anterior

Lateral ☐ Medial

Posterior

1 Tibialis anterior muscle (and tendon)
2 Tibia
3 Extensor hallucis longus muscle
4 Tibialis posterior muscle
5 Extensor digitorum longus muscle
   (and tendon)
6 Great saphenous vein
7 Superficial fibular (peroneal) nerve
8 Flexor digitorum longus muscle
   (and tendon)
9 Deep fibular (peroneal) nerve
10 Posterior tibial artery and vein
11 Anterior tibial artery and vein
12 Tibial nerve
13 Interosseous membrane of leg
14 Fibular (peroneal) artery and vein
15 Peroneus (fibularis) brevis muscle
16 Plantaris muscle (tendon)
17 Fibula
18 Flexor hallucis longus muscle
19 Peroneus (fibularis) longus muscle
   (and tendon)
20 Soleus muscle
21 Gastrocnemius muscle (tendon)
22 Small saphenous vein
23 Medial sural cutaneous nerve

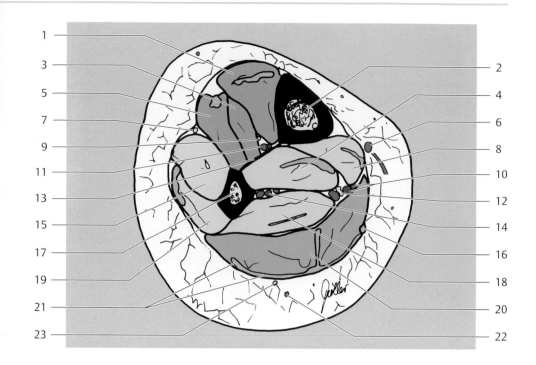

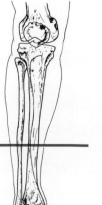

Anterior

Lateral ☐ Medial

Posterior

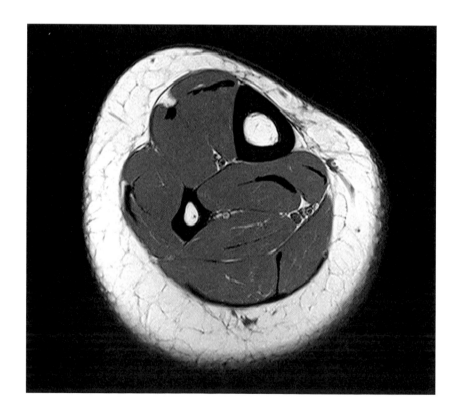

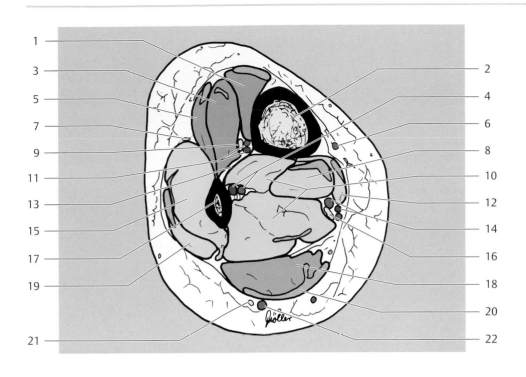

1 Tibialis anterior muscle (and tendon)
2 Tibia
3 Extensor hallucis longus muscle
4 Fibular (peroneal) artery and vein
5 Extensor digitorum longus muscle (and tendon)
6 Great saphenous vein
7 Superficial fibular (peroneal) nerve
8 Tibialis posterior muscle (and tendon)
9 Deep fibular (peroneal) nerve
10 Flexor hallucis longus muscle
11 Anterior tibial artery and vein
12 Flexor digitorum longus muscle (and tendon)
13 Interosseous membrane of leg
14 Posterior tibial artery and vein
15 Peroneus (fibularis) brevis muscle
16 Tibial nerve
17 Fibula
18 Soleus muscle
19 Peroneus (fibularis) longus muscle (and tendon)
20 Gastrocnemius muscle (tendon) and tendon of plantaris muscle
21 Sural nerve
22 Small saphenous vein

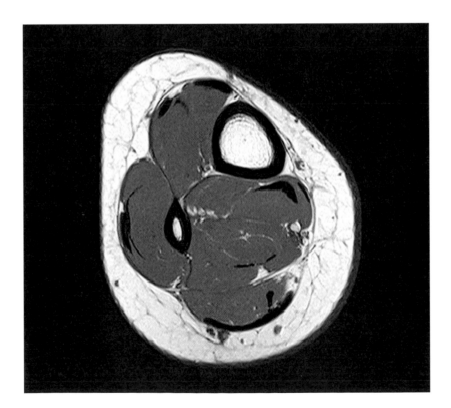

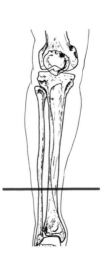

Anterior

Lateral   Medial

Posterior

1 Extensor hallucis longus muscle (and tendon)
2 Tibialis anterior muscle (and tendon)
3 Extensor digitorum longus muscle (and tendon)
4 Tibia
5 Anterior tibial artery and vein
6 Great saphenous vein
7 Deep fibular (peroneal) nerve
8 Flexor digitorum longus muscle (and tendon)
9 Superficial fibular (peroneal) nerve
10 Tibialis posterior muscle (and tendon)
11 Interosseous membrane of leg
12 Posterior tibial artery and vein
13 Fibular (peroneal) artery and veins
14 Tibial nerve
15 Fibula
16 Flexor hallucis longus muscle
17 Peroneus (fibularis) longus muscle (tendon)
18 Soleus muscle
19 Peroneus (fibularis) brevis muscle
20 Gastrocnemius muscle (tendon) and tendon of plantaris muscle
21 Sural nerve
22 Small saphenous vein

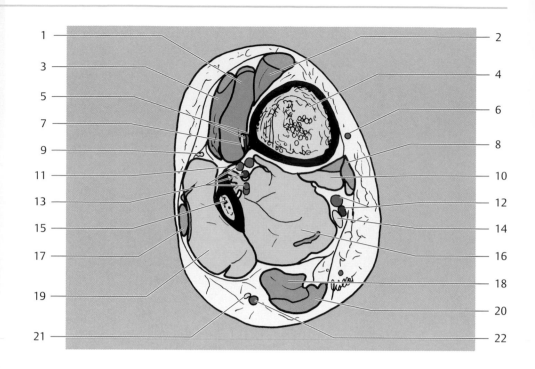

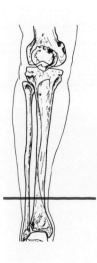

Anterior

Lateral □ Medial

Posterior

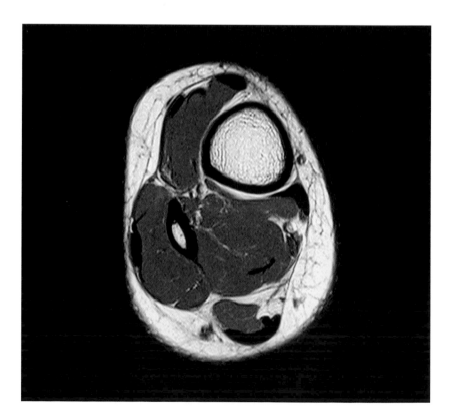

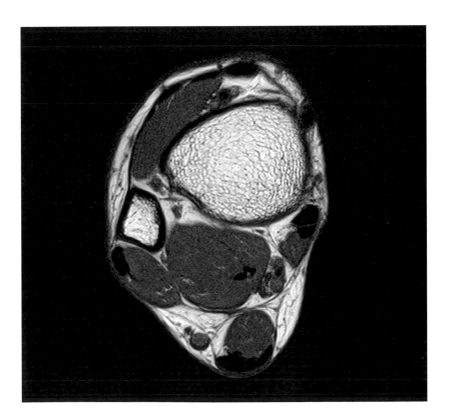

1 Extensor hallucis longus muscle
   (and tendon)
2 Tibialis anterior muscle (tendon)
3 Deep fibular (peroneal) nerve
4 Anterior tibial artery and vein
5 Extensor digitorum longus muscle
   (and tendon)
6 Great saphenous vein
7 Superficial fibular (peroneal) nerve
8 Tibia
9 Interosseous membrane of leg
10 Tibialis posterior muscle (tendon)
11 Fibular (peroneal) artery and vein
12 Flexor digitorum longus muscle
   (and tendon)
13 Fibula
14 Posterior tibial artery and vein
15 Peroneus (fibularis) longus muscle
   (tendon)
16 Tibial nerve
17 Peroneus (fibularis) brevis muscle
18 Flexor hallucis longus muscle
19 Sural nerve
20 Soleus muscle
21 Small saphenous vein
22 Triceps surae muscle (tendon) and
   plantaris muscle (tendon)

Anterior

Lateral ☐ Medial

Posterior

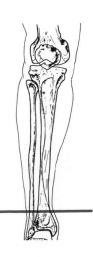

1 Extensor hallucis longus muscle (and tendon)
2 Tibialis anterior muscle (tendon)
3 Anterior tibial artery and veins
4 Great saphenous vein
5 Deep fibular (peroneal) nerve
6 Saphenous nerve
7 Extensor digitorum longus muscle (and tendon)
8 Tibia
9 Superficial fibular (peroneal) nerve
10 Tibialis posterior muscle (tendon)
11 Anterior tibiofibular ligament
12 Flexor digitorum longus muscle (and tendon)
13 Inferior tibiofibular joint
14 Posterior tibial artery and vein
15 Fibula
16 Tibial nerve
17 Posterior tibiofibular ligament
18 Flexor hallucis longus muscle (and tendon)
19 Peroneus (fibularis) longus muscle (tendon)
20 Soleus muscle
21 Fibular (peroneal) artery and vein
22 Triceps surae muscle (tendon) and plantaris muscle (tendon)
23 Peroneus (fibularis) brevis muscle (and tendon)
24 Sural nerve
25 Small saphenous vein

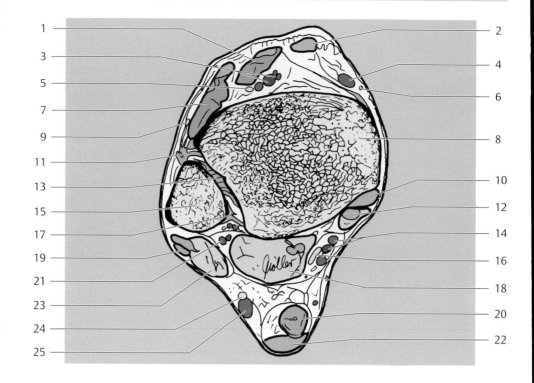

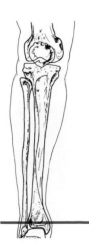

Anterior
Lateral ☐ Medial
Posterior

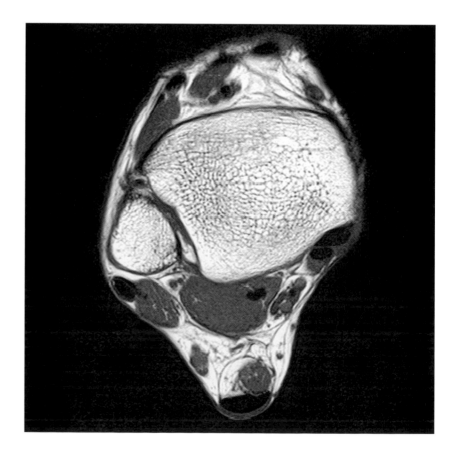

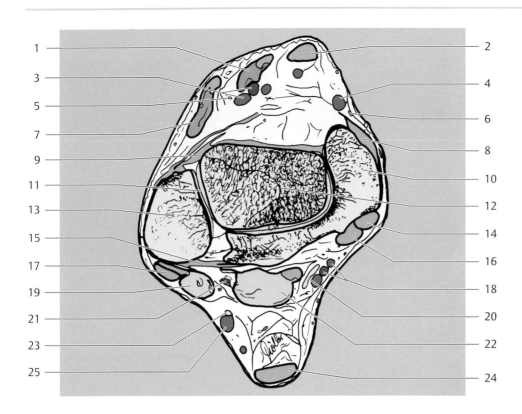

1 Extensor hallucis longus muscle (and tendon)
2 Tibialis anterior muscle (tendon)
3 Anterior tibial artery and vein
4 Great saphenous vein
5 Deep fibular (peroneal) nerve
6 Saphenous nerve
7 Extensor digitorum longus muscle (and tendon)
8 Deltoid ligament (tibionavicular and anterior tibiotalar parts)
9 Anterior tibiofibular ligament
10 Medial malleolus (tibia)
11 Tibiofibular syndesmosis
12 Talocrural joint
13 Lateral malleolus (fibula)
14 Tibialis posterior muscle (tendon)
15 Posterior tibiofibular ligament
16 Flexor digitorum longus muscle (tendon)
17 Peroneus (fibularis) longus muscle (tendon)
18 Posterior tibial artery and vein
19 Peroneus (fibularis) brevis muscle (and tendon)
20 Tibial nerve
21 Fibular (peroneal) artery and vein
22 Flexor hallucis longus muscle (and tendon)
23 Sural nerve
24 Triceps surae muscle (tendon) and plantaris muscle (tendon)
25 Small saphenous vein

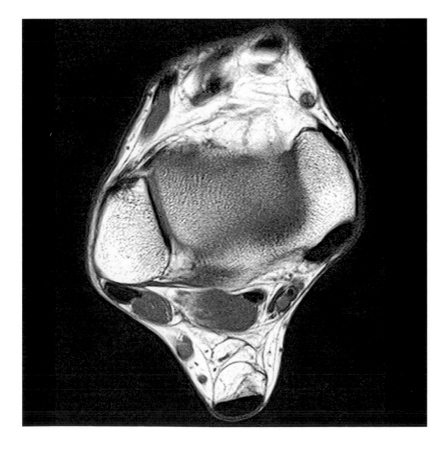

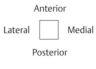

Anterior

Lateral ▢ Medial

Posterior

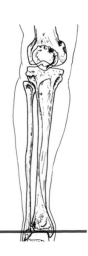

1 Extensor hallucis longus muscle (tendon)
2 Tibialis anterior muscle (tendon)
3 Extensor digitorum longus muscle (tendon)
4 Dorsalis pedis artery and vein
5 Lateral tarsal artery
6 Deep fibular nerve
7 Dorsal talonavicular ligament and joint capsule
8 Great saphenous vein
9 Extensor retinaculum
10 Deltoid ligament (tibionavicular and anterior tibiotalar parts)
11 Anterior talofibular ligament
12 Talus
13 Talocrural joint
14 Medial malleolus (tibia)
15 Lateral malleolus (fibula)
16 Tibialis posterior muscle (tendon)
17 Posterior talofibular ligament
18 Flexor digitorum longus muscle (tendon)
19 Posterior tibiofibular ligament
20 Flexor retinaculum
21 Peroneus (fibularis) longus muscle (tendon)
22 Posterior tibial artery and vein
23 Peroneus (fibularis) brevis muscle (and tendon)
24 Tibial nerve
25 Fibular (peroneal) artery and vein
26 Flexor hallucis longus muscle (and tendon)
27 Sural nerve
28 Calcaneal (Achilles) tendon
29 Small saphenous vein

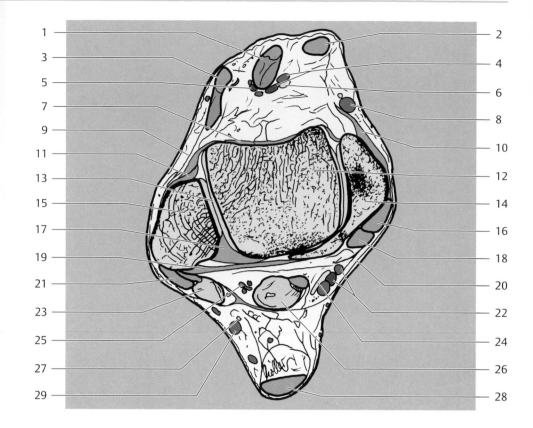

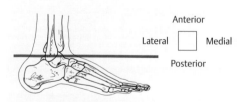

Anterior

Lateral ☐ Medial

Posterior

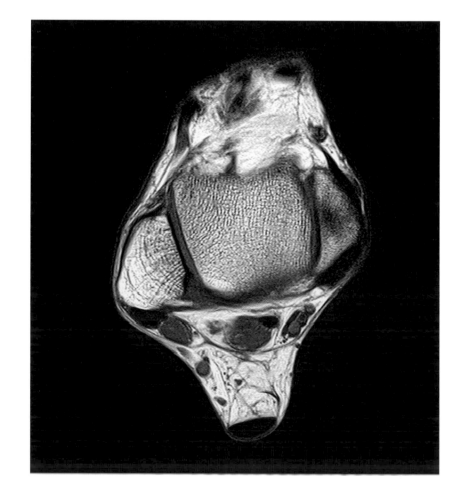

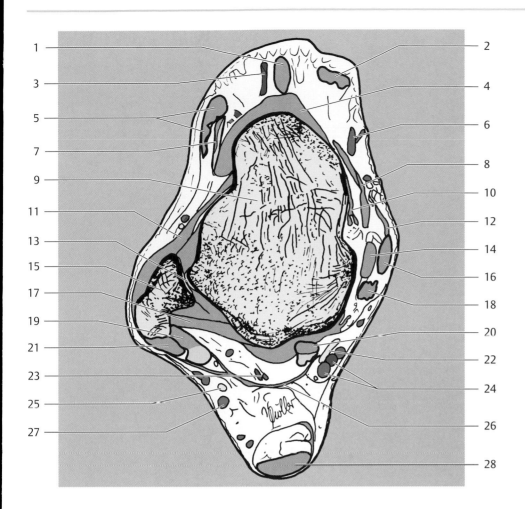

1 Extensor hallucis longus muscle (tendon)
2 Tibialis anterior muscle (tendon)
3 Dorsalis pedis artery
4 Dorsal talonavicular ligament
5 Extensor digitorum longus muscle (and tendon)
6 Great saphenous vein
7 Extensor digitorum brevis muscle (and tendon)
8 Deltoid ligament (tibionavicular part)
9 Talus
10 Deltoid ligament (anterior tibiotalar part)
11 Anterior talofibular ligament
12 Flexor retinaculum
13 Talocrural joint
14 Deltoid ligament (posterior tibiotalar part)
15 Lateral malleolus (fibula)
16 Tibialis posterior muscle (tendon)
17 Posterior talofibular ligament
18 Flexor digitorum longus muscle (tendon)
19 Peroneus (fibularis) brevis muscle (and tendon)
20 Flexor hallucis longus muscle (and tendon)
21 Peroneus (fibularis) longus muscle (tendon)
22 Tibial nerve
23 Fibular (peroneal) artery and vein
24 Posterior tibial artery and vein
25 Sural nerve
26 Superior peroneal retinaculum
27 Small saphenous vein
28 Calcaneal (Achilles) tendon

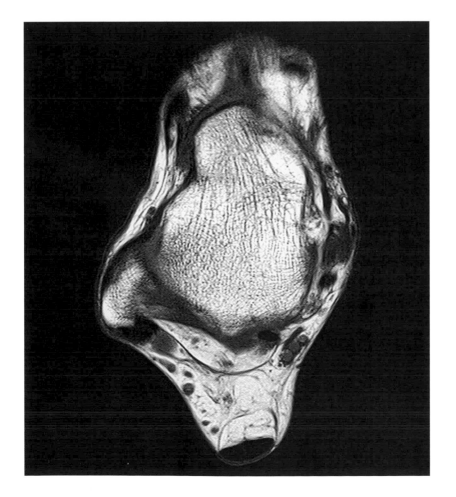

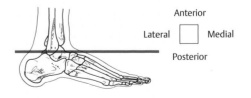

Anterior

Lateral Medial

Posterior

1　Dorsalis pedis artery
2　Extensor hallucis longus muscle (tendon)
3　Dorsal tarsal ligaments
4　Tibialis anterior muscle (tendon)
5　Extensor digitorum longus muscle (tendons)
6　Great saphenous vein
7　Extensor digitorum brevis muscle
8　Navicular
9　Dorsal talonavicular ligament
10　Talonavicular joint
11　Talus (head)
12　Deltoid ligament (tibionavicular part)
13　Talocalcaneal interosseous ligament
14　Tibialis posterior muscle (tendon)
15　Talus (neck)
16　Deltoid ligament (tibiocalcaneal part)
17　Talus (body)
18　Deltoid ligament (posterior tibiotalar part)
19　Calcaneofibular ligament
20　Flexor retinaculum
21　Peroneus (fibularis) brevis muscle (tendon)
22　Flexor digitorum longus muscle (tendon)
23　Peroneus (fibularis) longus muscle (tendon)
24　Tibial nerve
25　Superior fibular (peroneal) retinaculum
26　Flexor hallucis longus muscle (tendon)
27　Sural nerve
28　Posterior tibial artery and vein
29　Small saphenous vein
30　Calcaneal (Achilles) tendon

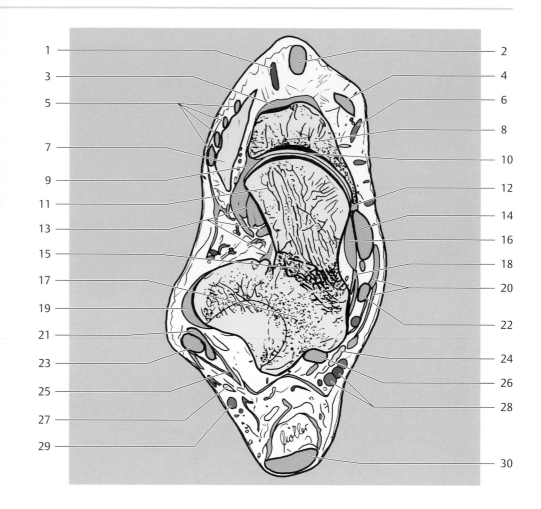

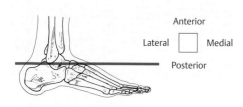

Anterior

Lateral　□　Medial

Posterior

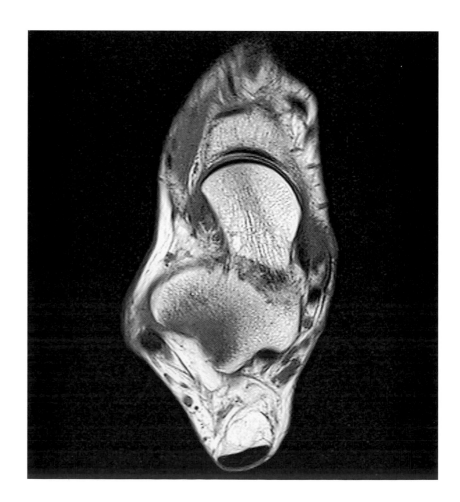

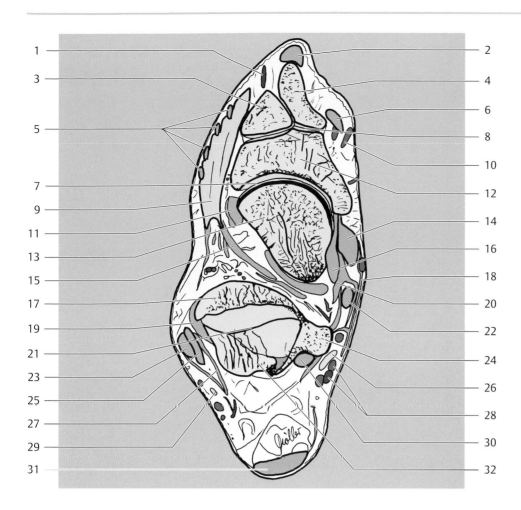

1 Dorsalis pedis artery
2 Extensor hallucis longus muscle (tendon)
3 Intermediate cuneiform
4 Medial cuneiform
5 Extensor digitorum longus muscle (tendons)
6 Tibialis anterior muscle (tendon)
7 Talonavicular joint
8 Cuneonavicular joint
9 Extensor digitorum brevis muscle
10 Great saphenous vein
11 Bifurcate ligament
12 Navicular
13 Talus (head)
14 Tibialis posterior muscle (tendon)
15 Talocalcaneal interosseous ligament
16 Deltoid ligament (tibiocalcaneal and tibionavicular parts)
17 Talus (body)
18 Flexor retinaculum
19 Calcaneofibular ligament
20 Talocalcaneal ligament (medial)
21 Subtalar (talocalcaneal) joint
22 Flexor digitorum longus muscle (tendon)
23 Peroneus (fibularis) longus muscle (tendon)
24 Talus (posterior process)
25 Peroneus (fibularis) brevis muscle (tendon)
26 Tibial nerve
27 Peroneal retinaculum
28 Posterior tibial artery and vein
29 Dorsal lateral cutaneous nerve
30 Flexor hallucis longus muscle (tendon)
31 Calcaneal (Achilles) tendon
32 Calcaneus

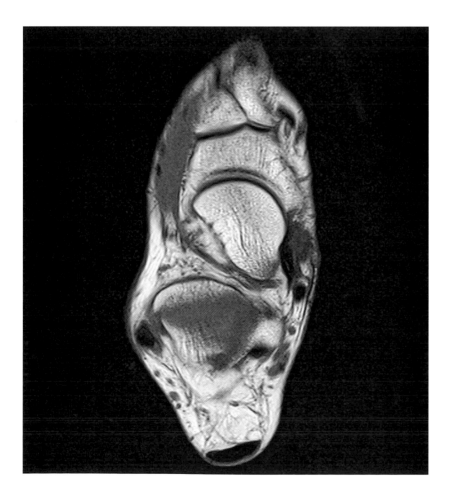

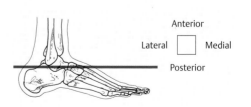

Anterior

Lateral ☐ Medial

Posterior

1 Extensor hallucis longus muscle (tendon)
2 Metatarsal I (base)
3 Dorsalis pedis artery
4 Tarsometatarsal I joint
5 Intermediate cuneiform
6 Medial cuneiform
7 Extensor digitorum longus muscle (tendons)
8 Tibialis anterior muscle (tendon)
9 Extensor digitorum brevis muscle
10 Great saphenous vein
11 Bifurcate ligament
12 Dorsal tarsal ligaments
13 Talus (head)
14 Navicular
15 Talocalcaneal interosseous ligament
16 Tibialis posterior muscle (tendon)
17 Peroneus brevis muscle (tendon)
18 Plantar calcaneonavicular ligament (spring ligament)
19 Peroneus longus muscle (tendon)
20 Flexor retinaculum
21 Calcaneus
22 Deltoid ligament (tibiocalcaneal part)
23 Inferior peroneal (fibular) retinaculum
24 Flexor digitorum longus muscle (tendon)
25 Lateral dorsal cutaneous nerve
26 Calcaneus (talar shelf)
27 Calcaneal (Achilles) tendon
28 Tibial nerve
29 Posterior tibial artery and vein
30 Flexor hallucis longus muscle (tendon)

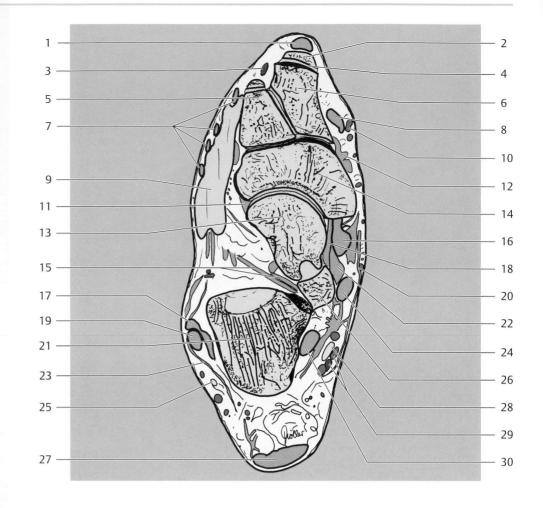

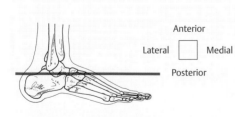

Anterior
Lateral ☐ Medial
Posterior

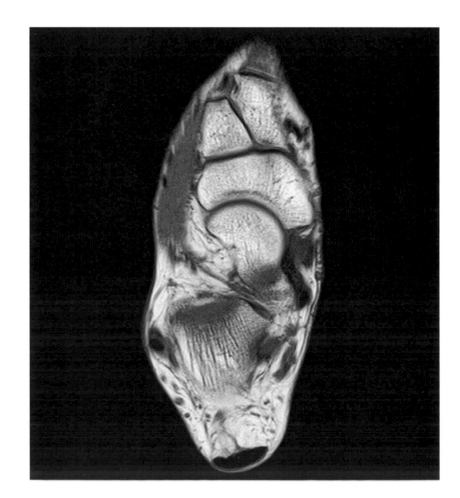

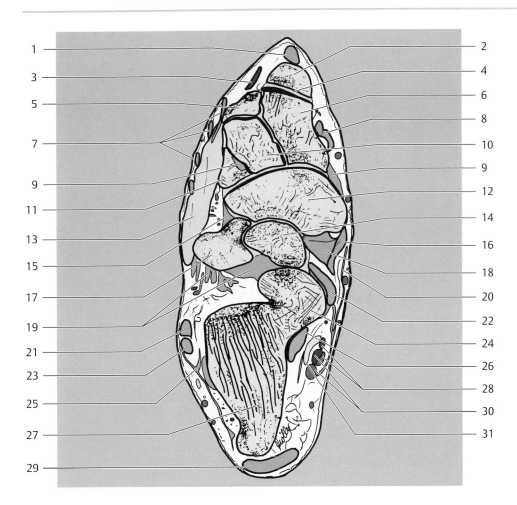

1 Extensor hallucis longus muscle
   (tendon)
2 Metatarsal I (base)
3 Dorsalis pedis artery
4 First tarsometatarsal joint
5 Metatarsal II (base)
6 Medial cuneiform
7 Extensor digitorum longus muscle
   (tendons)
8 Tibialis anterior muscle (tendon)
9 Dorsal tarsal ligaments
10 Intermediate cuneiform
11 Lateral cuneiform
12 Navicular
13 Extensor digitorum brevis muscle
14 Talus (head)
15 Bifurcate ligament
16 Deltoid ligament (tibionavicular part)
17 Calcaneus
18 Tibialis posterior muscle (tendon)
19 Talocalcaneal interosseous ligament
20 Flexor retinaculum
21 Peroneus (fibularis) brevis muscle
   (tendon)
22 Flexor digitorum longus muscle
   (tendon)
23 Peroneus (fibularis) longus muscle
   (tendon)
24 Calcaneus (talar shelf)
25 Inferior peroneal (fibular) retinaculum
26 Flexor hallucis longus muscle (tendon)
27 Calcaneal tuberosity
28 Medial plantar artery and vein
29 Calcaneal (Achilles) tendon
30 Lateral plantar artery and vein
31 Tibial nerve

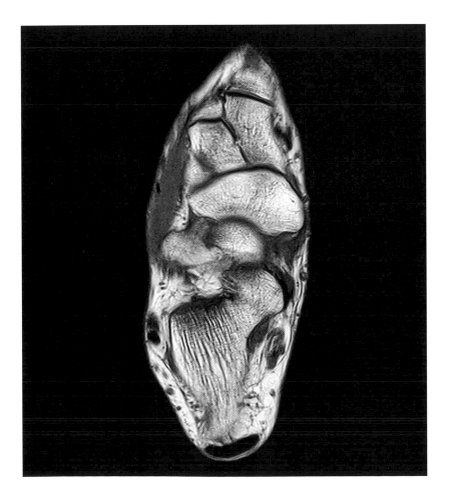

Anterior

Lateral ☐ Medial

Posterior

1 Extensor hallucis longus muscle
  (tendon)
2 Metatarsal I (base)
3 Dorsalis pedis artery
4 Metatarsal II (base)
5 Dorsal interosseous muscles
6 Cuneometatarsal interosseous
  ligaments
7 Extensor digitorum longus muscle
  (tendons)
8 Tibialis anterior muscle (tendon)
9 Intermediate cuneiform
10 Medial cuneiform
11 Lateral cuneiform
12 Dorsal tarsal ligaments
13 Extensor digitorum brevis muscle
14 Tibialis posterior muscle (tendon)
15 Cuboid
16 Plantar calcaneonavicular ligament
   (spring ligament, medioplantar part)
17 Navicular
18 Flexor digitorum longus muscle
   (tendon)
19 Plantar calcaneonavicular ligament
   (spring ligament)
20 Calcaneus (talar shelf)
21 Long plantar ligament
22 Medial plantar artery and nerve
23 Peroneus (fibularis) brevis muscle
   (tendon)
24 Flexor hallucis longus muscle (tendon)
25 Peroneus (fibularis) longus muscle
   (tendon)
26 Flexor retinaculum
27 Inferior peroneal (fibular) retinaculum
28 Lateral plantar artery and vein
29 Calcaneus (calcaneal tuberosity)
30 Quadratus plantae muscle
31 Calcaneal (Achilles) tendon

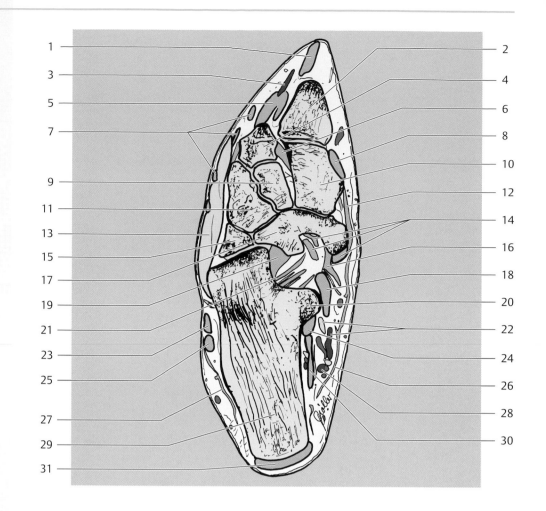

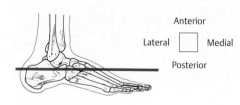

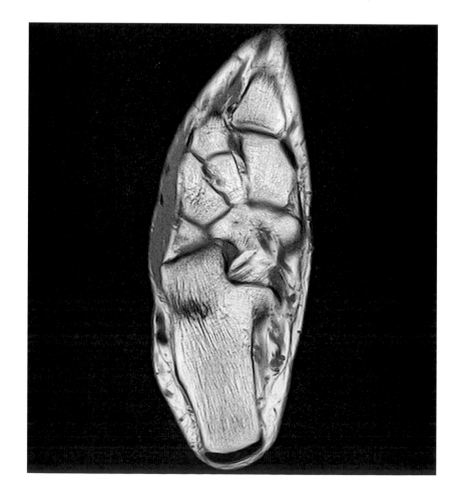

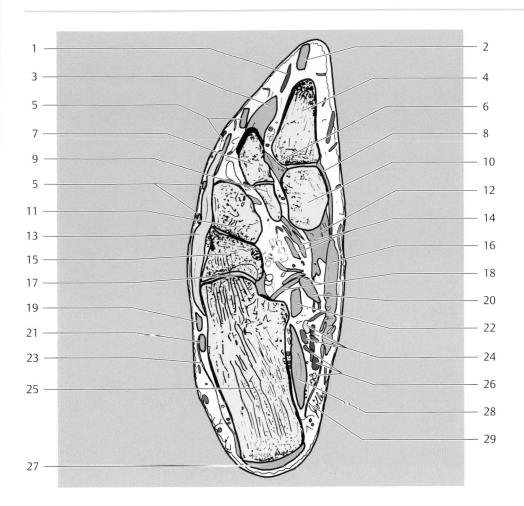

1 Dorsalis pedis artery
2 Extensor hallucis longus muscle (tendon)
3 Dorsal interosseous muscles
4 Metatarsal I (base)
5 Extensor digitorum longus muscle (tendons)
6 Cuneometatarsal interosseous ligaments
7 Metatarsal II (base)
8 Tibialis anterior muscle (tendon)
9 Intermediate cuneiform
10 Medial cuneiform
11 Lateral cuneiform
12 Plantar cuneonavicular ligament
13 Extensor digitorum brevis muscle
14 Tibialis posterior muscle (tendon)
15 Cuboid
16 Abductor hallucis muscle
17 Calcaneocuboid joint
18 Long plantar ligament
19 Peroneus (fibularis) brevis muscle (tendon)
20 Flexor digitorum longus muscle (tendon)
21 Peroneus (fibularis) longus muscle (tendon)
22 Flexor hallucis longus muscle (tendon)
23 Inferior fibular (peroneal) retinaculum
24 Medial plantar artery, vein, and nerve
25 Calcaneus
26 Lateral plantar artery, vein, and nerve
27 Calcaneal (Achilles) tendon (attachment)
28 Quadratus plantae muscle
29 Flexor retinaculum

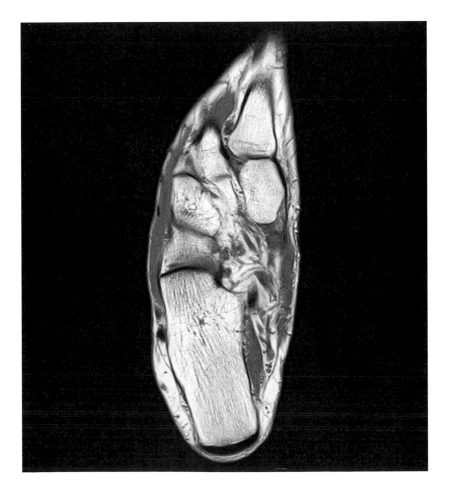

Anterior
Lateral | Medial
Posterior

1 Extensor digitorum longus muscle
   (tendons)
2 Proximal phalanx I
3 Dorsal and plantar interosseous
   muscles
4 Metacarpophalangeal joint
5 Adductor hallucis brevis muscle
   (oblique head)
6 Metatarsal I (head)
7 Peroneus (fibularis) longus muscle
   (tendon)
8 Joint capsule
9 Metatarsal IV (base)
10 Metatarsal II
11 Plantar arch
12 Plantar metatarsal artery, vein,
   and nerve
13 Lateral cuneiform
14 Flexor hallucis brevis muscle
   (medial head)
15 Cuboid
16 Flexor hallucis brevis muscle
   (lateral head)
17 Plantar digital V artery, vein, and nerve
18 Adductor hallucis brevis muscle
19 Abductor digiti minimi muscle
20 Flexor hallucis longus muscle (tendon)
21 Long plantar ligament
22 Flexor digitorum longus muscle
   (tendon)
23 Calcaneus (tuberosity)
24 Medial plantar artery, and nerve
25 Quadratus plantae muscle
26 Abductor hallucis muscle
27 Lateral plantar artery, vein, and nerve

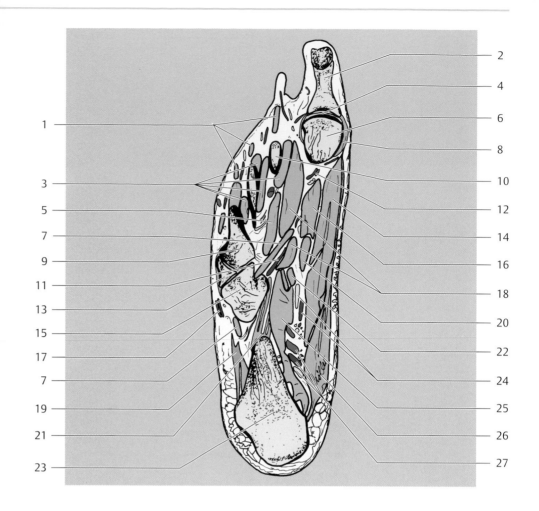

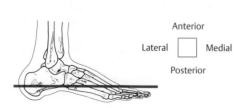

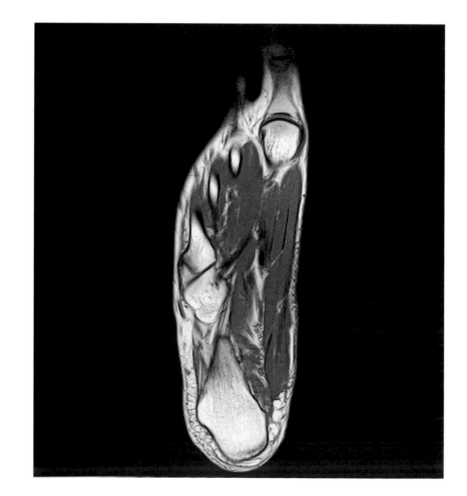

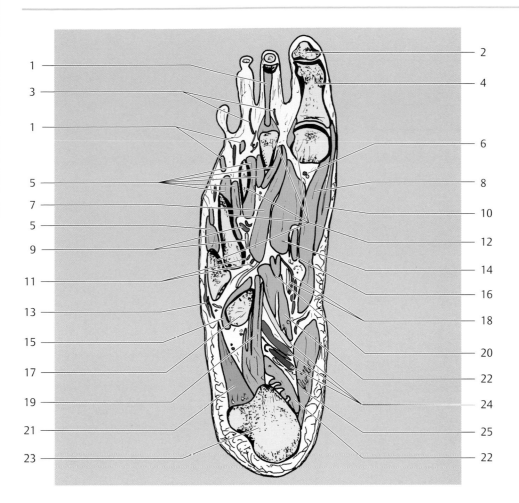

1 Extensor digitorum longus muscle (tendon)
2 Distal phalanx I
3 Plantar digital arteries
4 Proximal phalanx I
5 Dorsal and plantar interosseous muscles
6 Plantar metatarsal artery and nerve
7 Adductor hallucis brevis muscle
8 Flexor hallucis brevis muscle (medial head)
9 Lateral plantar artery and vein (superficial branch) and nerve
10 Abductor hallucis muscle (tendon)
11 Lateral plantar artery and vein (deep branch)
12 Metatarsals II–V
13 Fifth plantar digital artery, vein, and nerve
14 Flexor hallucis brevis muscle (lateral head)
15 Peroneus (fibularis) longus muscle (tendon)
16 Flexor hallucis longus muscle (tendon)
17 Cuboid
18 Medial plantar artery, vein, and nerve
19 Long plantar ligament
20 Flexor digitorum longus muscle (tendon)
21 Abductor digiti minimi muscle
22 Quadratus plantae muscle
23 Calcaneus (tuberosity)
24 Lateral plantar artery, vein, and nerve
25 Abductor hallucis muscle

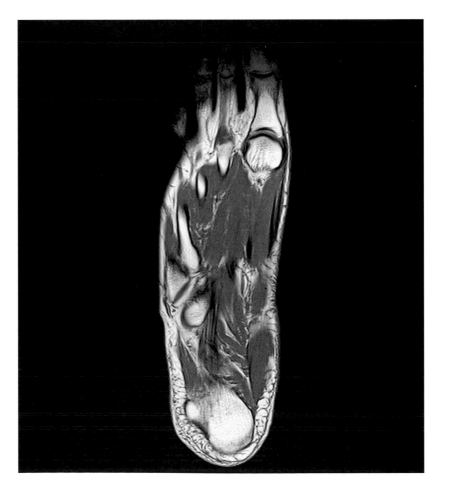

Anterior

Lateral ☐ Medial

Posterior

1 Distal phalanx IV
2 Adductor hallucis muscle (tendon attachment)
3 Distal interphalangeal joint
4 Abductor hallucis muscle (tendon attachment)
5 Middle phalanx IV
6 Common plantar digital artery, vein, and nerve
7 Proximal interphalangeal joint
8 Flexor hallucis brevis muscle (medial head)
9 Proximal phalanx IV
10 Flexor hallucis brevis muscle (lateral head)
11 Metacarpophalangeal IV joint
12 Flexor hallucis longus muscle (tendon)
13 Metatarsal IV
14 Adductor hallucis brevis muscle
15 Dorsal and plantar interosseous muscles
16 Medial plantar artery, and nerve (superficial branch)
17 Flexor digiti minimi brevis muscle
18 Lumbrical muscles
19 Opponens digiti minimi muscle
20 Medial plantar artery (deep branch)
21 Lateral plantar artery, vein, and nerve
22 Flexor digitorum longus muscle (tendons)
23 Abductor digiti minimi muscle
24 Flexor digitorum brevis muscle
25 Calcaneus (tuberosity)

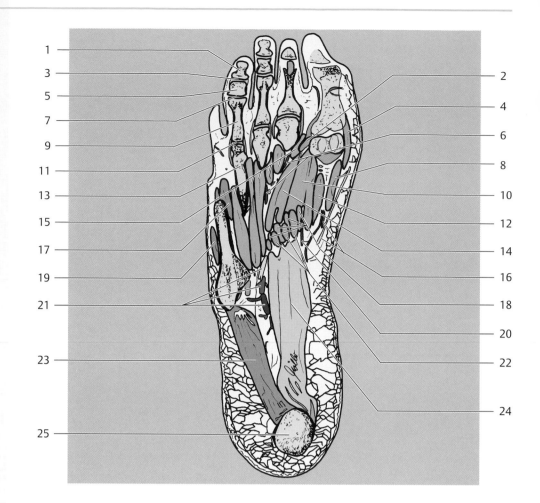

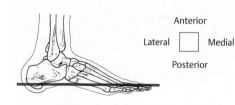

Anterior
Lateral | Medial
Posterior

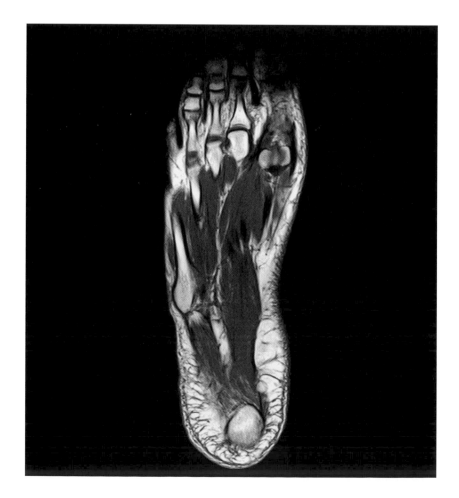

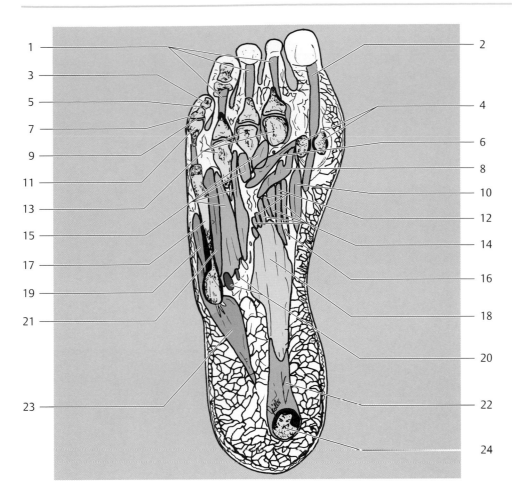

1 Flexor digitorum muscle (tendons)
2 Flexor hallucis longus muscle (tendon)
3 Distal phalanx V
4 Sesamoid bones
5 Fifth distal interphalangeal joint
6 Adductor hallucis muscle (transverse head)
7 Medial phalanx V
8 Adductor hallucis muscle (oblique head)
9 Fifth proximal interphalangeal joint
10 Flexor hallucis brevis muscle
11 Proximal phalanx V
12 Flexor digitorum longus muscle (tendons)
13 Metatarsals II–IV (heads)
14 Lumbrical muscles
15 Dorsal and plantar interosseous muscles
16 Medial plantar nerve (deep branch)
17 Metatarsal V
18 Flexor digitorum brevis muscle
19 Opponens digiti minimi muscle
20 Lateral plantar artery and vein
21 Flexor digiti minimi brevis muscle
22 Plantar aponeurosis
23 Abductor digiti minimi muscle
24 Calcaneus (tuberosity)

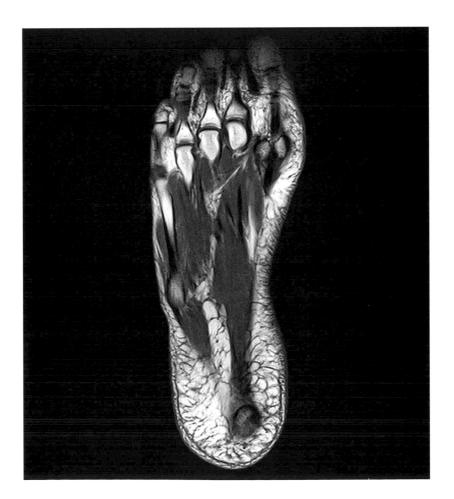

Anterior

Lateral ☐ Medial

Posterior

1 Small intestine
2 External oblique and internal oblique abdominal muscles
3 Anterior superior iliac spine
4 Transversus abdominis muscle
5 Uterus
6 Iliacus muscle
7 Ilium
8 Gluteus medius muscle
9 Femoral nerve
10 Iliopsoas muscle
11 Femoral artery and vein
12 Urinary bladder
13 Pubis
14 Tensor fasciae latae muscle
15 Lateral circumflex femoral artery (ascending branch)
16 Pectineus muscle
17 Rectus femoris muscle
18 Symphysis
19 Sartorius muscle
20 Adductor longus muscle
21 Vastus medialis muscle
22 Great saphenous vein
23 Vastus lateralis muscle

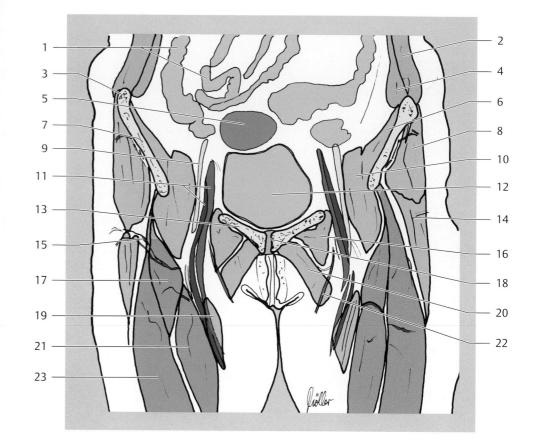

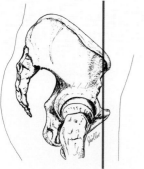

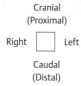

Cranial
(Proximal)

Right   Left

Caudal
(Distal)

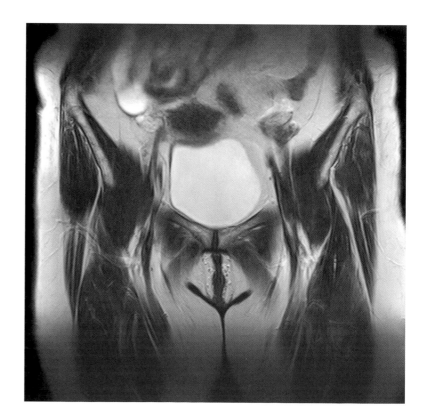

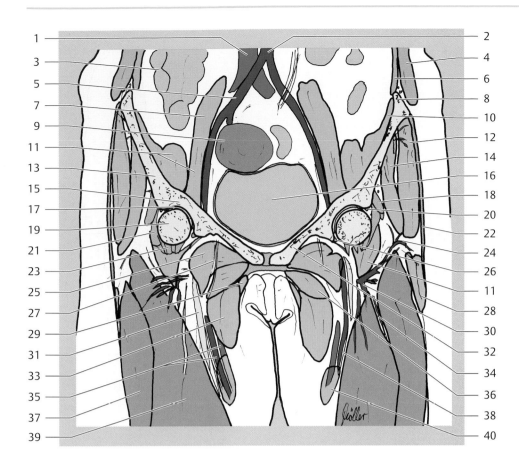

1 Inferior vena cava
2 Aorta (bifurcation)
3 Small intestine
4 External oblique and internal oblique abdominal muscles
5 (Right) common iliac artery
6 Transversus abdominis muscle
7 Psoas muscle
8 Anterior superior iliac spine
9 Uterus
10 Iliacus muscle
11 Iliopsoas muscle
12 Gluteus medius muscle
13 Ilium
14 Gluteus minimus muscle
15 Roof of acetabulum
16 Urinary bladder
17 Hip joint
18 Rectus femoris muscle (tendon)
19 Femur (head)
20 Superior glenoid labrum
21 Iliofemoral ligament (transverse part)
22 Iliotibial tract
23 Iliofemoral ligament (descending part)
24 Lateral circumflex femoral artery (ascending branch)
25 Pectineus muscle
26 Inferior glenoid labrum
27 Obturator nerve
28 Tensor fasciae latae muscle
29 Gracilis muscle
30 Deep artery of thigh
31 Femoral nerve
32 Pubis
33 Adductor longus muscle
34 Lateral circumflex femoral artery (descending branch)
35 Femoral artery and vein (superficial)
36 Adductor brevis muscle
37 Vastus lateralis muscle
38 Saphenous nerve
39 Vastus intermedius muscle
40 Sartorius muscle

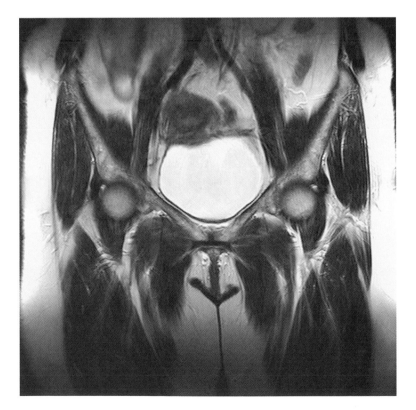

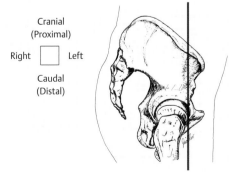

Cranial
(Proximal)

Right ☐ Left

Caudal
(Distal)

1 External oblique and internal oblique abdominal muscles
2 Lumbar vertebra IV
3 Transversus abdominis muscle
4 Psoas muscle
5 Small intestine
6 Anterior superior iliac spine
7 Lumbosacral trunk
8 Iliacus muscle
9 Sacral plexus
10 Left internal iliac artery
11 Ilium
12 Superior gluteal artery
13 Ovary
14 Sigmoid colon
15 Uterus
16 Gluteus medius muscle
17 Acetabulum
18 Gluteus minimus muscle
19 Urinary bladder
20 Hip joint
21 Femur (head)
22 Superior acetabular labrum
23 Obturator internus muscle
24 Iliofemoral ligament (transverse part)
25 Femur (neck)
26 Iliofemoral ligament (descending part)
27 Greater trochanter
28 Ligament of head of femur
29 Obturator externus muscle
30 Inferior acetabular labrum
31 Iliotibial tract
32 Lateral circumflex femoral artery (ascending branch)
33 Iliopsoas muscle
34 Joint capsule
35 Pectineus muscle
36 Obturator membrane
37 Pubis
38 Lateral circumflex femoral artery (descending branch)
39 Adductor brevis muscle
40 Obturator artery, vein, and nerve
41 Gracilis muscle
42 Vagina
43 Adductor longus muscle
44 Vastus intermedius muscle
45 Femur (shaft)
46 Deep femoral artery and vein
47 Vastus lateralis muscle
48 Superficial femoral artery, and vein, saphenous nerve
49 Vastus medialis muscle
50 Sartorius muscle

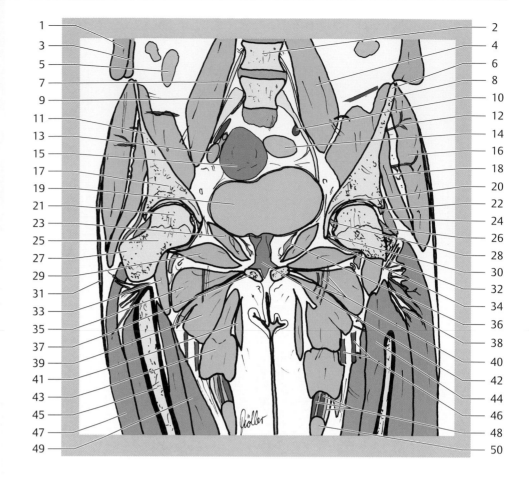

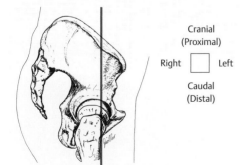

Cranial (Proximal)

Right | | Left

Caudal (Distal)

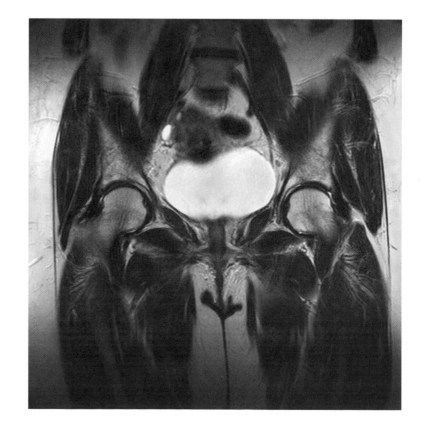

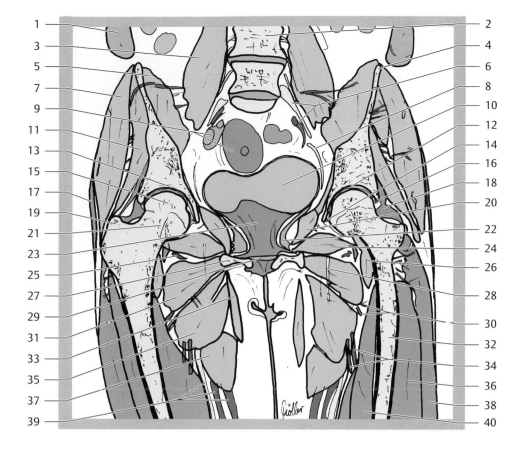

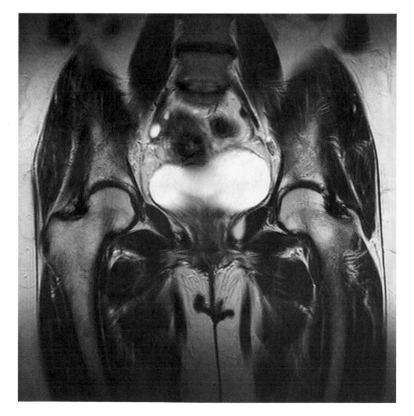

1 External oblique and internal oblique muscles of abdomen
2 Fourth lumbar vertebra
3 Psoas muscle
4 Anterior superior iliac spine
5 Iliacus muscle
6 Sacral plexus and (left) internal iliac artery and vein
7 Gluteus medius muscle
8 Obturator nerve
9 Ovary and uterus
10 Urinary bladder
11 Gluteus minimus muscle
12 Hip joint
13 Acetabulum (roof)
14 Inferior glenoid labrum
15 Femur (head)
16 Superior glenoid labrum
17 Iliotibial tract
18 Iliofemoral ligament
19 Greater trochanter
20 Obturator internus muscle
21 Femur (neck)
22 Levator ani muscle
23 Vagina
24 Obturator externus muscle
25 Medial circumflex femoral artery
26 Iliopsoas muscle
27 Pubis
28 Obturator nerve
29 Deep transverse perineal muscle
30 Lateral circumflex femoral artery and vein (descending branch) and femoral nerve (anterior cutaneous branch)
31 Pectineus muscle
32 Femur (shaft)
33 Gracilis muscle
34 Deep artery and vein of thigh
35 Adductor brevis muscle
36 Vastus intermedius muscle
37 Adductor longus muscle
38 Vastus lateralis muscle
39 (Superficial) Femoral artery and vein and saphenous nerve
40 Vastus medialis muscle

Cranial (Proximal)

Right Left

Caudal (Distal)

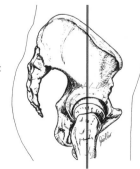

1 Lumbar plexus
2 Psoas muscle
3 Iliac crest
4 Superior gluteal artery and vein
5 Iliacus muscle
6 Sacrum
7 Sacral plexus
8 Sacro-iliac joint
9 Ilium
10 Gluteus medius muscle
11 Uterus
12 Inferior gluteal artery and vein
13 Vagina
14 Sigmoid colon
15 Acetabulum (roof)
16 Gluteus minimus muscle
17 Zona orbicularis
18 Gluteus maximus muscle
19 Greater trochanter
20 Urinary bladder
21 Levator ani muscle
22 Ischiofemoral ligament
23 Intertrochanteric crest
24 Femur (head)
25 Obturator externus muscle
26 Obturator internus muscle
27 Lesser trochanter
28 Medial circumflex femoral artery
     and vein
29 Adductor minimus muscle
30 Deep transverse perineal muscle
31 Pubis (inferior ramus)
32 Femur (shaft)
33 Adductor brevis muscle
34 Deep femoral artery and vein
35 Adductor magnus muscle
36 Vastus lateralis muscle
37 Gracilis muscle
38 Vastus intermedius muscle
39 Adductor brevis muscle

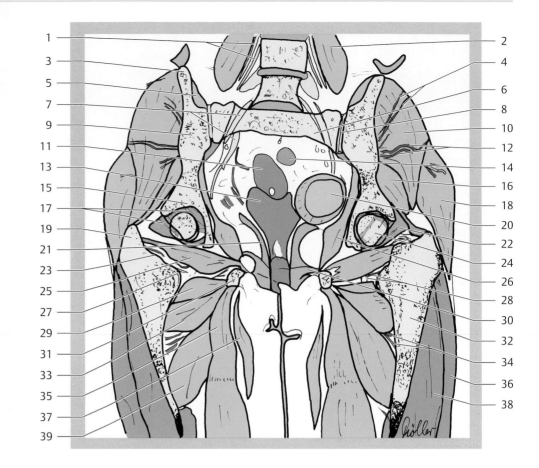

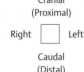
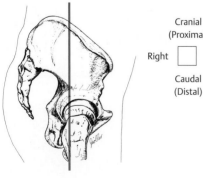

Cranial
(Proximal)

Right ☐ Left

Caudal
(Distal)

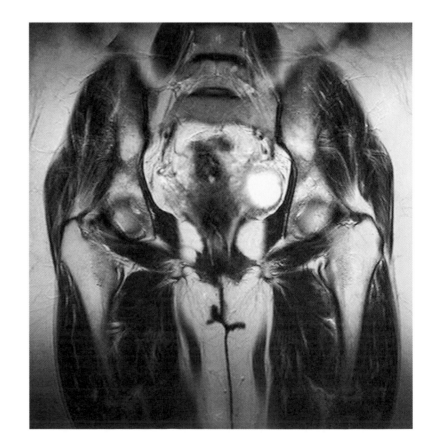

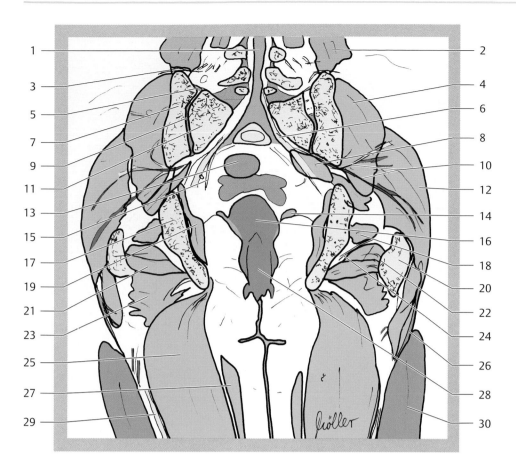

1 Spinal canal
2 Iliocostalis lumborum muscle
3 Superior cluneal nerves
4 Gluteus medius muscle
5 Sacro-iliac ligament
6 Sciatic nerve
7 Ilium
8 Piriformis muscle
9 Sacro-iliac joint
10 Inferior gluteal artery, vein, and nerve
11 Sacrum (lateral mass)
12 Gluteus maximus muscle
13 Sigmoid colon
14 Levator ani muscle
15 Pudendal nerve
16 Uterus
17 Ischium
18 Gemellus superior muscle
19 Obturator internus muscle
20 Greater trochanter
21 Gemellus inferior muscle
22 Intertrochanteric crest
23 Quadratus femoris muscle
24 Muscular nerve
25 Adductor magnus muscle
26 Iliotibial tract
27 Gracilis muscle
28 Vagina
29 Sciatic nerve
30 Vastus lateralis muscle

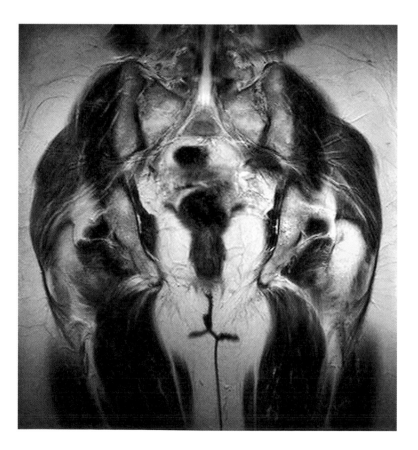

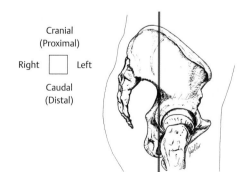

Cranial
(Proximal)

Right   Left

Caudal
(Distal)

1 Iliocostalis lumborum muscle
2 Multifidus muscle
3 Spinous process
4 Interspinal ligament
5 Ilium
6 Vertebral arch
7 Sacro-iliac joint
8 Superior gluteal artery, vein, and nerve
9 Rectum
10 Sacrum (lateral mass)
11 Inferior gluteal artery, vein, and nerve
12 Piriformis muscle
13 Ischial spine
14 Levator ani muscle
15 Obturator internus muscle
16 Sciatic nerve
17 Ischial tuberosity
18 Gluteus maximus muscle
19 Adductor magnus muscle (attachment)
20 Semitendinosus and biceps femoris muscles (common tendon attachment)
21 Biceps femoris muscle (long head)
22 Semitendinosus muscle
23 Adductor magnus muscle
24 Vastus lateralis muscle
25 Gracilis muscle

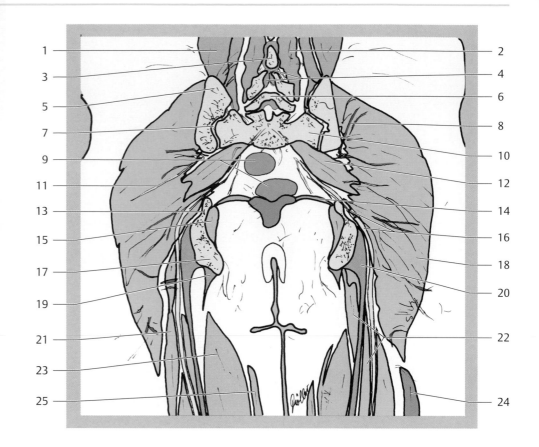

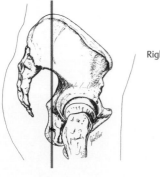

Cranial
(Proximal)

Right   Left

Caudal
(Distal)

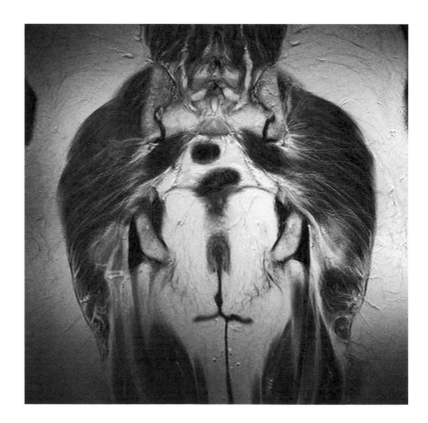

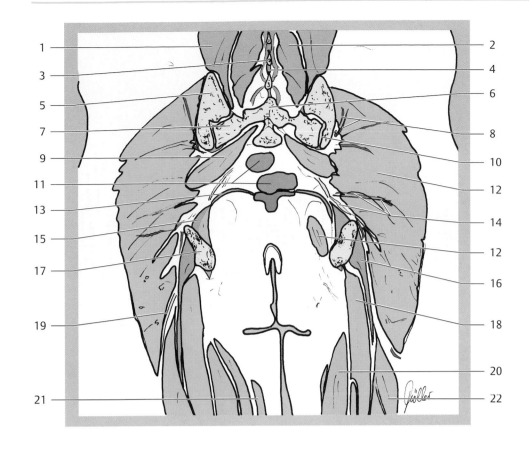

1 Iliocostalis lumborum muscle
2 Multifidus muscle
3 Spinous process (of vertebra)
4 Interspinal ligament
5 Ilium
6 Sacrum
7 Sacrum (lateral mass)
8 Superior gluteal artery, vein, and nerve
9 Piriformis muscle
10 Sacro-iliac joint
11 Rectum
12 Gluteus maximus muscle
13 Levator ani muscle
14 Inferior gluteal artery, vein, and nerve
15 Sacrotuberous ligament
16 Semitendinosus and biceps femoris
   muscles (common tendon attachment)
17 Ischial tuberosity
18 Semimembranosus muscle
19 Posterior cutaneous femoral nerve
20 Adductor magnus muscle
21 Gracilis muscle
22 Biceps femoris muscle (long head)

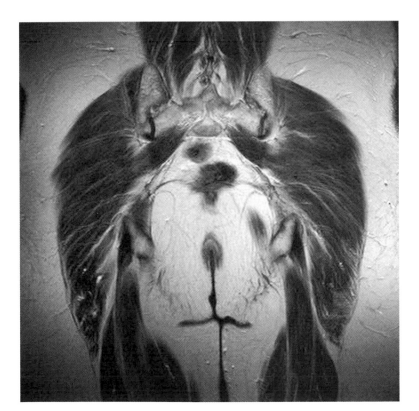

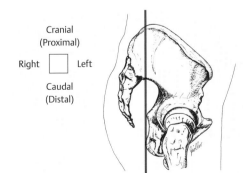

Cranial
(Proximal)

Right | Left

Caudal
(Distal)

1 External oblique and internal oblique abdominal muscles
2 Gluteus medius muscle
3 Transversus abdominis muscle
4 Gluteus maximus muscle
5 Anterior superior iliac spine
6 Greater trochanter
7 Sartorius muscle
8 Femur (neck)
9 Tensor fasciae latae muscle
10 Femur (shaft)
11 Lateral circumflex femoral artery and vein
12 Medial circumflex femoral artery and vein
13 Rectus femoris muscle
14 Vastus intermedius muscle

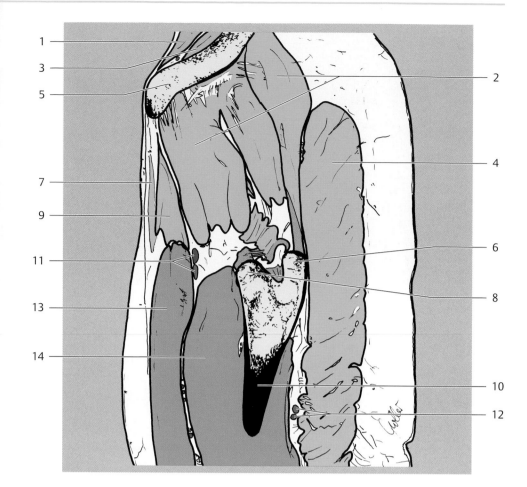

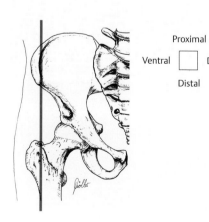

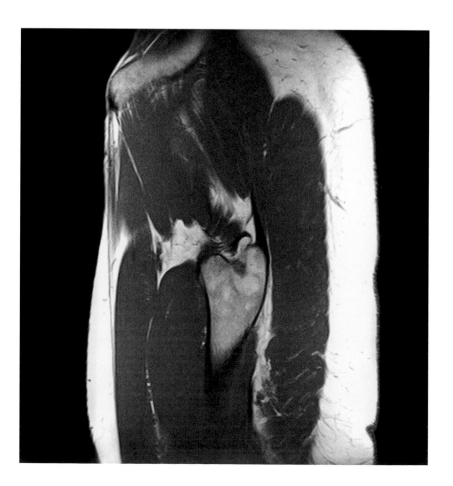

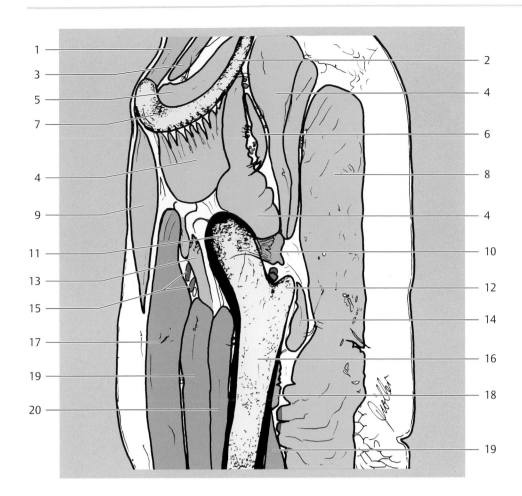

1 External oblique and internal oblique abdominal muscles
2 Ilium (wing)
3 Transversus abdominis muscle
4 Gluteus medius muscle
5 Iliopsoas muscle
6 Gluteus minimus muscle
7 Anterior superior iliac spine
8 Gluteus maximus muscle
9 Sartorius muscle
10 Obturator internus muscle and gemellus muscles
11 Femur (neck)
12 Greater trochanter
13 Iliopsoas muscle
14 Quadratus femoris muscle
15 Lateral circumflex femoral artery and vein
16 Femur (shaft)
17 Rectus femoris muscle
18 Adductor magnus muscle (tendon attachment)
19 Vastus intermedius muscle
20 Vastus medialis muscle

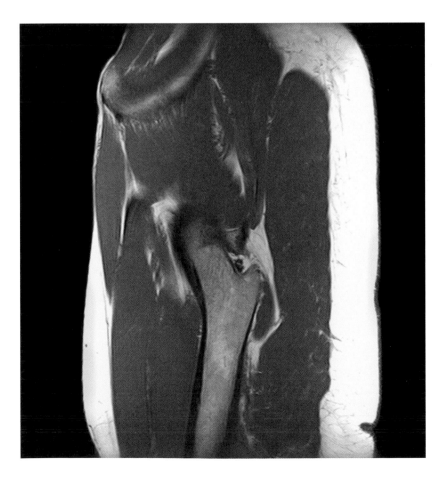

Proximal
Ventral □ Dorsal
Distal

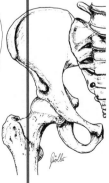

1 Small intestine
2 Gluteus medius muscle
3 Rectus abdominis muscle
4 Superior gluteal artery and vein
5 Iliopsoas muscle
6 Gluteus minimus muscle
7 Ilium (roof of acetabulum)
8 Superficial circumflex iliac artery
9 Hip joint
10 Gluteus maximus muscle
11 Superior glenoid labrum
12 Obturator internus muscle and
   gemellus muscles
13 Femur (head)
14 Medial circumflex femoral artery and
   veins
15 Sartorius muscle
16 Quadratus femoris muscle
17 Lateral circumflex femoral artery
   (ascending branch)
18 Lesser trochanter
19 Rectus femoris muscle
20 Biceps femoris muscle (long head)
21 Lateral circumflex femoral artery and
   veins (descending branch)
22 Adductor brevis muscle
23 Vastus intermedius muscle
24 Perforating artery and vein
25 Femur (shaft)
26 Adductor magnus muscle

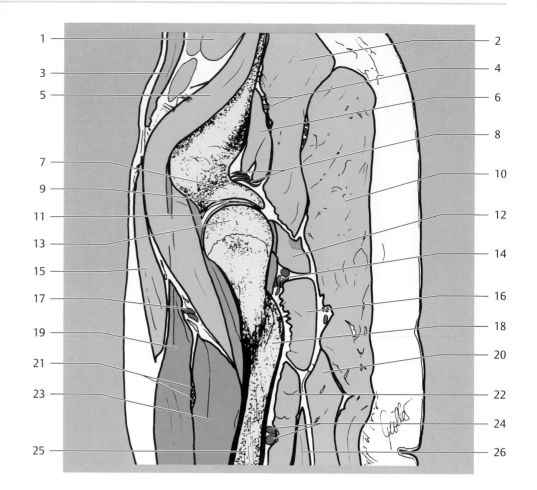

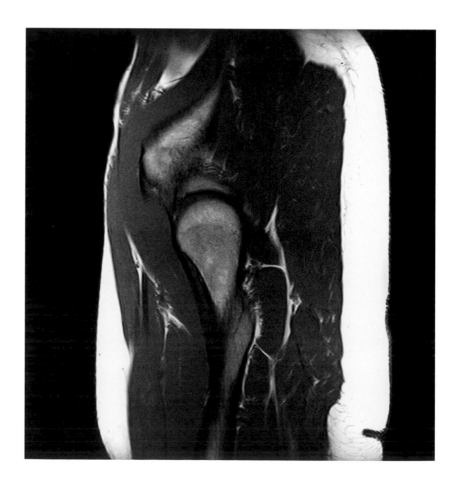

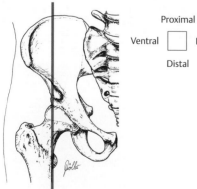

Proximal

Ventral   Dorsal

Distal

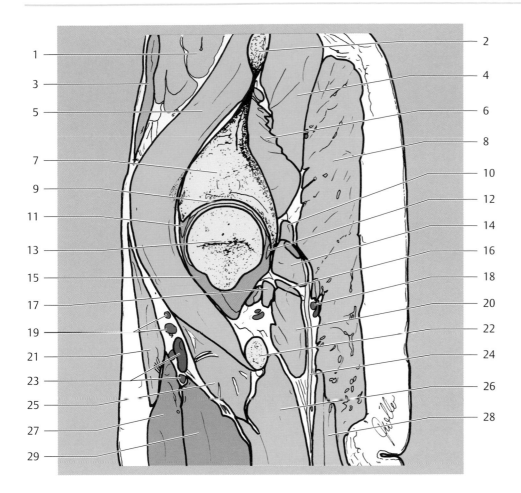

1 Small intestine
2 Ilium
3 Rectus abdominis muscle
4 Gluteus medius muscle
5 Iliopsoas muscle
6 Gluteus minimus muscle
7 Ilium (roof of acetabulum)
8 Gluteus maximus muscle
9 Hip joint
10 Piriformis muscle
11 Superior glenoid labrum
12 Inferior glenoid labrum
13 Femur (head)
14 Obturator internus muscle and
   gemellus muscles
15 Joint capsule
16 Adductor minimus muscle
17 Obturator externus muscle
18 Inferior gluteal artery and vein
19 Lateral circumflex femoral artery and
   vein (ascending branch)
20 Quadratus femoris muscle
21 Sartorius muscle
22 Lesser trochanter
23 Lateral circumflex femoral artery and
   vein (descending branch)
24 Sciatic nerve
25 Pectineus muscle
26 Adductor magnus muscle
27 Rectus femoris muscle
28 Biceps femoris muscle
29 Vastus medialis muscle

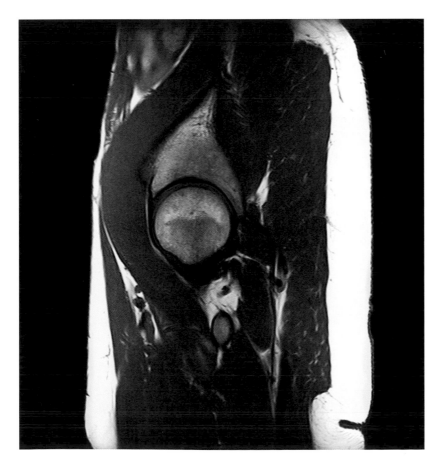

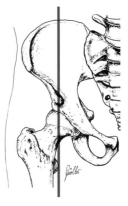

Proximal

Ventral ☐ Dorsal

Distal

1 Small intestine
2 Gluteus medius muscle
3 Rectus abdominis muscle
4 Ilium
5 Iliopsoas muscle
6 Superior gluteal artery and vein
7 Ilium (roof of acetabulum)
8 Gluteus minimus muscle
9 Hip joint
10 Gluteus maximus muscle
11 Superior glenoid labrum
12 Superior gluteal artery and vein,
   inferior gluteal nerve
13 Femur (head)
14 Sciatic nerve
15 Joint capsule
16 Piriformis muscle
17 Obturator externus muscle
18 Obturator internus muscle and
   gemellus muscles
19 Lateral circumflex femoris artery and
   vein (ascending branch)
20 Obturator internus muscle (tendon)
21 Pectineus muscle
22 Gemellus inferior muscle
23 Sartorius muscle
24 Inferior glenoid labrum
25 Adductor magnus muscle
26 Ischium
27 Deep artery and vein of thigh
28 Semimembranosus and semitendinosus
   muscles (tendon attachment)
29 Perforating artery
30 Quadratus femoris muscle
31 Adductor brevis muscle
32 Biceps femoris muscle (and tendon)
33 Vastus medialis muscle

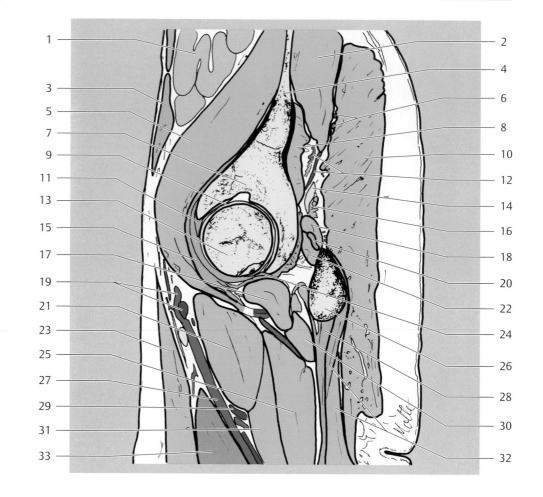

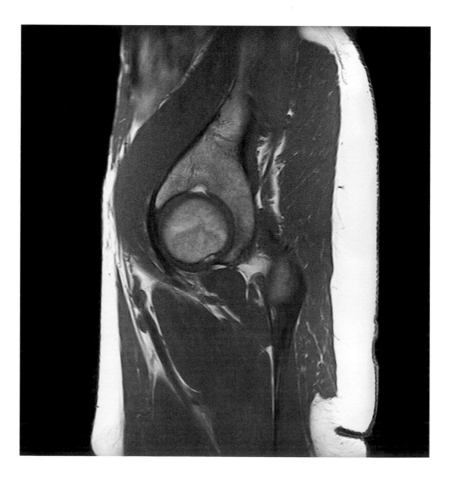

Proximal

Ventral   Dorsal

Distal

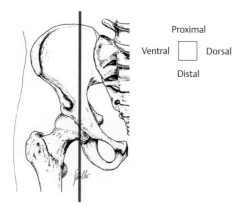

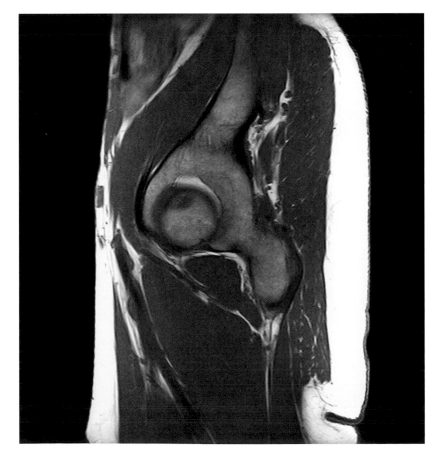

1 Small intestine
2 Gluteus medius muscle
3 Ilium
4 Gluteus maximus muscle
5 Psoas muscle
6 Superior gluteal artery, vein, and nerve
7 Iliacus muscle
8 Piriformis muscle
9 Rectus abdominis muscle
10 Sciatic nerve
11 Ilium (roof of acetabulum)
12 Gemellus superior muscle
13 Acetabular fossa
14 Inferior glenoid labrum
15 Fovea
16 Gemellus inferior muscle
17 Femur (head)
18 Obturator externus muscle
19 Superior glenoid labrum
20 Ischium
21 Lateral circumflex femoral artery and vein
22 Adductor minimus muscle
23 Ischiofemoral ligament
24 Quadratus femoris muscle
25 Lateral circumflex femoral artery
26 Adductor magnus muscle
27 Pectineus muscle
28 Biceps femoris muscle
29 Superficial femoral artery and vein
30 Adductor brevis muscle
31 Sartorius muscle
32 Deep artery and vein of thigh
33 Vastus medialis muscle

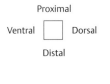

Proximal
Ventral ☐ Dorsal
Distal

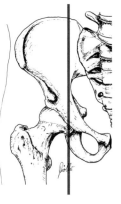

1 Small intestine
2 Ilium
3 Iliopsoas muscle
4 Superior gluteal artery and veins
5 Rectus abdominis muscle
6 Sciatic nerve
7 Internal iliac artery and vein
8 Piriformis muscle
9 Ilium (joint socket)
10 Gemellus superior muscle
11 Pectineus muscle
12 Gluteus maximus muscle
13 Obturator externus muscle
14 Inferior gluteal artery and vein
15 Femoral artery and vein
16 Obturator internus muscle
17 Adductor minimus muscle
18 Gemellus inferior muscle
19 Adductor magnus muscle
20 Sacrotuberous ligament
21 Adductor brevis muscle
22 Ischial tuberosity
23 Adductor longus muscle
24 Biceps femoris muscle
   (common tendon)
25 (Superficial) Femoral artery and vein
26 Biceps femoris muscle
27 Sartorius muscle

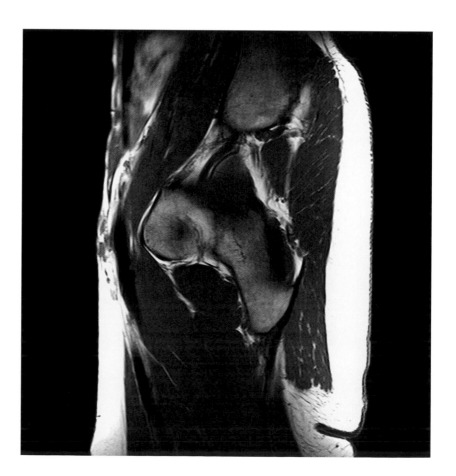

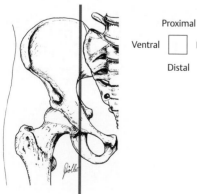

Proximal

Ventral ☐ Dorsal

Distal

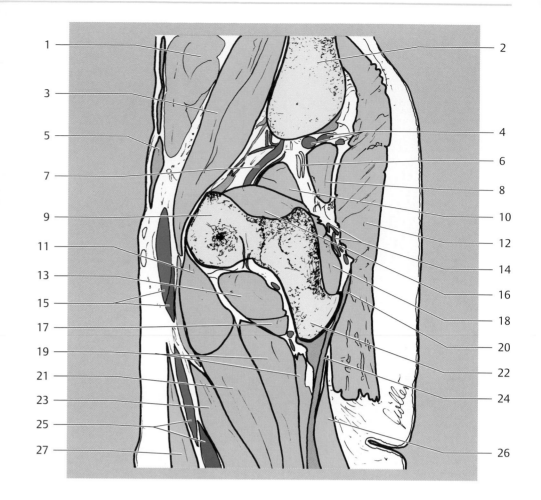

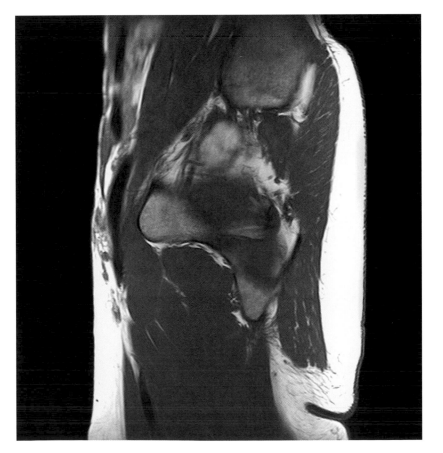

1 Psoas muscle
2 Ilium (wing)
3 Small intestine (ileum)
4 Sacral plexus
5 Iliacus muscle
6 Piriformis muscle
7 Rectus abdominis muscle
8 Gluteus maximus muscle
9 Obturator artery and nerve
10 Gemellus superior muscle
11 Obturator internus muscle
12 Superior gluteal artery and vein and inferior gluteal nerve
13 Femoral artery and vein
14 Gemellus inferior muscle
15 Pubis
16 Sacrotuberous ligament
17 Pectineus muscle
18 Adductor minimus muscle
19 Obturator externus muscle
20 Ischial tuberosity
21 Adductor brevis muscle
22 Adductor magnus muscle
23 Adductor longus muscle
24 Semimembranosus muscle
25 (Superficial) Femoral artery
26 Semitendinosus muscle
27 Sartorius muscle

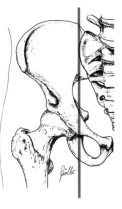

Proximal
Ventral | | Dorsal
Distal

1 Tendon of quadriceps femoris muscle
2 Suprapatellar fat pad
3 Base of patella
4 Patella (body)
5 Lateral patellar retinaculum
6 Medial patellar retinaculum
7 Patella (apex)
8 Infrapatellar fat pad
9 Femoral nerve (anterior cutaneous branches)
10 Patellar ligament

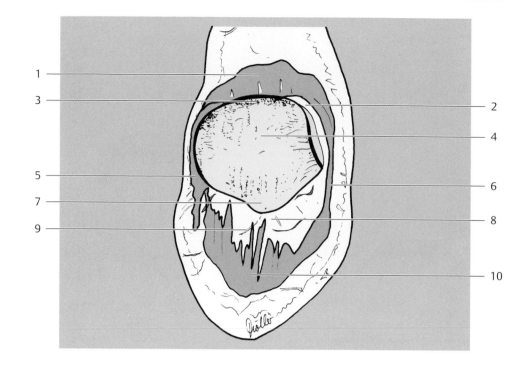

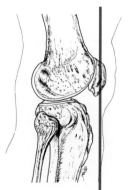

Proximal

Lateral ☐ Medial

Distal

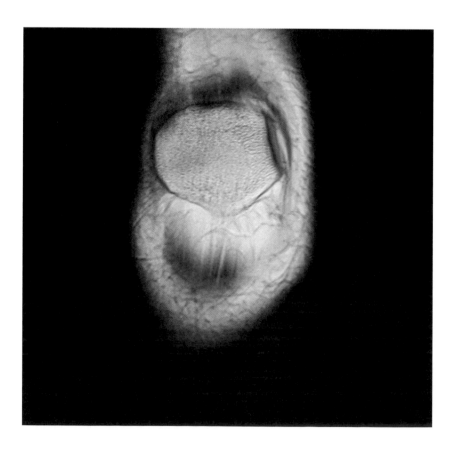

1 Tendon of quadriceps femoris muscle
2 Vastus medialis muscle
3 Vastus lateralis muscle (tendon)
4 Suprapatellar fat pad
5 Patella
6 Descending genicular artery
7 Lateral patellar retinaculum
8 Joint capsule (knee)
9 Femoropatellar joint
10 Medial patellar retinaculum
11 Femur (lateral condyle)
12 Femur (medial condyle)
13 Inferior lateral genicular artery
14 Saphenous nerve (infrapatellar branch)
15 Patellar ligament
16 Infrapatellar fat pad

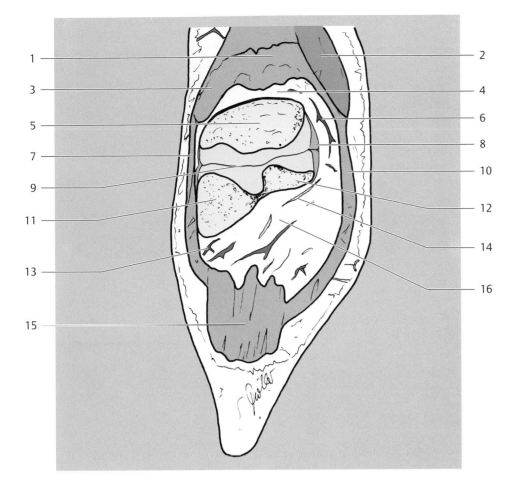

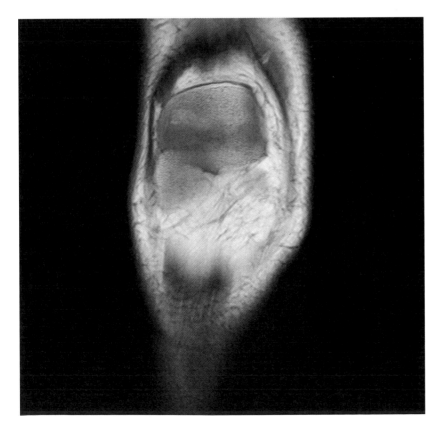

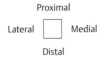

Proximal

Lateral ⬚ Medial

Distal

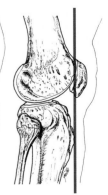

1 Tendon of quadriceps femoris muscle
2 Vastus medialis muscle
3 Vastus lateralis muscle
4 Suprapatellar fat pad
5 Genicular anastomosis
6 Suprapatellar bursa
7 Iliotibial tract
8 Medial patellar retinaculum
9 Femur (lateral condyle)
10 Femur (medial condyle)
11 Lateral patellar retinaculum
12 Infrapatellar fat pad
13 Patellar ligament
14 Tibia (tuberosity)

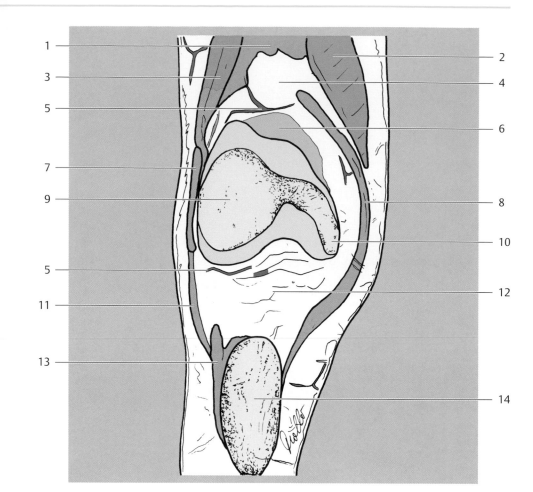

Proximal

Lateral ☐ Medial

Distal

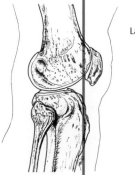

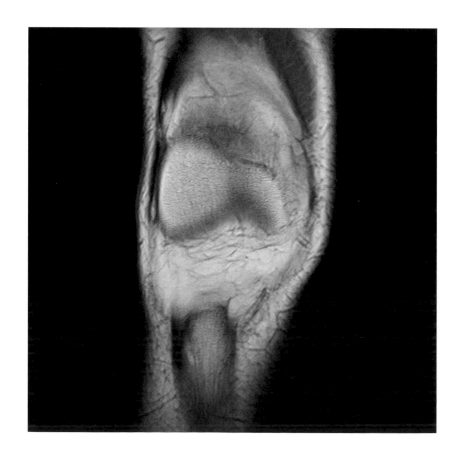

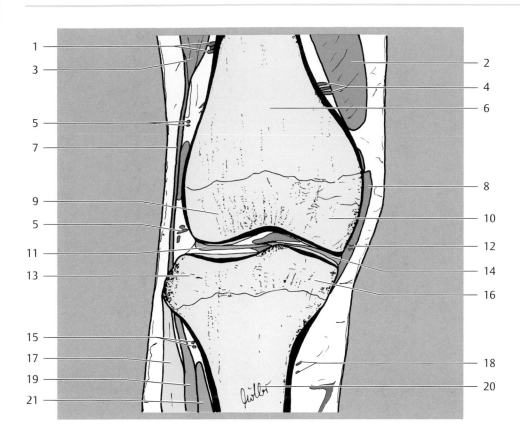

1 Superior lateral genicular artery and veins
2 Vastus medialis muscle
3 Vastus lateralis muscle
4 Superior medial genicular artery and veins
5 Genicular anastomosis
6 Femur (shaft)
7 Iliotibial tract
8 Medial collateral ligament
9 Lateral femoral condyle
10 Medial femoral condyle
11 Lateral meniscus (anterior horn)
12 Descending genicular vein (articular branches)
13 Lateral tibial condyle
14 Medial meniscus (anterior horn)
15 Inferior lateral genicular artery and vein
16 Medial tibial condyle
17 Peroneus (fibularis) longus muscle
18 Inferior medial genicular artery and vein
19 Extensor digitorum longus muscle
20 Tibia (shaft)
21 Tibialis anterior muscle

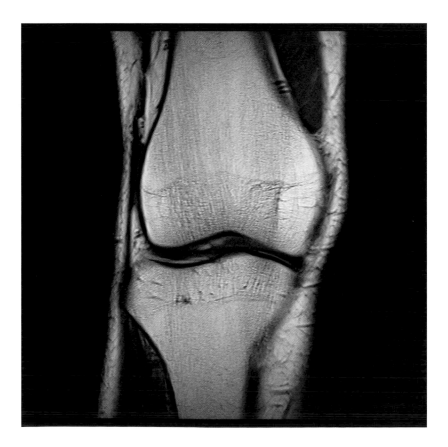

Proximal

Lateral   Medial

Distal

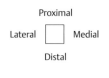
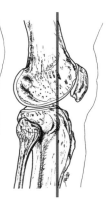

1 Vastus lateralis muscle
2 Femur (shaft)
3 Superior lateral genicular artery and veins
4 Vastus medialis muscle
5 Iliotibial tract
6 Superior medial genicular artery and vein
7 Lateral femoral condyle
8 Medial collateral ligament
9 Popliteus muscle (tendon)
10 Intercondylar fossa
11 Transverse ligament of knee
12 Anterior cruciate ligament
13 Lateral meniscus (intermediate portion)
14 Medial femoral condyle
15 Lateral tibial condyle
16 Medial meniscus (intermediate portion)
17 Anterior ligament of fibular head
18 Medial intercondylar tubercle
19 Peroneus (fibularis) longus muscle
20 Medial tibial condyle
21 Inferior lateral genicular artery and vein
22 Inferior medial genicular artery and vein
23 Extensor digitorum longus muscle
24 Pes anserinus (superficial)
25 Anterior tibial recurrent artery and vein
26 Tibia (shaft)
27 Tibialis anterior muscle

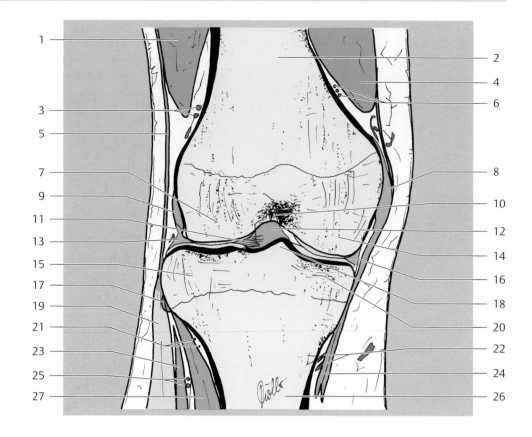

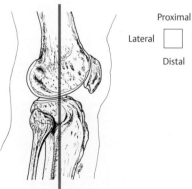

Proximal

Lateral ☐ Medial

Distal

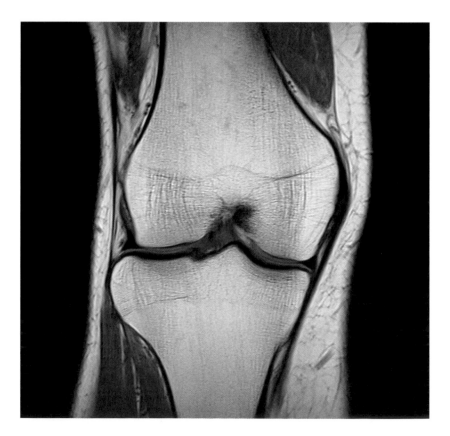

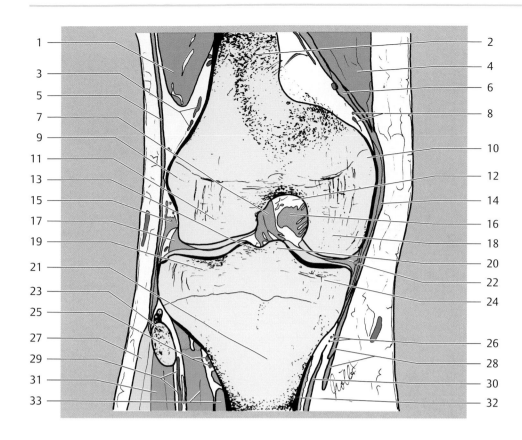

1 Vastus lateralis muscle
2 Femur (shaft)
3 Superior lateral genicular artery and vein
4 Vastus medialis muscle
5 Iliotibial tract
6 Adductor magnus muscle (tendon)
7 Anterior cruciate ligament
8 Superior medial genicular artery and vein
9 Lateral epicondyle
10 Medial epicondyle
11 Lateral femoral condyle
12 Intercondylar fossa
13 Lateral intercondylar tubercle
14 Medial collateral ligament
15 Popliteus muscle (tendon)
16 Posterior cruciate ligament
17 Lateral meniscus (intermediate portion)
18 Medial femoral condyle
19 Lateral tibial condyle
20 Medial intercondylar tubercle
21 Tibia (shaft)
22 Medial meniscus (intermediate portion)
23 Fibula (head)
24 Medial tibial condyle
25 Inferior lateral genicular artery and vein
26 Inferior medial genicular artery and vein
27 Peroneus (fibularis) longus muscle
28 Pes anserinus (superficial)
29 Anterior tibial recurrent artery and vein
30 Semimembranosus muscle (tibial attachment, deep pes anserinus)
31 Extensor digitorum longus muscle
32 Popliteus muscle (tibial attachment)
33 Tibialis anterior muscle

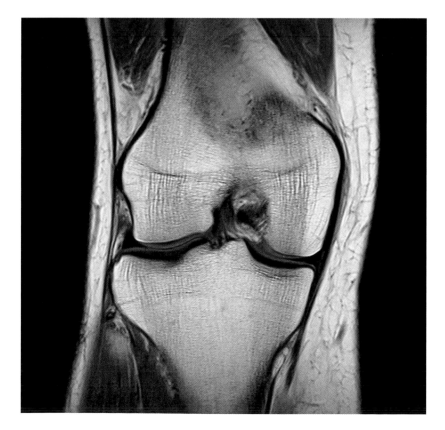

Proximal

Lateral ☐ Medial

Distal

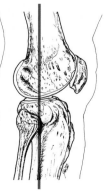

1 Vastus lateralis muscle
2 Popliteal artery
3 Superior lateral genicular artery
4 Sartorius muscle
5 Medial genicular artery
6 Vastus medialis muscle
7 Gastrocnemius muscle
   (lateral head, femoral attachment)
8 Superior medial genicular artery and
   vein
9 Plantaris muscle (tendon)
10 Gastrocnemius muscle (medial head)
11 Iliotibial tract
12 Adductor magnus muscle
   (tendon attachment)
13 Lateral femoral condyle
14 Medial collateral ligament
15 Anterior cruciate ligament
16 Medial femoral condyle
17 Popliteus muscle (tendon)
18 Intercondylar fossa
19 Lateral intercondylar tubercle
20 Posterior cruciate ligament
21 Lateral meniscus (posterior horn)
22 Medial intercondylar tubercle
23 Fibular collateral ligament
24 Medial meniscus (posterior horn)
25 Lateral tibial condyle
26 Medial tibial condyle
27 Tibiofibular joint
28 Pes anserinus (superficial)
29 Fibula (head)
30 Inferior medial genicular artery and vein
31 Inferior lateral genicular artery and vein
32 Semitendinosus muscle (tendon)
33 Peroneus (fibularis) longus muscle
34 Semimembranous muscle
   (tibial attachment, deep pes anserinus)
35 Tibialis posterior muscle
36 Popliteus muscle

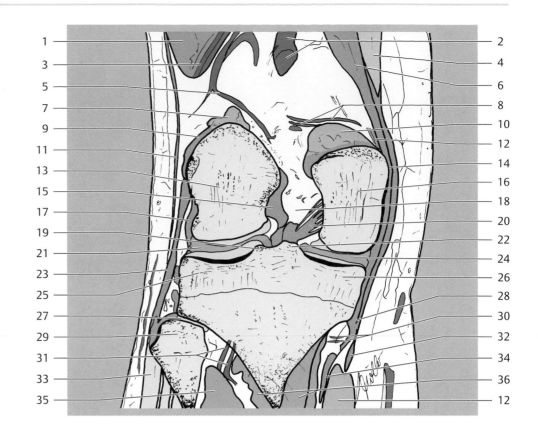

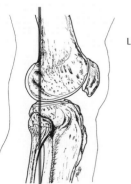

Proximal

Lateral ☐ Medial

Distal

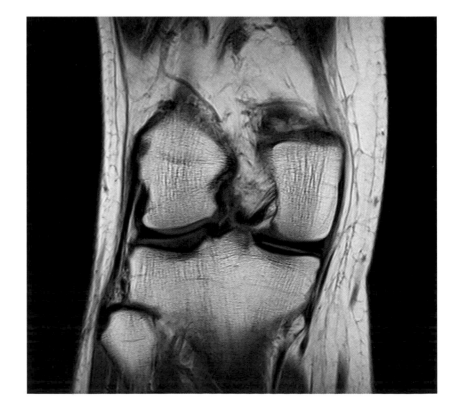

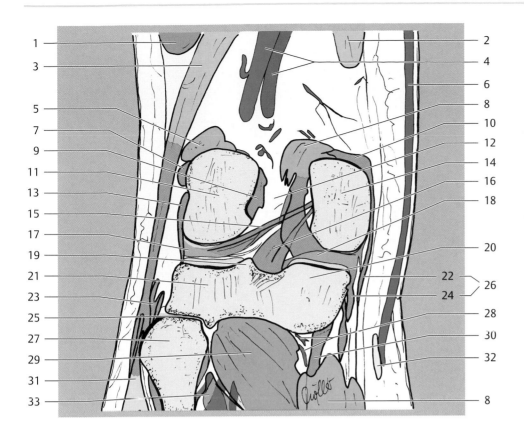

1 Vastus lateralis muscle
2 Sartorius muscle
3 Biceps femoris muscle
4 Popliteal artery and vein
5 Gastrocnemius muscle (lateral head, femoral attachment)
6 Great saphenous vein
7 Plantaris muscle (tendon attachment)
8 Gastrocnemius muscle (medial head, femoral attachment)
9 Anterior cruciate ligament
10 Joint capsule
11 Femur (lateral condyle)
12 Intercondylar fossa
13 Popliteus muscle (tendon)
14 Femur (medial condyle)
15 Posterior meniscofemoral ligament (Ligament of Wrisberg)
16 Posterior cruciate ligament
17 Lateral meniscus (posterior horn)
18 Medial meniscus (posterior horn)
19 Lateral intercondylar tuberosity
20 Tibia (medial head)
21 Tibia (lateral head)
22 Gracilis muscle (tendon)
23 Collateral fibular ligament
24 Semitendinosus muscle (tendon)
25 Tibiofibular joint (proximal)
26 Pes anserinus (superficial)
27 Fibula (head)
28 Inferior medial genicular artery and vein
29 Popliteus muscle
30 Semimembranosus muscle (tibial attachment, pes anserinus profundus)
31 Peroneus longus muscle
32 Saphenous nerve
33 Tibialis posterior muscle

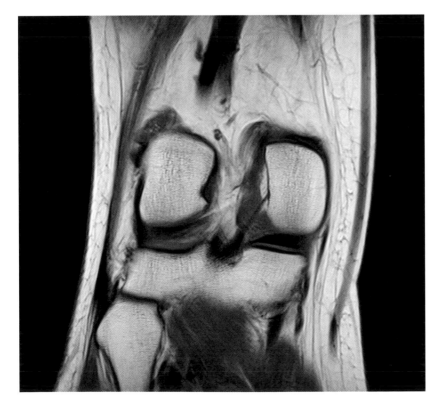

Proximal
Lateral ☐ Medial
Distal

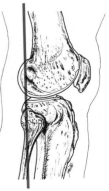

1 Biceps femoris muscle
2 Gracilis muscle
3 Gastrocnemius muscle (lateral head)
4 Popliteal artery and vein
5 Sural arteries and veins
6 Gastrocnemius muscle
  (medial head, femoral attachment)
7 Plantaris muscle
8 Saphenous nerve (branch)
9 Lateral femoral condyle
10 Medial femoral condyle
11 Iliotibial tract
12 Joint capsule
13 Arcuate popliteal ligament
14 Oblique popliteal ligament
15 Lateral tibial condyle
16 Semitendinosus muscle (tendon)
17 Popliteus muscle
18 Medial tibial condyle
19 Fibular collateral ligament
20 Saphenous nerve
21 Fibular collateral ligament
22 Semimembranosus muscle (tibial
   attachment, deep pes anserinus)
23 Fibula (head)
24 Gastrocnemius muscle (medial head)
25 Common fibular (peroneal) nerve
26 Tibial nerve
27 Posterior tibial artery
   (circumflex fibular branch)
28 Plantaris muscle (tendon)
29 Soleus muscle

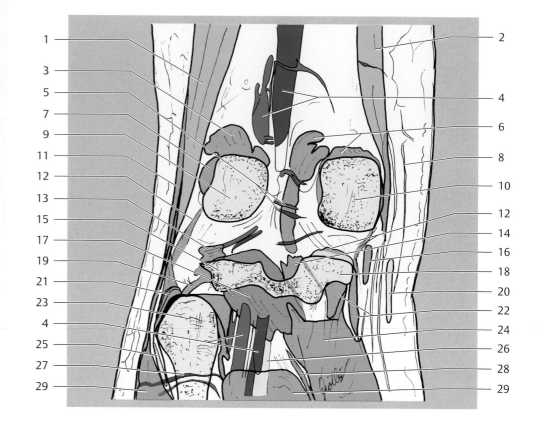

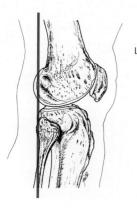

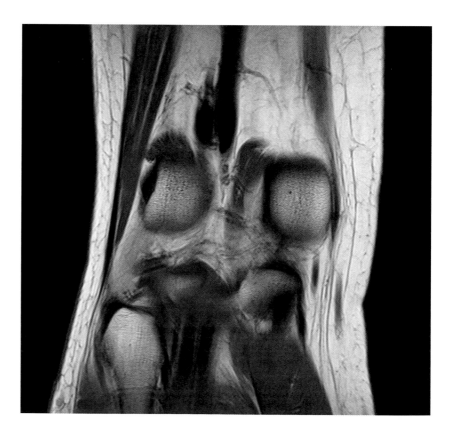

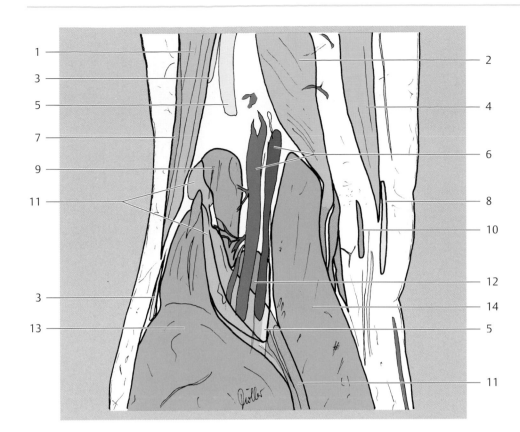

1 Biceps femoris muscle
2 Semimembranosus muscle
3 Common fibular (peroneal) nerve
4 Gracilis muscle
5 Tibial nerve
6 Popliteal artery and vein
7 Iliotibial tract
8 Saphenous nerve
9 Gastrocnemius muscle (lateral head)
10 Semitendinosus muscle (tendon)
11 Plantaris muscle (and tendon)
12 Popliteus muscle
13 Soleus muscle
14 Gastrocnemius muscle (medial head)

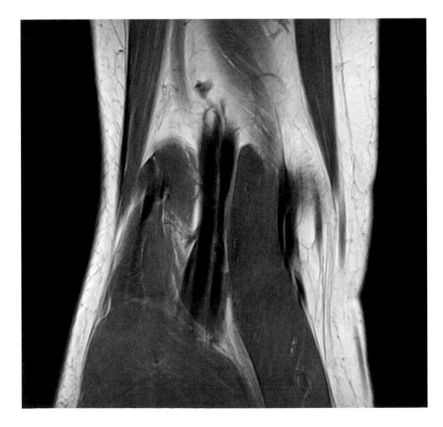

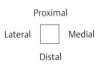

Proximal

Lateral   Medial

Distal

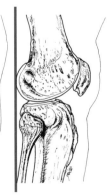

1 Vastus lateralis muscle
2 Iliotibial tract
3 Lateral patellar retinaculum
4 Biceps femoris muscle
5 Joint capsule
6 Femur (lateral condyle)
7 Lateral meniscus
 (intermediate portion)
8 Superior lateral genicular artery and vein
9 Tibia (lateral head)
10 Lateral collateral ligament
11 Anterior ligament of fibular head
12 Common peroneal nerve
13 Fibula (head)
14 Posterior ligament of fibular head
15 Extensor digitorum longus muscle
16 Tibiofibular joint (proximal)
17 Peroneus (fibularis) longus muscle
18 Soleus muscle

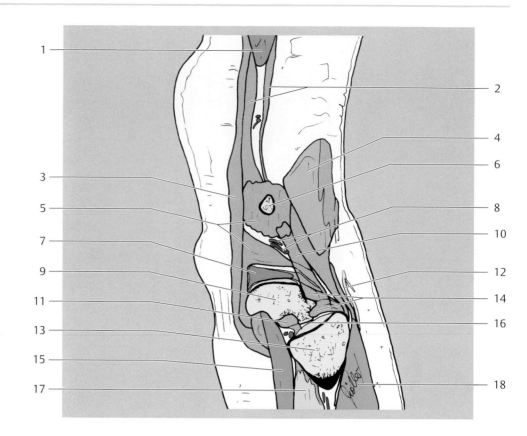

Proximal

Ventral ☐ Dorsal

Distal

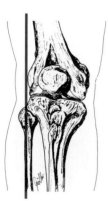

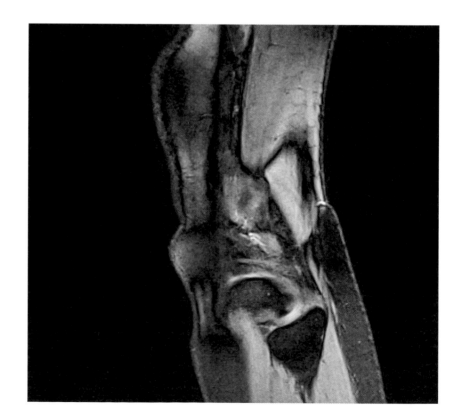

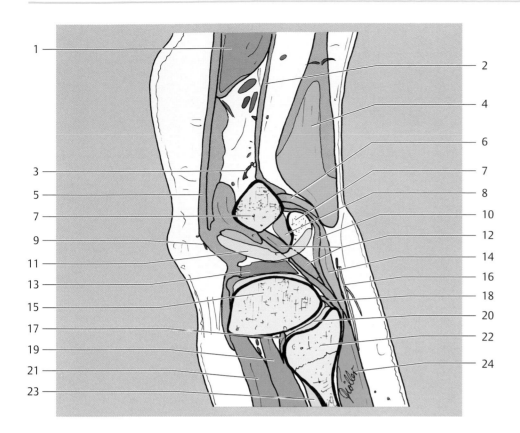

1 Vastus lateralis muscle
2 Iliotibial tract
3 Blood vessels to genicular anastomosis
4 Biceps femoris muscle
5 Lateral patellar retinaculum
6 Gastrocnemius muscle (lateral head)
7 Femur (lateral condyle)
8 Lateral joint recess
9 Inferior lateral genicular artery
10 Joint capsule
11 Femur (lateral condyle, joint cartilage)
12 Popliteus muscle (tendon)
13 Lateral meniscus
   (intermediate portion)
14 Plantaris muscle
   (and tendon attachment)
15 Lateral tibial condyle
16 Common fibular (peroneal) nerve
17 Anterior ligament of fibular head
18 Posterior ligament of fibular head
19 Extensor digitorum longus muscle
20 Tibiofibular joint
21 Tibialis anterior muscle
22 Fibula (head)
23 Peroneus (fibularis) longus muscle
24 Soleus muscle

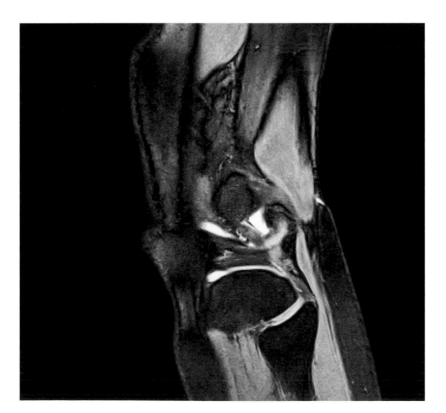

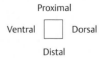

Proximal

Ventral ☐ Dorsal

Distal

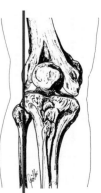

1 Vastus lateralis muscle
2 Biceps femoris muscle (long head)
3 Vastus intermedius muscle
4 Biceps femoris muscle (short head)
5 Lateral patellar retinaculum (longitudinal)
6 Superior lateral genicular artery and vein
7 Lateral patellar retinaculum (transverse)
8 Gastrocnemius muscle (lateral head)
9 Femur (lateral condyle)
10 Common fibular (peroneal) nerve
11 Knee joint
12 Lateral meniscus (posterior horn)
13 Lateral meniscus (anterior horn)
14 Plantaris muscle
15 Inferior lateral genicular artery and vein
16 Popliteus muscle (with tendon)
17 Lateral tibial condyle
18 Tibiofibular joint (proximal)
19 Anterior tibial artery
20 Fibula (head)
21 Tibialis posterior muscle
22 Soleus muscle
23 Tibialis anterior muscle
24 Peroneus (fibularis) longus muscle

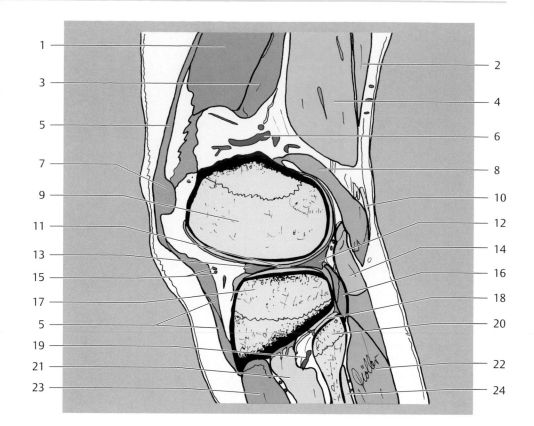

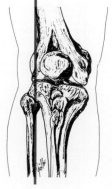

Proximal

Ventral □ Dorsal

Distal

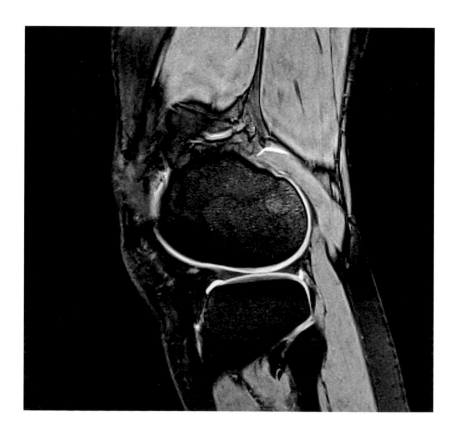

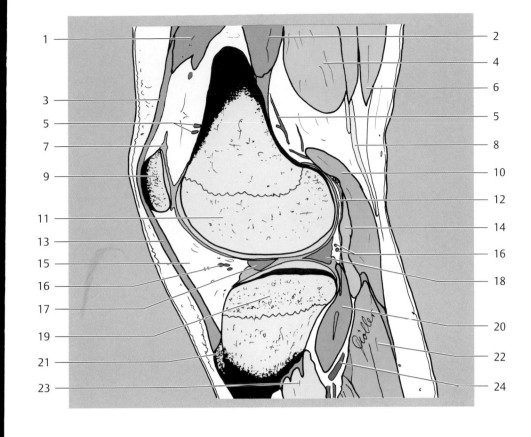

1 Vastus lateralis muscle
2 Vastus intermedius muscle
3 Quadriceps tendon
4 Biceps femoris muscle (short head)
5 Superior lateral genicular artery
  and vein
6 Biceps femoris muscle (long head)
7 Suprapatellar bursa
8 Common fibular (peroneal) nerve
9 Patella
10 Gastrocnemius muscle (lateral head)
11 Femur (lateral condyle)
12 Joint capsule
13 Patellar ligament
14 Plantaris muscle
15 Infrapatellar (Hoffa) fat pad
16 Inferior lateral genicular artery
   and vein
17 Lateral meniscus (anterior horn)
18 Lateral meniscus (posterior horn)
19 Lateral condyle of tibia
20 Popliteus muscle
21 Tibial tuberosity
22 Soleus muscle
23 Tibialis posterior muscle
24 Anterior tibial artery

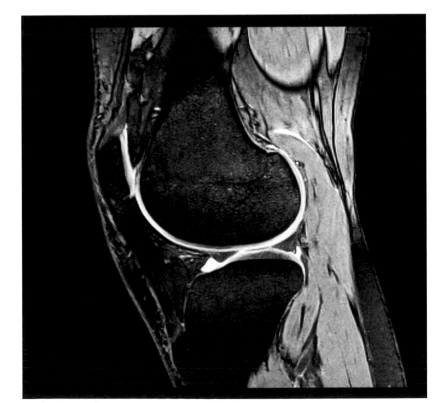

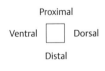

Proximal

Ventral ☐ Dorsal

Distal

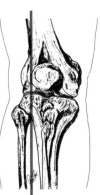

1 Vastus lateralis muscle
2 Semimembranosus muscle
3 Vastus intermedius muscle
4 Biceps femoris muscle
5 Femur (shaft)
6 Sciatic nerve
7 Tendon of quadriceps femoris muscle
8 Superior lateral genicular artery
   and vein
9 Suprapatellar bursa
10 Joint capsule
11 Patella
12 Femur (lateral condyle)
13 Infrapatellar (Hoffa) fat pad
14 Gastrocnemius muscle (lateral head)
15 Patellar ligament
16 Lateral meniscus (posterior horn)
17 Inferior lateral genicular artery
   and vein
18 Plantaris muscle
19 Transverse genicular ligament
20 Popliteus muscle
21 Lateral meniscus (anterior horn)
22 Anterior tibial artery
23 Tibia (head)
24 Soleus muscle
25 Tibial tuberosity
26 Tibialis posterior muscle

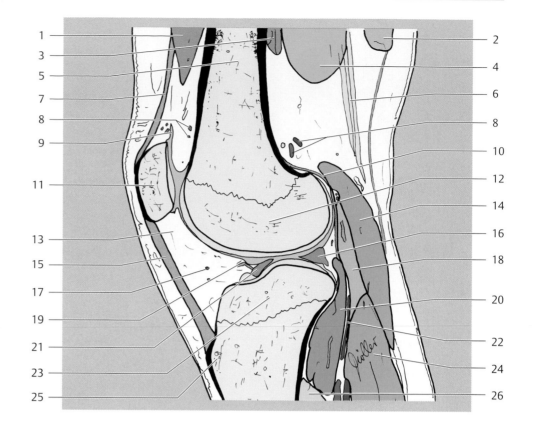

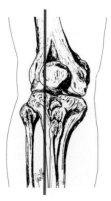

Proximal

Ventral [ ] Dorsal

Distal

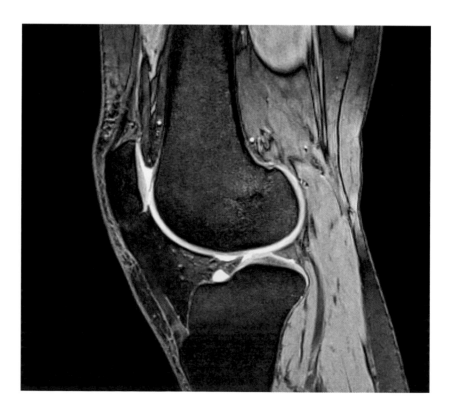

1 Vastus medialis muscle
2 Biceps femoris muscle
3 Quadriceps tendon
4 Semimembranosus muscle
5 Suprapatellar bursa
6 Femur (shaft)
7 Patellar anastomosis
8 Superior lateral genicular artery and vein
9 Patella
10 Popliteal vein
11 Femur (lateral condyle)
12 Joint capsule
13 Subcutaneous prepatellar bursa
14 Anterior cruciate ligament (femoral attachment)
15 Infrapatellar (Hoffa) fat pad
16 Tibial nerve
17 Transverse ligament of knee
18 Popliteal artery
19 Inferior lateral genicular artery and vein
20 Oblique popliteal ligament
21 Subcutaneous infrapatellar bursa
22 Lateral meniscus (posterior horn, inner attachment)
23 Patellar ligament
24 Plantaris muscle
25 Posterior cruciate ligament (tibial origin)
26 Gastrocnemius muscle (lateral head)
27 Tibia (head)
28 Popliteus muscle
29 Deep infrapatellar bursa
30 Soleus muscle
31 Tibial tuberosity

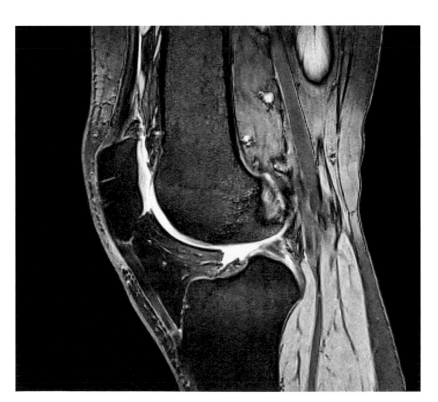

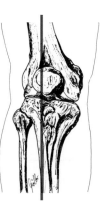

Proximal
Ventral ☐ Dorsal
Distal

1 Femur (shaft)
2 Vastus medialis muscle
3 Quadriceps muscle
4 Semimembranosus muscle
5 Suprapatellar bursa
6 Popliteal artery
7 Patellar anastomosis
8 Popliteal vein
9 Patella
10 Joint capsule
11 Subcutaneous prepatellar bursa
12 Femur (intercondylar part)
13 Anterior cruciate ligament
14 Oblique popliteal ligament
15 Infrapatellar (Hoffa) fat pad
16 Tibial nerve
17 Inferior lateral genicular artery
   and vein
18 Posterior cruciate ligament
19 Subcutaneous infrapatellar bursa
20 Medial intercondylar tubercle
21 Transverse ligament of knee
22 Plantaris muscle
23 Patellar ligament
24 Gastrocnemius muscle (lateral head)
25 Tibia (head)
26 Popliteus muscle
27 Deep infrapatellar bursa
28 Soleus muscle

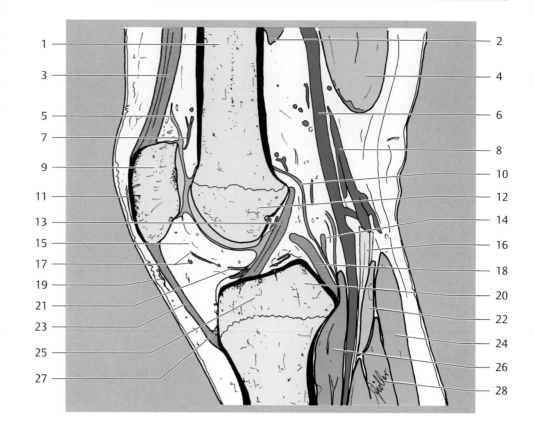

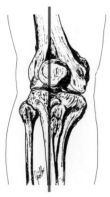

Proximal

Ventral [ ] Dorsal

Distal

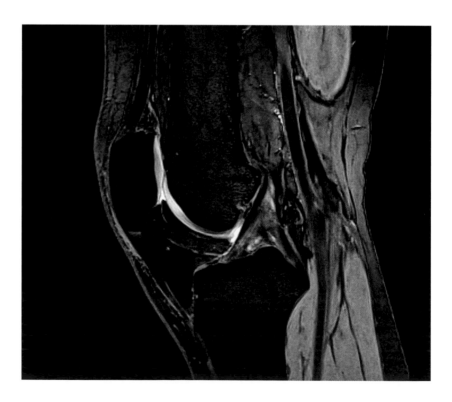

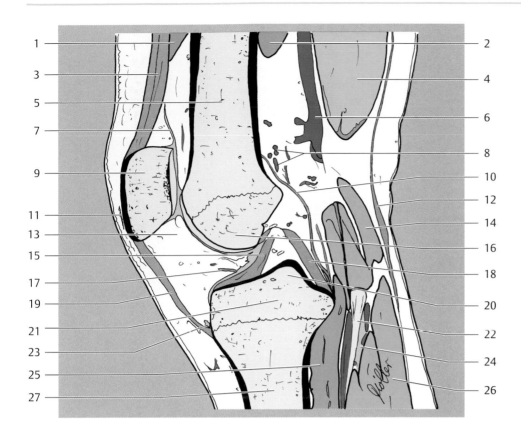

1 Rectus femoris muscle
2 Vastus medialis muscle
3 Tendon of quadriceps femoris muscle
4 Semimembranosus muscle
5 Femur (shaft)
6 Popliteal artery
7 Suprapatellar bursa
8 Superior medial genicular artery and vein
9 Patella
10 Joint capsule
11 Prepatellar bursa (subcutaneous)
12 Deep fascia of leg
13 Infrapatellar (Hoffa) fat pad
14 Gastrocnemius muscle (medial head)
15 Anterior cruciate ligament
16 Femur (medial condyle)
17 Transverse genicular ligament
18 Posterior cruciate ligament
19 Patellar ligament
20 Medial intercondylar tuberosity
21 Tibia (head)
22 Tibial nerve
23 Deep infrapatellar bursa
24 Plantaris muscle
25 Popliteus muscle
26 Gastrocnemius muscle (lateral head)
27 Tibia (shaft)

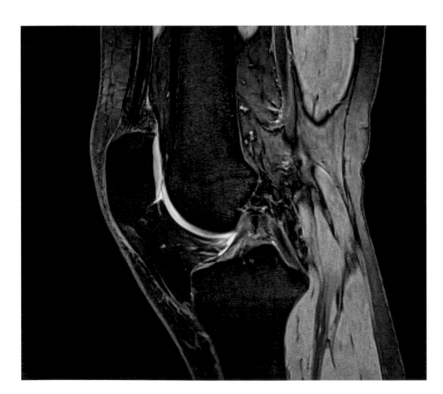

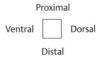

Proximal

Ventral ☐ Dorsal

Distal

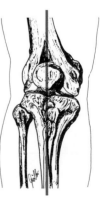

1 Rectus femoris muscle
2 Vastus medialis muscle
3 Quadriceps tendon
4 Superficial femoral artery
5 Suprapatellar bursa
6 Semimembranosus muscle
7 Patellar anastomosis
8 Femur (shaft)
9 Patella
10 Superior medial genicular artery
    and vein
11 Subcutaneous prepatellar bursa
12 Joint capsule
13 Infrapatellar (Hoffa) fat pad
14 Femur (medial condyle)
15 Transverse ligament of knee
16 Posterior cruciate ligament
17 Patellar ligament
18 Gastrocnemius muscle (medial head)
19 Medial intercondylar tubercle
    of tibial condyle
20 Posterior meniscofemoral ligament
    (Ligament of Wrisberg)
21 Deep infrapatellar bursa
22 Inferior medial genicular artery
    and vein
23 Popliteus muscle
24 Tibial nerve
25 Tibia (shaft)
26 Gastrocnemius muscle (lateral head)

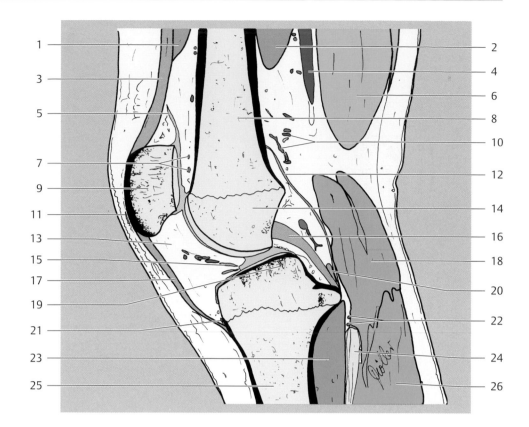

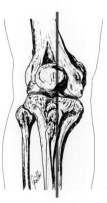

Proximal

Ventral ☐ Dorsal

Distal

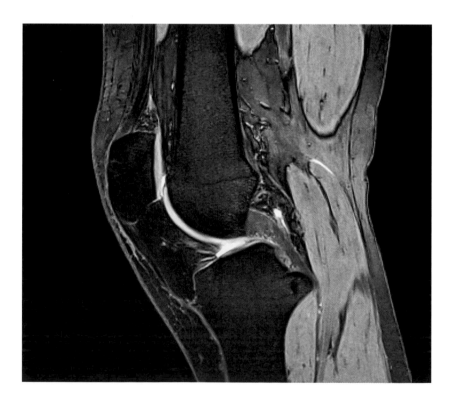

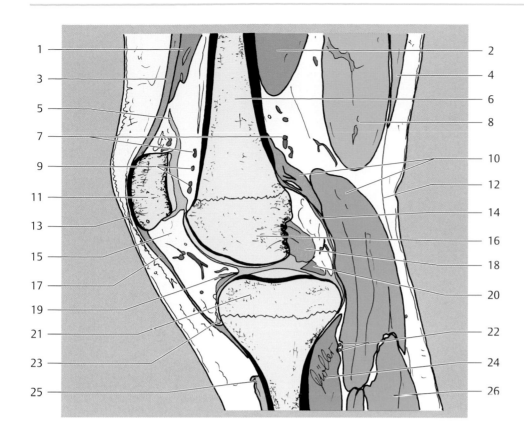

1 Rectus femoris muscle
2 Vastus medialis muscle
3 Quadriceps tendon
4 Semitendinosus muscle
5 Suprapatellar bursa
6 Femur (shaft)
7 Superior medial genicular arteries
8 Semimembranosus muscle
9 Patellar anastomosis
10 Gastrocnemius muscle (medial head and tendon attachment)
11 Patella
12 Deep fascia of leg
13 Subcutaneous prepatellar bursa
14 Joint capsule
15 Infrapatellar (Hoffa) fat pad
16 Femur (medial condyle)
17 Patellar ligament
18 Posterior cruciate ligament (attachment)
19 Transverse ligament of knee
20 Medial meniscus (posterior horn, inner attachment)
21 Medial tibial condyle
22 Inferior medial genicular artery and vein
23 Deep infrapatellar bursa
24 Popliteus muscle
25 Sartorius muscle (attachment, part of superficial pes anserinus)
26 Gastrocnemius muscle (lateral head)

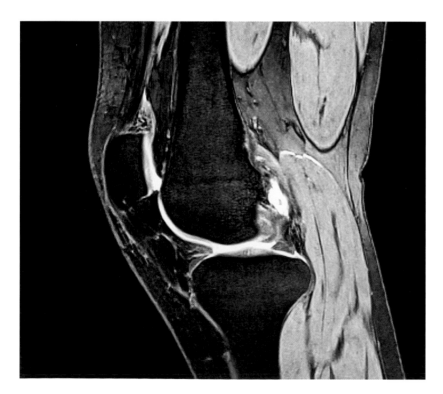

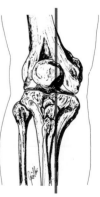

Proximal

Ventral ☐ Dorsal

Distal

1 Rectus femoris muscle
2 Vastus medialis muscle
3 Femur (shaft)
4 Semitendinosis muscle
5 Quadriceps tendon
6 Semimembranosus muscle
7 Suprapatellar bursa
8 Superior medial genicular artery and vein
9 Patella
10 Deep fascia of leg
11 Subcutaneous prepatellar bursa
12 Posterior cruciate ligament (attachment)
13 Infrapatellar (Hoffa) fat pad
14 Joint capsule
15 Femur (medial condyle)
16 Medial meniscus (posterior horn)
17 Patellar ligament
18 Gastrocnemius muscle (medial head)
19 Transverse ligament of knee
20 Inferior medial genicular artery and vein
21 Deep infrapatellar bursa
22 Popliteus muscle
23 Medial condyle of tibia
24 Gastrocnemius muscle (lateral head)
25 Sartorius muscle (tendon attachment, part of superficial pes anserinus)

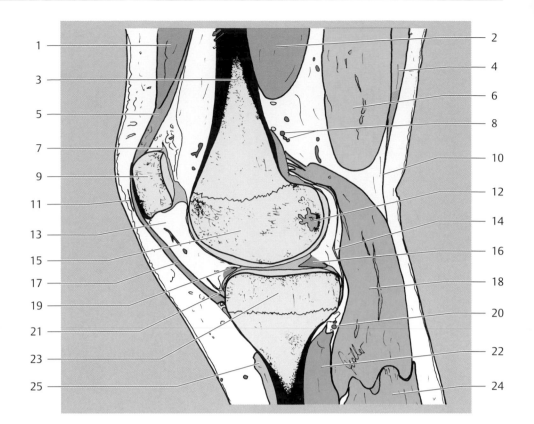

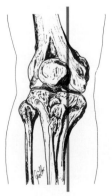

Proximal

Ventral ☐ Dorsal

Distal

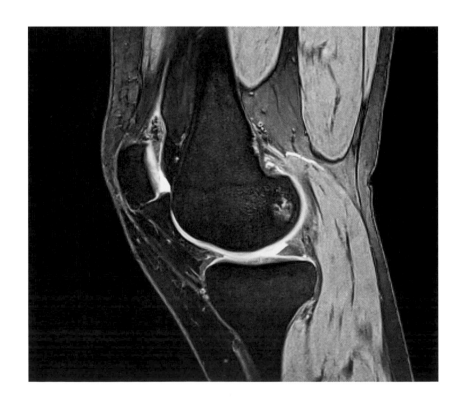

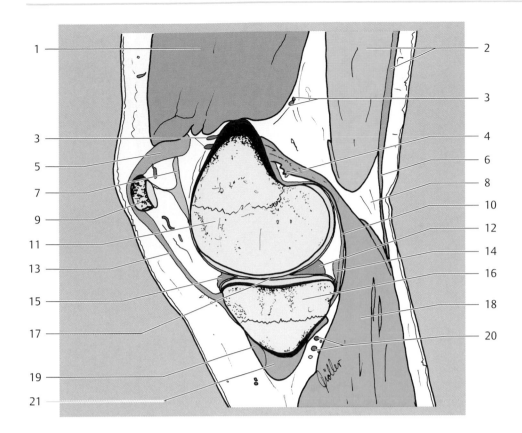

1 Vastus medialis muscle
2 Semimembranosus muscle and semitendinosus muscle (tendon)
3 Superior medial genicular artery and vein
4 Medial subtendinous bursa of gastrocnemius
5 Medial patellar retinaculum
6 Deep fascia of leg
7 Suprapatellar bursa
8 Popliteal fossa
9 Patella
10 Joint capsule
11 Femur (medial condyle)
12 Medial meniscus (posterior horn)
13 Medial patellar retinaculum
14 Oblique popliteal ligament
15 Medial meniscus (anterior horn)
16 Medial tibial condyle
17 Knee joint
18 Gastrocnemius muscle (medial head)
19 Sartorius muscle (attachment, part of superficial pes anserinus)
20 Inferior medial genicular artery and vein
21 Pes anserinus (superficial part)

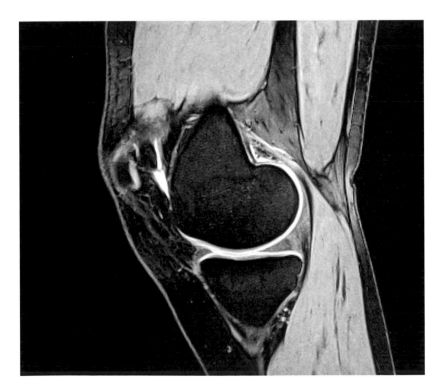

Proximal
Ventral ☐ Dorsal
Distal

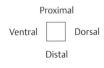
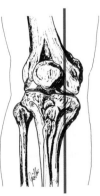

1 Vastus medialis muscle
2 Saphenous nerve
3 Adductor magnus muscle (tendon)
4 Sartorius muscle
5 Superior medial genicular artery
  and vein
6 Semimembranosus muscle
  (and tendon)
7 Femur (medial condyle)
8 Joint capsule
9 Medial patellar retinaculum
10 Semitendinosus muscle (tendon)
11 Medial meniscus (anterior horn)
12 Medial meniscus (posterior horn)
13 Medial meniscus (intermediate portion)
14 Pes anserinus (deep part)
15 Medial tibial condyle
16 Pes anserinus (superficial part)
17 Sartorius muscle (attachment, part of
   superficial pes anserinus)
18 Anserine bursa
19 Gracilis muscle (attachment, part of
   superficial pes anserinus)
20 Gastrocnemius muscle (medial head)

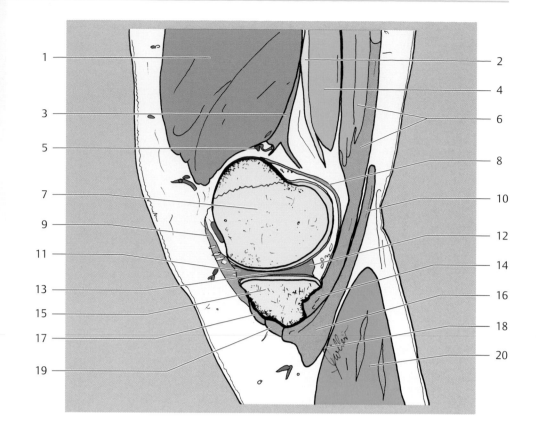

Proximal
Ventral ☐ Dorsal
Distal

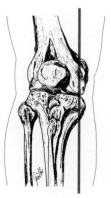

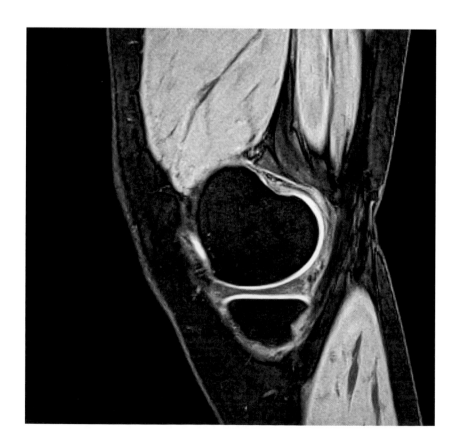

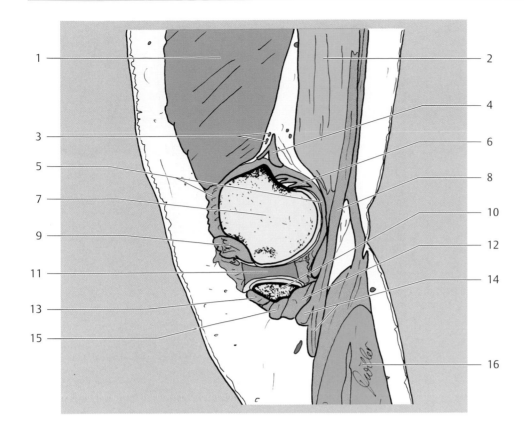

1 Vastus medialis muscle
2 Sartorius muscle
3 Superior medial genicular artery and vein
4 Adductor magnus muscle (tendon)
5 Joint capsule
6 Gastrocnemius muscle (medial head, tendon attachment)
7 Femur (medial condyle)
8 Semitendinosus muscle (tendon)
9 Medial patellar retinaculum
10 Tibia (medial condyle, medial head)
11 Medial meniscus (intermediate portion)
12 Semimembranosus muscle (tendon attachment, pes anserinus profundus)
13 Sartorius muscle (tendon attachment, part of the pes anserinus superficialis)
14 Pes anserinus superficialis
15 Gracilis muscle (tendon attachment, part of pes anserinus superficialis)
16 Gastrocnemius muscle (medial head)

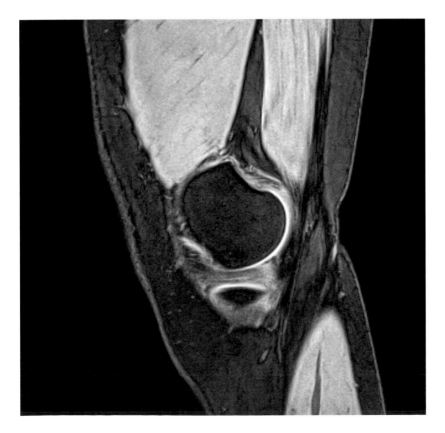

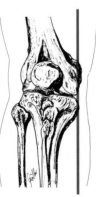

Proximal

Ventral ☐ Dorsal

Distal

1 Flexor hallucis longus muscle
2 Tibialis posterior muscle
3 Fibular artery (communicating branch) and vein
4 Posterior tibial artery (communicating branch) and vein
5 Fibular artery
6 Tibia
7 Fibula
8 Talocrural joint (upper ankle joint)
9 Dorsal capsule
10 Deltoid ligament
11 Talus
12 Tibialis posterior muscle (tendon)
13 Posterior talofibular ligament
14 Flexor digitorum longus muscle (tendon)
15 Peroneus (fibularis) brevis muscle (tendon)
16 Subtalar joint
17 Peroneus (fibularis) longus muscle (tendon)
18 Medial plantar artery, vein, and nerve
19 Calcaneus
20 Flexor hallucis longus muscle (tendon)
21 Sural nerve with accompanying vessels
22 Lateral plantar artery, vein, and nerve
23 Abductor digiti minimi muscle
24 Quadratus plantae muscle
25 Flexor digitorum brevis muscle
26 Abductor hallucis muscle
27 Plantar aponeurosis

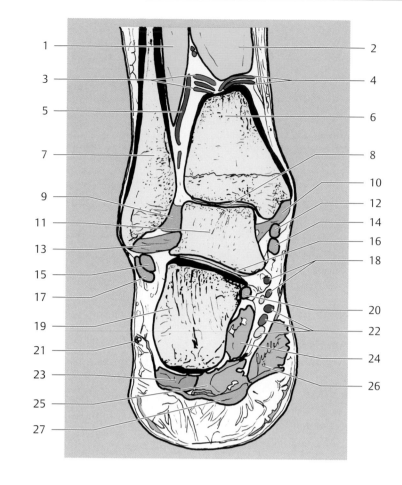

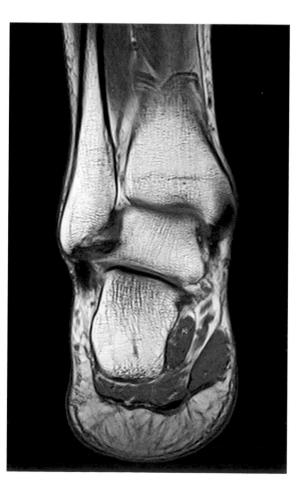

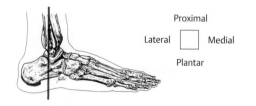

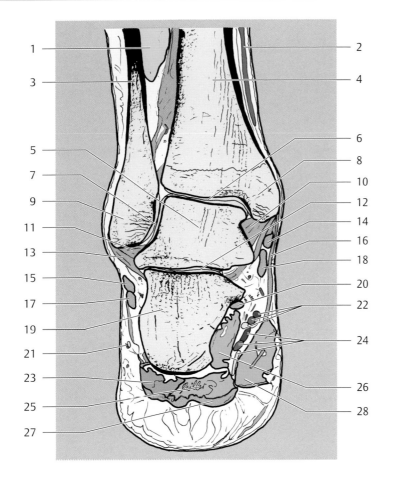

1 Flexor hallucis longus muscle
2 Great saphenous vein
3 Fibula
4 Tibia
5 Talus
6 Talocrural joint (upper ankle joint)
7 Talofibular joint
8 Medial malleolus
9 Lateral malleolus
10 Deltoid ligament (posterior tibiotalar part)
11 Posterior talofibular ligament
12 Subtalar joint
13 Calcaneofibular ligament
14 Tibialis posterior muscle (tendon)
15 Peroneus (fibularis) brevis muscle (tendon)
16 Flexor retinaculum
17 Peroneus (fibularis) longus muscle (tendon)
18 Flexor digitorum longus muscle (tendon)
19 Calcaneus
20 Flexor hallucis longus muscle (tendon)
21 Sural nerve with accompanying vessels
22 Medial plantar artery, vein, and nerve
23 Abductor digiti minimi muscle
24 Lateral plantar artery, vein, and nerve
25 Flexor digitorum brevis muscle
26 Quadratus plantae muscle
27 Plantar aponeurosis
28 Abductor hallucis muscle

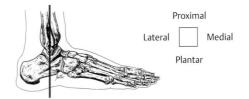

Proximal

Lateral ▢ Medial

Plantar

1 Extensor digitorum longus muscle
2 Great saphenous vein
3 Tibia
4 Medial malleolus
5 Talocrural joint
6 Deltoid ligament
  (posterior tibiotalar part)
7 Talus
8 Deltoid ligament (tibiocalcaneal part)
9 Fibula (lateral malleolus)
10 Tibialis posterior muscle (tendon)
11 Calcaneofibular ligament
12 Flexor retinaculum
13 Peroneus (fibularis) brevis muscle
  (tendon)
14 Flexor digitorum longus muscle
  (tendon)
15 Peroneus (fibularis) longus muscle
  (tendon)
16 Flexor hallucis longus muscle (tendon)
17 Sural nerve with accompanying vessels
18 Quadratus plantae muscle
19 Calcaneus
20 Medial plantar artery, vein, and nerve
21 Long plantar ligament
22 Abductor hallucis muscle
23 Abductor digiti minimi muscle
24 Lateral plantar artery, vein, and nerve
25 Flexor digitorum brevis muscle
26 Plantar aponeurosis

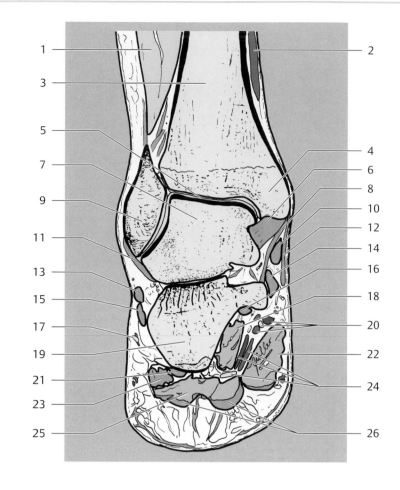

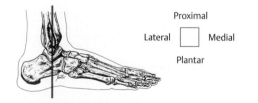

Proximal

Lateral ☐ Medial

Plantar

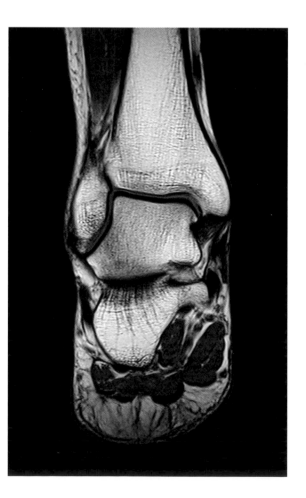

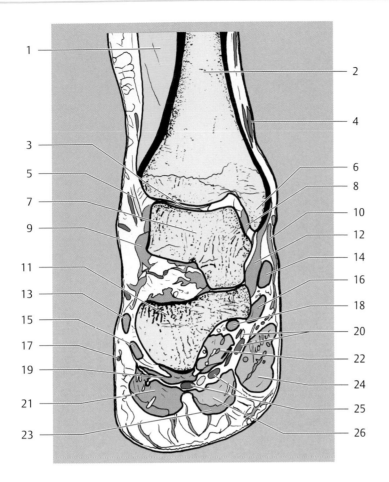

1 Extensor digitorum longus muscle
2 Tibia
3 Talocrural joint (upper ankle joint)
4 Great saphenous vein
5 Dorsal cutaneous nerve
6 Medial malleolus
7 Talus
8 Deltoid ligament
  (posterior tibiotalar part)
9 Anterior talofibular ligament
10 Flexor retinaculum
11 Calcaneus
12 Deltoid ligament (tibiocalcaneal part)
13 Peroneus (fibularis) brevis muscle
  (tendon)
14 Tibialis posterior muscle (tendon)
15 Peroneus (fibularis) longus muscle
  (tendon)
16 Flexor digitorum longus muscle (tendon)
17 Sural nerve with accompanying blood
  vessels
18 Flexor hallucis longus muscle (tendon)
19 Long plantar ligament
20 Medial plantar artery, vein, and nerve
21 Abductor digiti minimi muscle
22 Quadratus plantae muscle
23 Plantar aponeurosis
24 Abductor hallucis muscle
25 Lateral plantar artery, vein, and nerve
26 Flexor digitorum brevis muscle

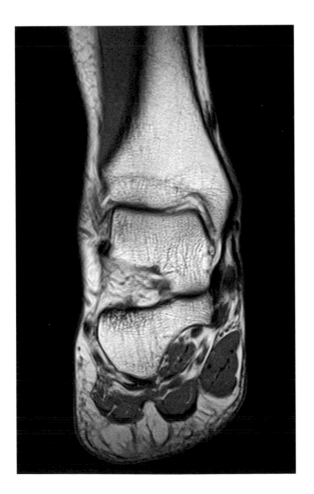

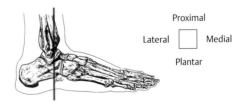

1 Extensor digitorum longus muscle
  (and tendon)
2 Extensor hallucis longus muscle
3 Deep fibular nerve
4 Posterior tibial artery
5 Tibia
6 Great saphenous vein
7 Talus
8 Deltoid ligament (tibiocalcaneal part)
9 Talocalcaneal interosseous ligament
10 Deltoid ligament (tibionavicular part)
11 Calcaneus
12 Tibialis posterior muscle (tendon)
13 Quadratus plantae muscle
14 Plantar calcaneonavicular ligament
   (spring ligament)
15 Peroneus (fibularis) brevis muscle
   (tendon)
16 Flexor digitorum longus muscle (tendon)
17 Peroneus (fibularis) longus muscle
   (tendon)
18 Flexor hallucis longus muscle (tendon)
19 Lateral dorsal cutaneous nerve
20 Abductor hallucis muscle
21 Long plantar ligament
22 Medial plantar artery, vein, and nerve
23 Abductor digiti minimi muscle
24 Lateral plantar artery, vein, and nerve
25 Plantar aponeurosis
26 Flexor digitorum brevis muscle

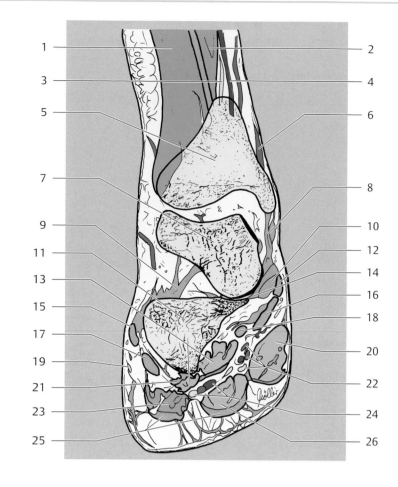

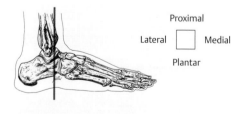

Proximal

Lateral   Medial

Plantar

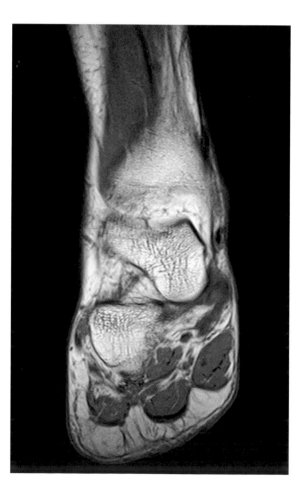

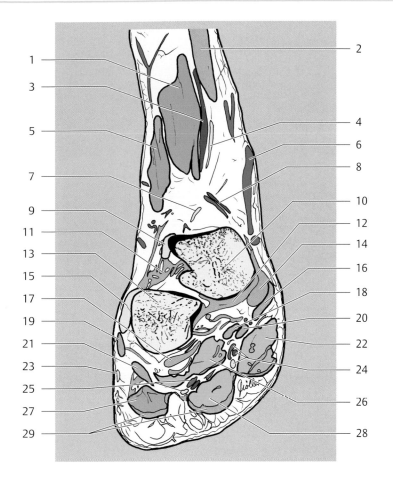

1 Extensor hallucis longus muscle
2 Tibialis anterior muscle (tendon)
3 Anterior tibial artery
4 Deep fibular (peroneal) nerve
5 Extensor digitorum longus muscle
6 Great saphenous vein
7 Deep fibular (peroneal) nerve
   (cutaneous branch)
8 Tarsal artery (medial)
9 Extensor hallucis brevis muscle
   (tendon)
10 Talus
11 Talocalcaneal interosseous ligament
12 Plantar calcaneonavicular ligament
   (spring ligament)
13 Calcaneus
14 Deltoid ligament (tibionavicular part)
15 Extensor digitorum brevis muscle
16 Tibialis posterior muscle (tendon)
17 Long plantar ligament
18 Flexor hallucis longus muscle (tendon)
19 Peroneus (fibularis) brevis muscle
   (tendon)
20 Flexor digitorum longus muscle
   (tendon)
21 Peroneus (fibularis) longus muscle
   (tendon)
22 Abductor hallucis muscle
23 Lateral dorsal cutaneous nerve
24 Medial plantar artery, vein, and nerve
25 Lateral plantar artery, vein, and nerve
26 Quadratus plantae muscle
27 Abductor digiti minimi muscle
28 Flexor digitorum brevis muscle
29 Plantar aponeurosis

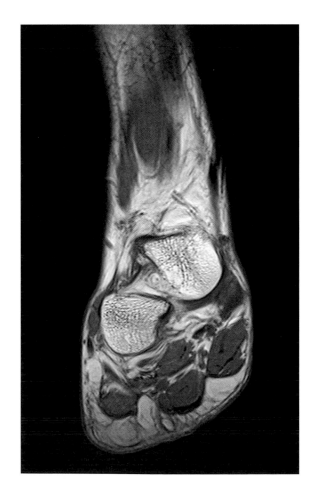

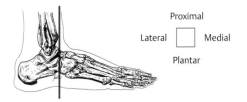

Proximal

Lateral ☐ Medial

Plantar

1 Extensor hallucis longus muscle (tendon)
2 Tibialis anterior muscle (tendon)
3 Extensor digitorum longus muscle (tendon)
4 Anterior tibial artery
5 Deep fibular (peroneal) nerve (medial branch)
6 Deltoid ligament (anterior tibiotalar part)
7 Extensor hallucis brevis muscle
8 Great saphenous vein
9 Deep fibular (peroneal) nerve (lateral branch)
10 Talus
11 Calcaneus and bifurcate ligament
12 Navicular
13 Extensor digitorum brevis muscle
14 Plantar calcaneonavicular ligament (spring ligament)
15 Cuboid
16 Tibialis posterior muscle (tendon)
17 Adductor hallucis muscle (oblique head)
18 Flexor hallucis longus muscle (tendon)
19 Quadratus plantae muscle
20 Flexor digitorum longus muscle (tendon)
21 Peroneus (fibularis) brevis muscle (tendon)
22 Abductor hallucis muscle
23 Peroneus (fibularis) longus muscle (tendon)
24 Medial plantar artery, vein, and nerve
25 Lateral dorsal cutaneous nerve
26 Long plantar ligament
27 Abductor digiti minimi muscle
28 Lateral plantar artery, vein, and nerve
29 Plantar aponeurosis
30 Flexor digitorum brevis muscle

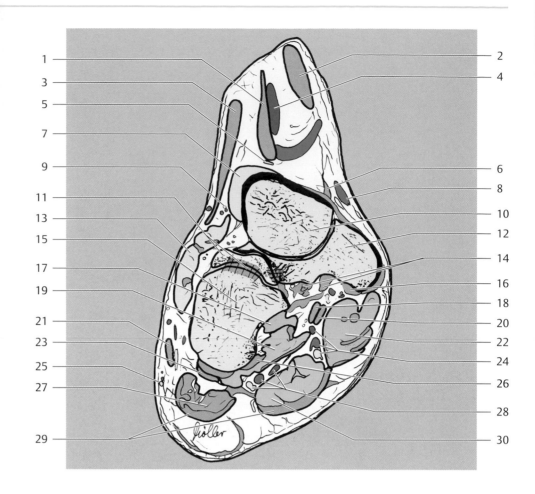

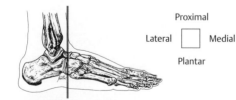

Proximal

Lateral ☐ Medial

Plantar

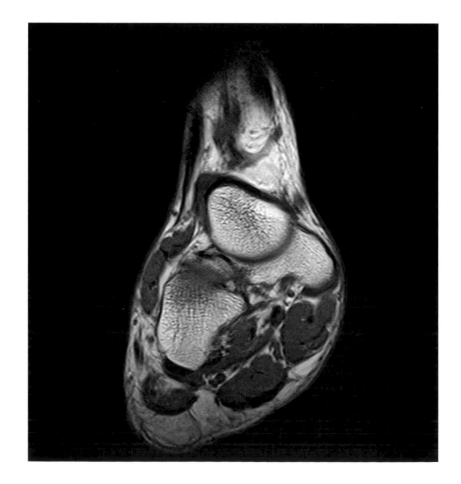

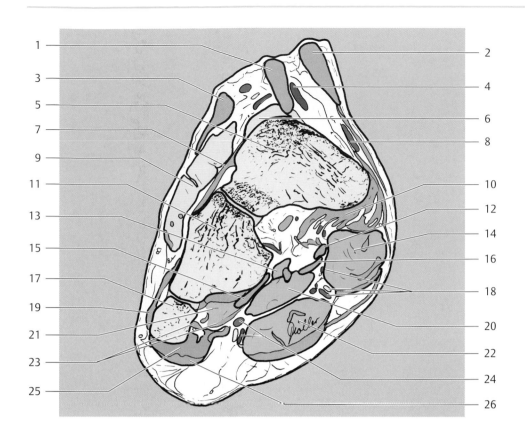

1 Extensor hallucis longus muscle (tendon)
2 Tibialis anterior muscle (tendon)
3 Extensor digitorum longus muscle (tendon)
4 Anterior tibial artery
5 Navicular
6 Extensor hallucis brevis muscle
7 Dorsal tarsal ligaments
8 Great saphenous vein
9 Extensor digitorum brevis muscle
10 Tibialis posterior muscle (tendon)
11 Cuboid
12 Flexor hallucis longus muscle (tendon)
13 Adductor hallucis muscle (oblique head)
14 Abductor hallucis muscle
15 Peroneus (fibularis) longus muscle (tendon)
16 Flexor digitorum longus muscle (tendon)
17 Metatarsal V (base)
18 Medial plantar artery, vein, and nerve
19 Peroneus (fibularis) brevis muscle (tendon)
20 Quadratus plantae muscle
21 Plantar interossei muscles
22 Flexor digitorum brevis muscle
23 Long plantar ligament
24 Lateral plantar artery, vein, and nerve
25 Abductor digiti minimi muscle
26 Plantar aponeurosis

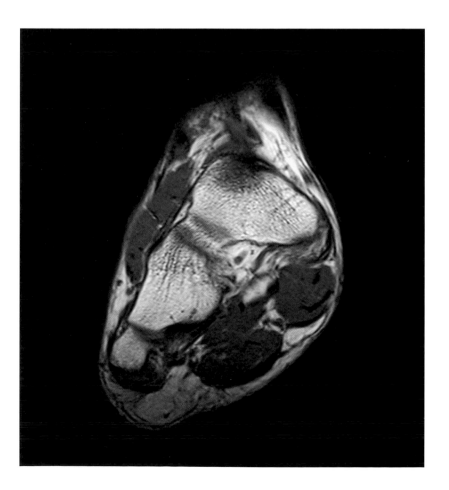

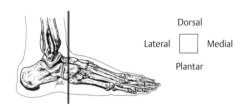

Dorsal

Lateral Medial

Plantar

1 Extensor hallucis longus muscle (tendon)
2 Anterior tibial artery
3 Extensor hallucis brevis muscle (tendon)
4 Tibialis anterior muscle (tendon)
5 Extensor digitorum longus muscle (tendon)
6 Intermediate cuneiform
7 Extensor digitorum brevis muscle
8 Great saphenous vein
9 Deep fibular (peroneal) nerve (lateral branch)
10 Medial cuneiform
11 Lateral cuneiform
12 Tibialis posterior muscle (tendon attachment)
13 Dorsal tarsal ligaments
14 Lateral plantar nerve (deep branch)
15 Cuboid
16 Abductor hallucis muscle
17 Metatarsal IV (base)
18 Medial plantar septum
19 Peroneus (fibularis) longus muscle (tendon)
20 Adductor hallucis muscle (oblique head) and deep plantar arch
21 Long plantar ligament
22 Flexor hallucis longus muscle (tendon)
23 Quadratus plantae muscle
24 Flexor hallucis brevis muscle
25 Metatarsal V (base)
26 Medial plantar artery, vein, and nerve
27 Plantar interossei muscles
28 Flexor digitorum longus muscle (tendon)
29 Flexor digiti minimi brevis muscle
30 Flexor digitorum brevis muscle
31 Abductor digiti minimi muscle
32 Lateral plantar artery, vein, and nerve
33 Plantar aponeurosis

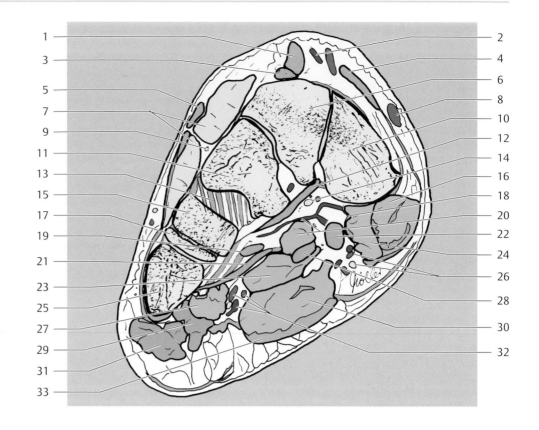

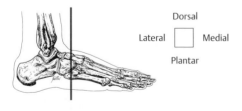

Dorsal

Lateral ☐ Medial

Plantar

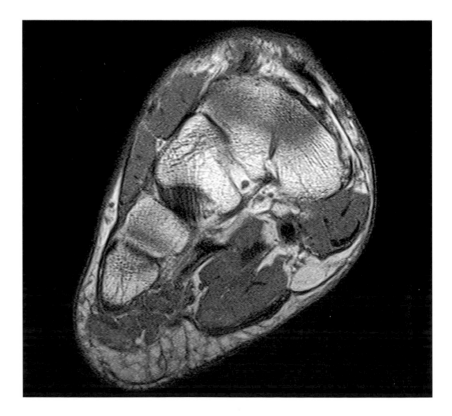

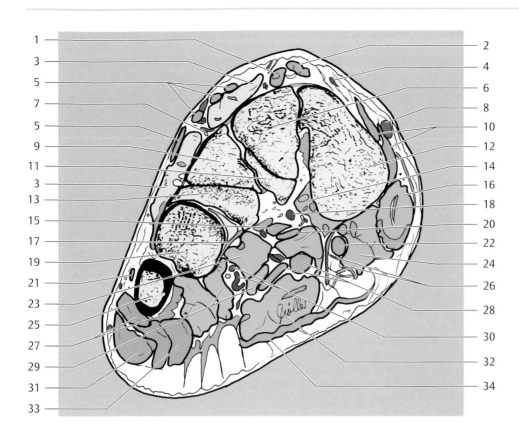

1 Extensor hallucis brevis muscle
   (tendon)
2 Extensor hallucis longus muscle
   (tendon)
3 Extensor digitorum brevis muscle
4 Anterior tibial artery
5 Extensor digitorum longus muscle
   (tendons)
6 Intermediate cuneiform
7 Deep fibular (peroneal) nerve
   (lateral branch)
8 Great saphenous vein
9 Lateral cuneiform
10 Tibialis anterior muscle (tendon)
11 Metatarsal II (base)
12 Medial cuneiform
13 Metatarsal III (base)
14 Flexor hallucis brevis muscle
   (lateral head)
15 Peroneus (fibularis) longus muscle
   (tendon)
16 Abductor hallucis muscle
17 Long plantar ligament
18 Deep plantar arch
19 Metatarsal IV (base)
20 Adductor hallucis muscle
   (oblique head and tendon)
21 Extensor digiti minimi brevis muscle
   (tendon)
22 Flexor hallucis longus muscle (tendon)
23 Flexor hallucis brevis muscle (lateral
   head)
24 Flexor hallucis brevis muscle
   (medial head)
25 Metatarsal V (base)
26 Medial plantar artery, vein, and nerve
   (superficial branch)
27 Opponens digiti minimi muscle
28 Flexor digitorum longus muscle (tendon)
29 Plantar interossei muscles
30 Lateral plantar artery, vein, and nerve
31 Abductor digiti minimi muscle
32 Flexor digitorum brevis muscle
33 Flexor digiti minimi brevis muscle
34 Plantar aponeurosis

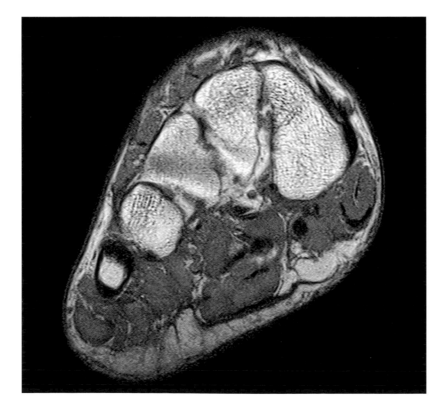

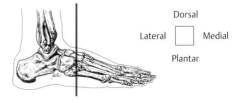

Dorsal

Lateral ☐ Medial

Plantar

1 Extensor hallucis brevis muscle (tendon)
2 Extensor hallucis longus muscle (tendon)
3 Metatarsal II (base)
4 Metatarsal I (base)
5 Extensor digitorum longus muscle (tendons)
6 Metatarsal III (base)
7 Extensor digitorum brevis muscle (tendons)
8 Plantar metatarsal arteries
9 Plantar interossei muscles
10 Perforating vein (of first dorsal interosseous muscle)
11 Extensor digiti minimi brevis muscle (tendon)
12 Peroneus (fibularis) longus muscle (attachment)
13 Lateral plantar nerve (deep branch) and plantar metatarsal arteries
14 Abductor hallucis muscle
15 Metatarsal V (base)
16 Flexor hallucis brevis muscle (lateral head)
17 Opponens digiti minimi muscle
18 Adductor hallucis muscle (oblique head)
19 Flexor digiti minimi brevis muscle
20 Flexor hallucis longus muscle (tendon)
21 Abductor digiti minimi muscle
22 Flexor digitorum longus muscle (and tendons)
23 Proper plantar digital artery, vein, and nerve
24 Plantar aponeurosis
25 Flexor digitorum brevis muscle (and tendons)

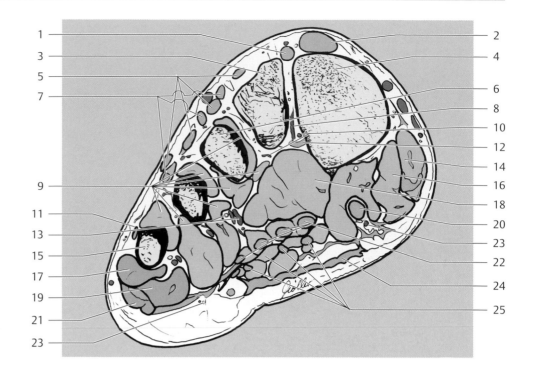

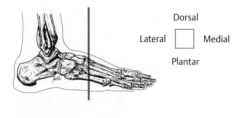

Dorsal

Lateral Medial

Plantar

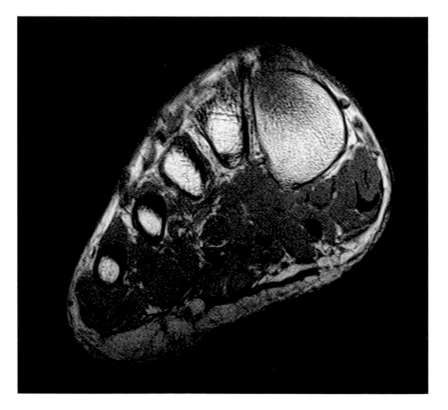

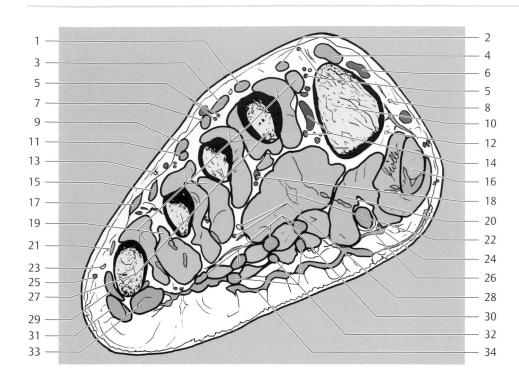

1 Extensor digitorum longus II muscle (tendon)
2 Extensor hallucis brevis muscle (tendon)
3 Extensor digitorum brevis II muscle (tendon)
4 Extensor hallucis longus muscle (tendon)
5 Dorsal metatarsal arteries and veins
6 Dorsal venous arch of foot
7 Extensor digitorum longus III muscle (tendon)
8 Dorsal digital nerve I
9 Extensor digitorum longus IV muscle (tendon)
10 Metatarsal I (base)
11 Extensor digitorum brevis III muscle (tendon)
12 Plantar digital nerve I
13 Dorsal digital nerve of foot
14 Plantar metatarsal artery and vein (deep branch of dorsal interosseous I muscle)
15 Extensor digitorum brevis IV muscle (tendon)
16 Abductor hallucis muscle
17 Extensor digitorum longus V muscle (tendon)
18 Plantar metatarsal arteries and veins
19 Dorsal and plantar interossei muscles
20 Flexor hallucis brevis muscle (lateral head)
21 Extensor digitorum brevis V muscle (tendon)
22 Adductor hallucis muscle (oblique head)
23 Dorsal digital cutaneous nerve of foot
24 Plantar digital artery and vein proper and proper plantar digital nerve
25 Small saphenous vein (branch)
26 Flexor hallucis longus muscle (tendon)
27 Metatarsals II–V
28 Lateral plantar nerve (deep branch) and plantar metatarsal arteries
29 Opponens digiti minimi muscle
30 Flexor digitorum longus muscle (and tendons)
31 Abductor digiti minimi muscle (and tendon)
32 Flexor digitorum brevis muscle (and tendons)
33 Extensor digiti minimi brevis muscle
34 Plantar aponeurosis

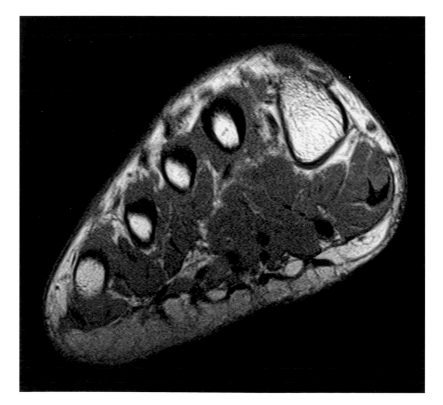

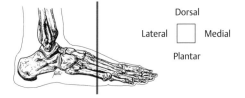

Dorsal

Lateral ☐ Medial

Plantar

1 Extensor digitorum longus muscle II (tendon)
2 Dorsal venous arch of foot
3 Extensor digitorum brevis muscle II (tendon)
4 Extensor hallucis longus muscle (tendon)
5 Extensor digitorum longus muscle III (tendon)
6 Extensor hallucis brevis muscle (tendon)
7 Extensor digitorum brevis muscle III (tendon)
8 Dorsal metatarsal arteries and veins
9 Extensor digitorum brevis muscle IV (tendon)
10 Metatarsal I
11 Extensor digitorum brevis muscle IV (tendon)
12 Plantar metatarsal artery and vein (perforating branch of first dorsal interosseous muscle)
13 Extensor digitorum longus muscle V (tendons)
14 Abductor hallucis muscle
15 Extensor digitorum brevis muscle V (tendon)
16 Proper plantar digital arteries, veins, and nerve
17 Dorsal digital cutaneous nerve of foot
18 Adductor hallucis muscle (oblique head)
19 Small saphenous vein
20 Flexor hallucis brevis muscle (lateral head)
21 Metatarsals
22 Flexor hallucis longus muscle (tendon)
23 Dorsal and plantar interossei muscles
24 Lateral plantar nerve (deep branch) and plantar metatarsal arteries
25 Abductor digiti minimi muscle (attachment)
26 Flexor digitorum longus and brevis muscles (tendons)
27 Extensor digiti minimi brevis muscle (tendon)
28 Adductor hallucis muscle (transverse head)

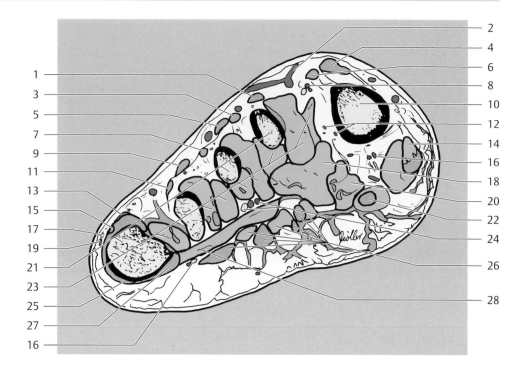

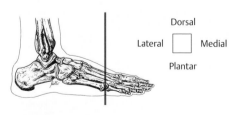

Dorsal

Lateral ☐ Medial

Plantar

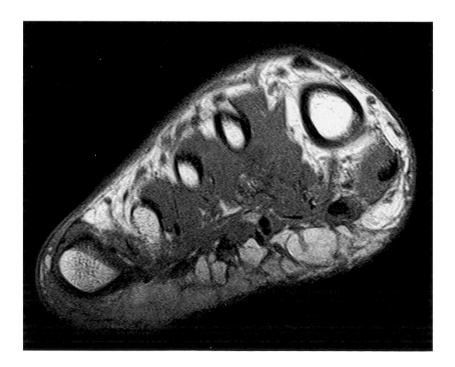

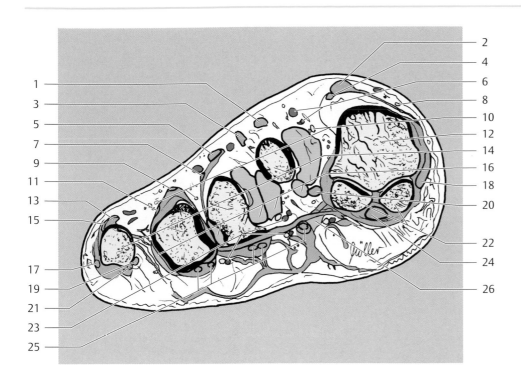

1 Extensor digitorum longus II muscle (tendon)
2 Extensor hallucis longus muscle (tendon)
3 Extensor digitorum brevis II muscle (tendon)
4 Extensor hallucis brevis muscle (tendon)
5 Extensor digitorum longus III muscle (tendon)
6 Dorsal metatarsal arteries and veins
7 Extensor digitorum brevis III muscle (tendon)
8 Medial dorsal cutaneous nerve I
9 Extensor digitorum longus IV muscle (tendon)
10 Dorsal digital nerves of foot
11 Extensor digitorum brevis IV muscle (tendon)
12 Metatarsal I (head)
13 Extensor digiti minimi longus muscle (tendon)
14 Metatarsals II–V
15 Extensor digiti minimi brevis muscle (tendon)
16 Dorsal and plantar interossei muscles
17 Abductor digiti minimi muscle (tendon attachment)
18 Abductor hallucis muscle (tendon)
19 Flexor digiti minimi longus muscle (tendon)
20 Adductor hallucis muscle (tendon)
21 Flexor digiti minimi brevis muscle (tendon)
22 Sesamoid bones
23 Plantar digital artery and vein proper and proper plantar digital nerve
24 Flexor hallucis longus muscle (tendon)
25 Flexor digitorum longus and brevis muscles (tendons)
26 Adductor hallucis muscle (transverse head)

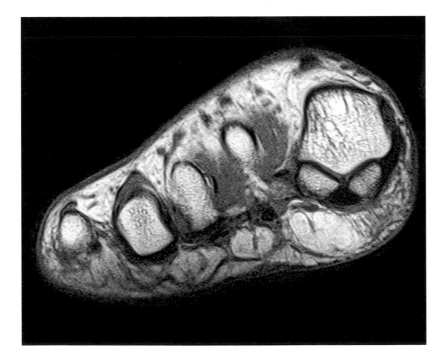

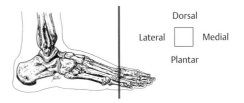

Dorsal

Lateral ☐ Medial

Plantar

1 Extensor digitorum longus II muscle (tendon)
2 Joint capsule
3 Extensor digitorum brevis II muscle (tendon)
4 Extensor hallucis brevis muscle (tendon)
5 Dorsal digital nerves of foot
6 Extensor hallucis longus muscle (tendon)
7 Extensor digitorum longus III muscle (tendon)
8 Metatarsal I (head)
9 Extensor digitorum brevis III muscle (tendon)
10 Collateral ligament
11 Dorsal metatarsal arteries and veins
12 Abductor hallucis muscle (tendon)
13 Extensor digitorum longus IV muscle (tendon)
14 Sesamoid ligaments
15 Extensor digitorum brevis IV muscle (tendon)
16 Adductor hallucis muscle (tendon)
17 Abductor digiti minimi muscle (tendon attachment)
18 Flexor hallucis longus muscle (tendon)
19 Proximal phalanx V
20 Plantar digital artery and vein proper and proper plantar digital nerve
21 Metatarsals II–IV (heads)
22 Plantar ligaments
23 Flexor digiti minimi brevis muscle (tendon)
24 Flexor digitorum longus muscle (tendon)
25 Flexor digiti minimi longus muscle (tendon)
26 Flexor digitorum brevis (tendon)
27 Plantar interossei muscles (tendons)
28 Deep transverse metatarsal ligament

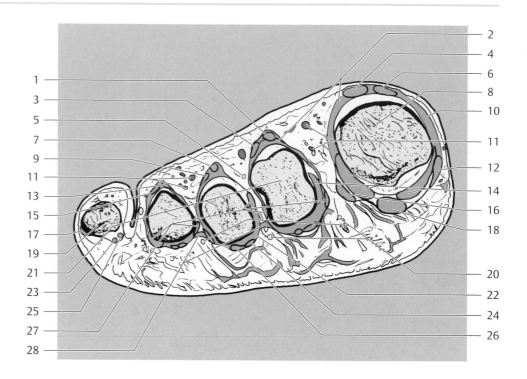

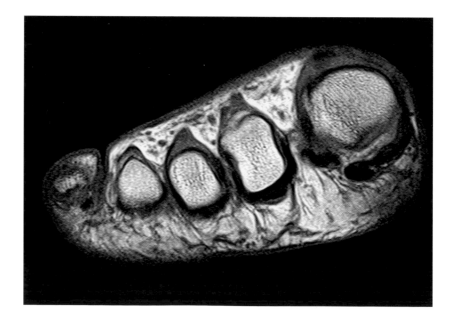

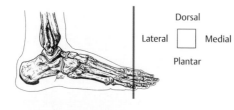

Dorsal

Lateral ▢ Medial

Plantar

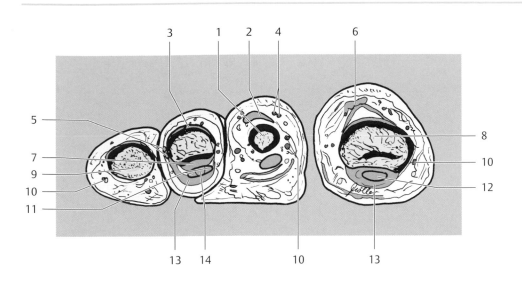

1 Proximal phalanx II
2 Extensor digitorum II muscle (aponeurosis)
3 Extensor digitorum III muscle (aponeurosis)
4 Dorsal digital artery, vein, and nerve of foot
5 Collateral ligament
6 Extensor hallucis muscle (aponeurosis)
7 Mesotendon
8 Proximal phalanx I
9 Proximal interphalangeal joint IV
10 Plantar digital artery and vein proper and proper plantar digital nerve
11 Flexor digitorum longus muscle (tendon)
12 Flexor hallucis longus muscle (tendon)
13 Synovial sheath and joint capsule with capsule ligaments
14 Flexor digitorum brevis muscle (tendon)

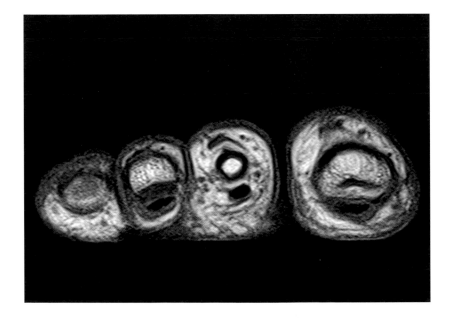

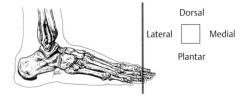

Dorsal
Lateral   Medial
Plantar

1 Dorsal metatarsal ligaments
2 Distal phalanx IV
3 Dorsal interosseous muscle
4 Distal interphalangeal joint IV
5 Metatarsal III (base)
6 Middle phalanx IV
7 Lateral cuneiform
8 Proximal interphalangeal joint IV
9 Cuneocuboid interosseous ligament
10 Proximal phalanx IV
11 Extensor digitorum brevis muscle
12 Metatarsophalangeal joint IV
13 Cuboid
14 Flexor digitorum longus muscle
   (tendon)
15 Bifurcate ligament
16 Extensor digitorum muscle (tendon)
17 Calcaneocuboid joint
18 Plantar interosseous muscle
19 Calcaneus
20 Metatarsal IV
21 Extensor digitorum longus muscle
22 Flexor digiti minimi brevis muscle
23 Anterior lateral malleolar artery
24 Tarsometatarsal joint IV
25 Fibula
26 Metatarsal V (base)
27 Peroneus (fibularis) brevis muscle
   (tendon)
28 Lateral plantar artery, vein, and nerve
29 Calcaneofibular ligament
30 Abductor digiti minimi muscle (foot)
31 Peroneus (fibularis) longus muscle
   (tendon)

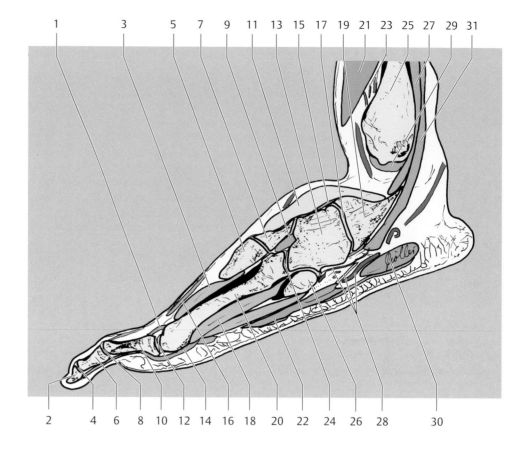

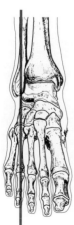

Proximal
Dorsal

Anterior ☐ Posterior

Distal
Plantar

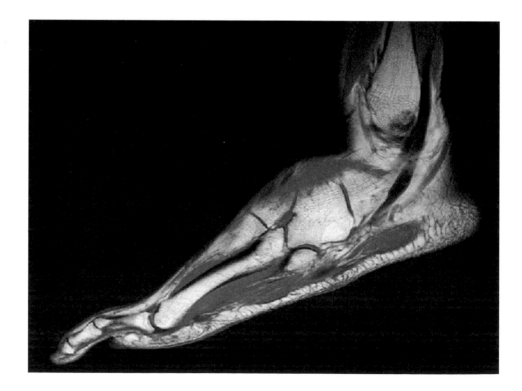

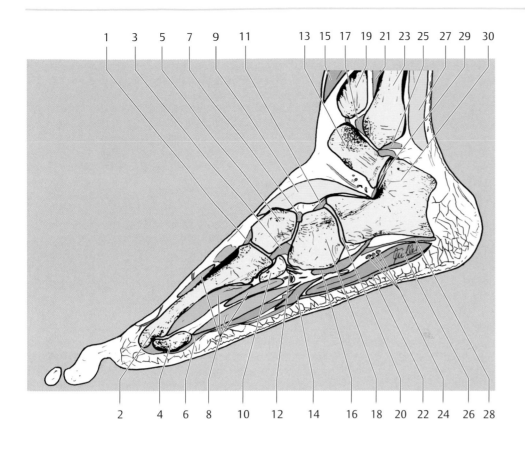

1 Dorsal metatarsal ligaments
2 Metatarsal III
3 Cuneocuboid interosseous ligament
4 Metatarsal IV (head)
5 Lateral cuneiform
6 Flexor digitorum longus muscle
7 Dorsal tarsal ligaments
8 Dorsal and plantar interossei muscles
9 Extensor digitorum brevis muscle
10 Metatarsal IV (base)
11 Bifurcate ligament
12 Deep plantar arch
13 Talus
14 Flexor digiti minimi brevis muscle
15 Extensor digitorum longus muscle
16 Peroneus (fibularis) longus muscle (tendon)
17 Anterior talofibular ligament
18 Cuboid
19 Tibia
20 Calcaneocuboid joint
21 Tibiofibular syndesmosis (anterior tibiofibular ligament)
22 Plantar aponeurosis
23 Fibula
24 Lateral plantar artery, vein, and nerve
25 Posterior talofibular ligament
26 Abductor digiti minimi muscle (foot)
27 Peroneus (fibularis) brevis muscle
28 Long plantar ligament
29 Subtalar joint
30 Calcaneus

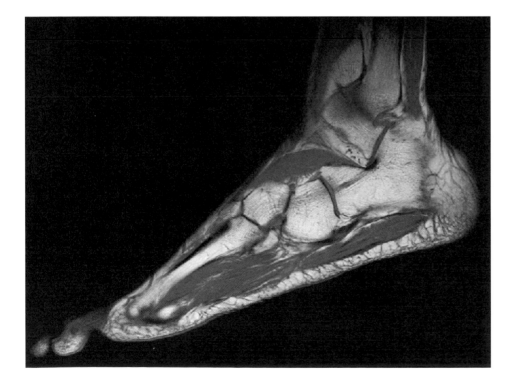

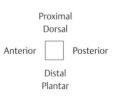

Proximal
Dorsal
Anterior ☐ Posterior
Distal
Plantar

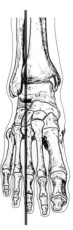

1 Interossei muscles
2 Distal phalanx III
3 Metatarsal II (base)
4 Distal interphalangeal joint III
5 Metatarsal III (base)
6 Middle phalanx III
7 Intermediate cuneiform
8 Proximal interphalangeal joint III (PIP)
9 Lateral cuneiform
10 Extensor digiti III muscle (tendon)
11 Extensor digitorum brevis muscle
12 Proximal phalanx III
13 Calcaneocuboid joint
14 Metatarsophalangeal joint III
15 Lateral tarsal artery
16 Flexor digitorum longus muscle (tendon)
17 Talocalcaneal interosseous ligament
18 Metatarsal III (head)
19 Talus
20 Lumbrical muscle
21 Extensor digitorum longus muscle
22 Flexor digitorum longus muscle (tendon)
23 Dorsalis pedis artery
24 Adductor hallucis muscle (oblique head)
25 Tibia
26 Deep plantar arch
27 Talocrural joint
28 Peroneus (fibularis) longus muscle (tendon)
29 Subtalar joint (posterior inferior ankle joint)
30 Cuboid
31 Posterior talofibular ligament
32 Lateral plantar artery, vein, and nerve
33 Flexor hallucis longus muscle
34 Long plantar ligament
35 Peroneus (fibularis) brevis muscle
36 Plantar aponeurosis
37 Small saphenous vein
38 Abductor digiti minimi muscle
39 Calcaneus

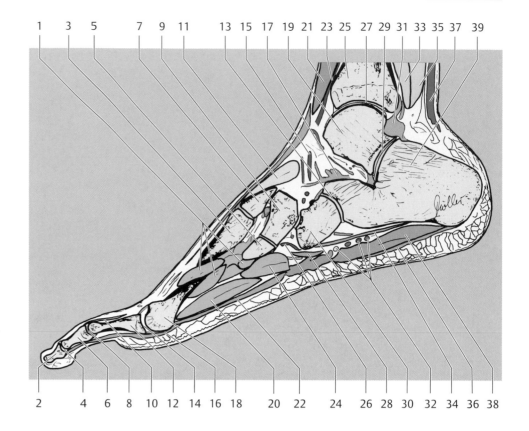

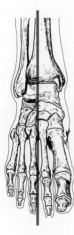

Proximal
Dorsal

Anterior   Posterior

Distal
Plantar

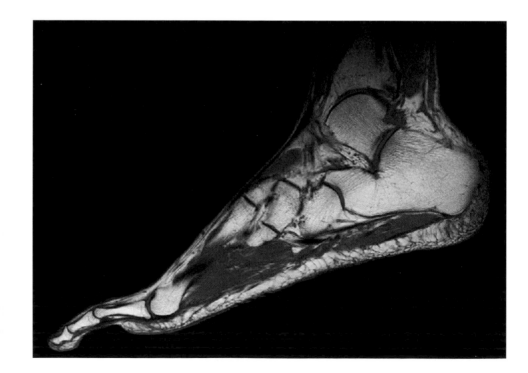

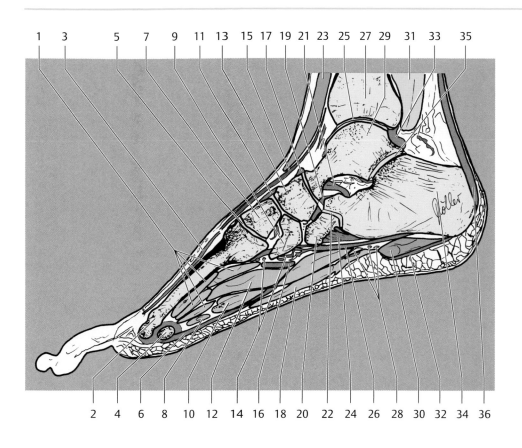

1 3   5   7   9   11 13 15 17 19 21 23 25 27 29 31 33   35

2   4   6   8   10   12   14   16   18   20   22   24   26   28   30   32   34   36

1 Plantar interossei muscles
2 Metatarsal II
3 Extensor digiti II muscle (tendon)
4 Metatarsal II (head)
5 Tarsometatarsal joint II
6 Flexor digitorum longus muscle (tendon)
7 Intermediate cuneiform
8 Adductor hallucis muscle (transverse head)
9 Lateral cuneiform
10 Lumbrical muscle
11 Dorsal tarsal ligaments
12 Adductor hallucis muscle (oblique head)
13 Navicular
14 Deep plantar arch
15 Dorsalis pedis artery
16 Peroneus (fibularis) longus muscle (tendon)
17 Dorsal talonavicular ligament
18 Flexor digitorum brevis muscle
19 Bifurcate ligament
20 Cuboid
21 Talocalcaneal interosseous ligament
22 Calcaneocuboid joint
23 Extensor digitorum longus muscle
24 Plantar calcaneonavicular ligament (spring ligament)
25 Talocrural joint
26 Long plantar ligament
27 Tibia
28 Lateral plantar artery, vein, and nerve
29 Talus
30 Abductor digiti minimi muscle
31 Flexor hallucis longus muscle
32 Plantar aponeurosis
33 Posterior talofibular ligament
34 Calcaneus
35 Subtalar joint
36 Calcaneal (Achilles) tendon

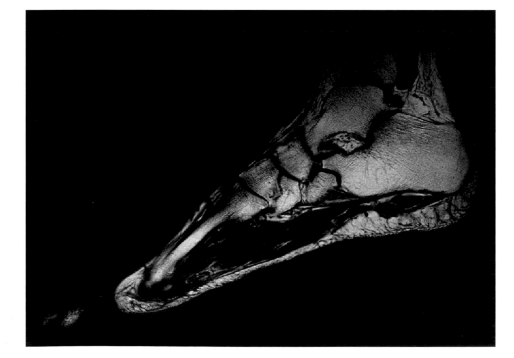

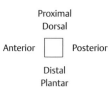

Proximal
Dorsal

Anterior ☐ Posterior

Distal
Plantar

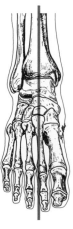

1 Dorsal and plantar interossei muscles
2 Proximal, middle, and distal phalanges II
3 Metatarsal I (base)
4 Extensor digitorum muscle (tendon)
5 Cuneonavicular joint
6 Metatarsal II (head)
7 Navicular
8 Adductor hallucis muscle (transverse head)
9 Talonavicular joint
10 Flexor digitorum longus muscle (tendon)
11 Talonavicular ligament
12 Adductor hallucis muscle (oblique head)
13 Medial tarsal artery
14 Medial cuneiform
15 Talocalcaneal interosseous ligament
16 Intermediate cuneiform
17 Anterior medial malleolar artery
18 Peroneus (fibularis) longus muscle (tendon)
19 Talus
20 Deep plantar arch
21 Extensor hallucis longus muscle (tendon)
22 Quadratus plantae muscle
23 Tibia
24 Plantar calcaneonavicular ligament (spring ligament)
25 Talocrural joint
26 Flexor digitorum brevis muscle
27 Tibialis posterior muscle
28 Plantar aponeurosis
29 Flexor hallucis longus muscle
30 Lateral plantar artery, vein, and nerve
31 Posterior talofibular ligament
32 Abductor digiti minimi muscle
33 Calcaneal (Achilles) tendon
34 Subtalar joint
35 Pre-Achilles fat pad
36 Calcaneus

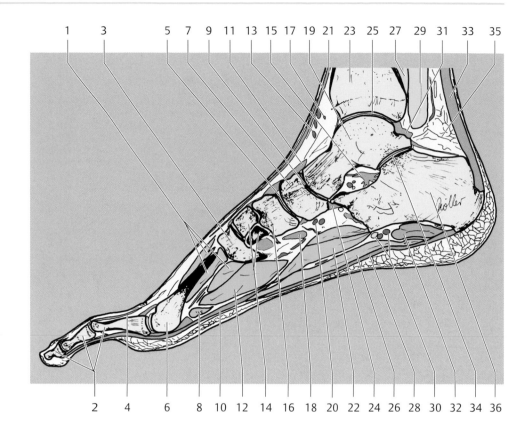

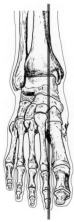

Proximal
Dorsal

Anterior ☐ Posterior

Distal
Plantar

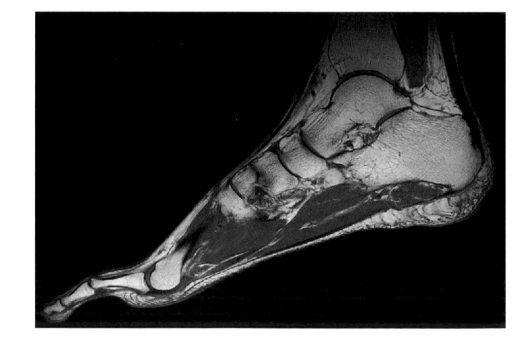

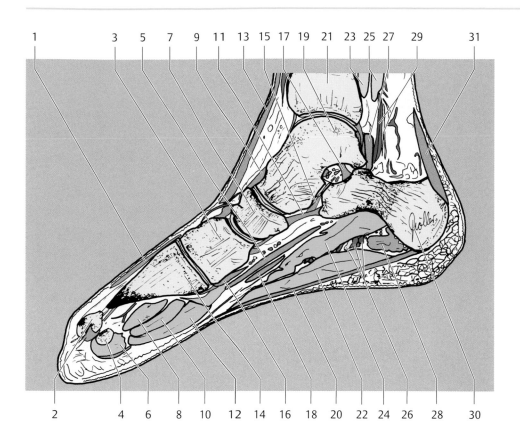

1 Extensor hallucis longus muscle (tendon)
2 Metatarsal I (head)
3 Medial cuneiform
4 Lateral sesamoid
5 Flexor hallucis longus muscle (tendon)
6 Lumbrical muscles
7 Navicular
8 Plantar interosseous muscle
9 Dorsal talonavicular ligament
10 Abductor hallucis muscle (oblique head)
11 Plantar calcaneonavicular ligament (spring ligament)
12 Adductor hallucis muscle (oblique head)
13 Tibialis anterior muscle (tendon)
14 Metatarsal I (base)
15 Plantar talonavicular ligament
16 Peroneus (fibularis) longus muscle (tendon attachment)
17 Talocalcaneal interosseous ligament
18 Flexor digitorum longus muscle (tendon)
19 Talus
20 Plantar aponeurosis
21 Tibia
22 Flexor digitorum brevis muscle
23 Tibialis posterior muscle
24 Quadratus plantae muscle
25 Flexor hallucis longus muscle
26 Lateral plantar artery, vein, and nerve
27 Posterior talofibular ligament
28 Abductor digiti minimi muscle
29 Medial plantar artery, vein, and nerve
30 Calcaneus (tuberosity)
31 Calcaneal (Achilles) tendon

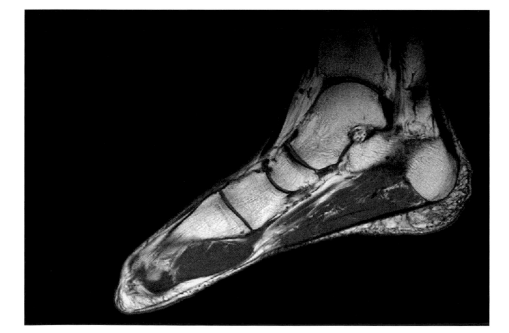

Proximal
Dorsal

Anterior ☐ Posterior

Distal
Plantar

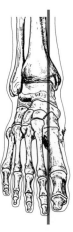

1 Extensor hallucis longus muscle (tendon)
2 Distal phalanx I
3 Metatarsal I
4 Proximal phalanx I
5 Medial cuneiform
6 Sesamoid bone
7 Tibialis anterior muscle
8 Flexor hallucis brevis muscle (lateral head)
9 Navicular
10 Plantar aponeurosis
11 Talonavicular ligament
12 Flexor hallucis longus muscle (tendon)
13 Calcaneus
14 Flexor hallucis brevis muscle (medial head)
15 Talus
16 Tibialis posterior muscle (tendon)
17 Tibia
18 Plantar calcaneonavicular ligament (spring ligament)
19 Tibialis posterior muscle
20 Medial plantar artery, vein, and nerve
21 Flexor digitorum longus muscle (tendon)
22 Lateral plantar artery, vein, and nerve
23 Deltoid ligament (posterior tibiotalar part)
24 Abductor hallucis muscle
25 Flexor hallucis longus muscle (tendon)
26 Quadratus plantae muscle
27 Flexor digitorum longus muscle (tendon)
28 Plantar aponeurosis (calcaneal attachment)
29 Calcaneal anastomosis
30 Calcaneus (tuberosity)
31 Calcaneal (Achilles) tendon

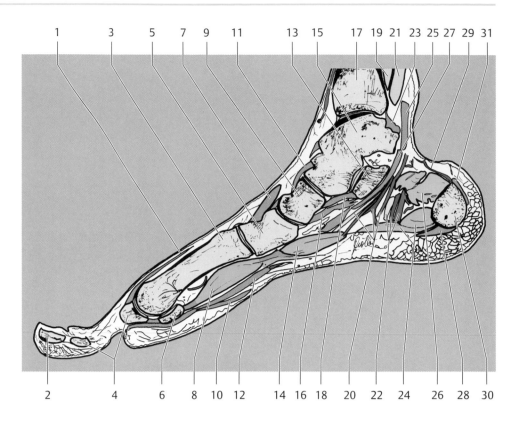

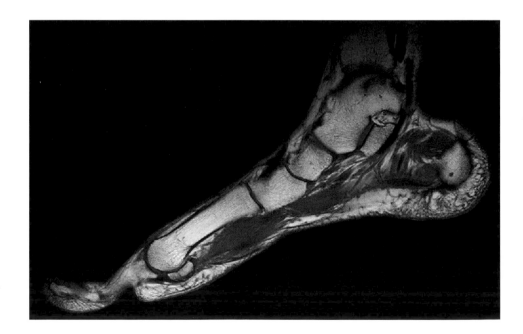

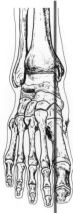

Proximal
Dorsal

Anterior ☐ Posterior

Distal
Plantar

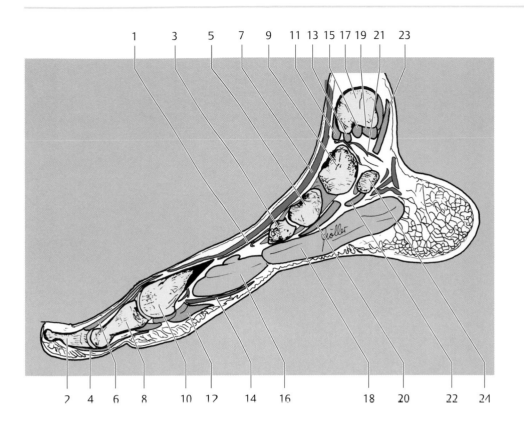

1 Medial tarsal arteries
2 Distal phalanx I
3 Medial cuneiform
4 Flexor hallucis longus muscle (tendon)
5 Navicular
6 Extensor hallucis longus muscle (tendon)
7 Dorsalis pedis vein (to great saphenous vein)
8 Proximal phalanx I
9 Talus
10 Metatarsal I (head)
11 Deltoid ligament (anterior tibiotalar part)
12 Plantar aponeurosis
13 Deltoid ligament (tibionavicular part)
14 Medial plantar artery and nerve (superficial branch)
15 Deltoid ligament (tibiocalcaneal part)
16 Flexor hallucis brevis muscle
17 Tibia (medial malleolus)
18 Abductor hallucis muscle
19 Deltoid ligament (posterior tibiotalar part)
20 Tibialis posterior muscle (tendon)
21 Posterior tibial artery (medial malleolar branches)
22 Flexor hallucis longus muscle (tendon)
23 Flexor digitorum longus muscle (tendon)
24 Calcaneus

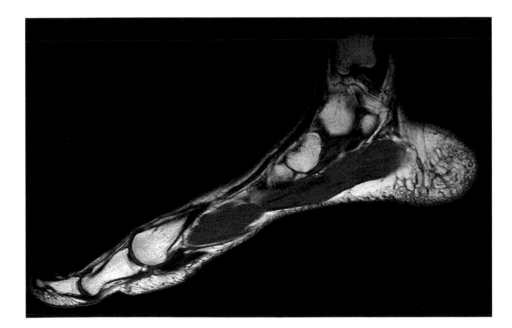

Proximal
Dorsal

Anterior   Posterior

Distal
Plantar

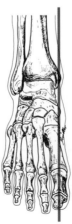

Index

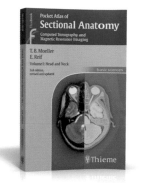
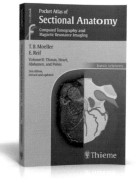
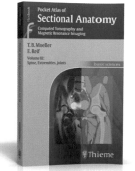
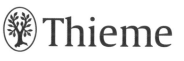

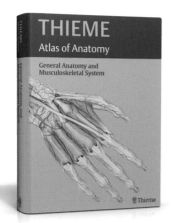
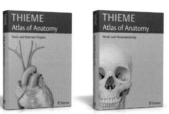
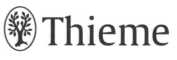
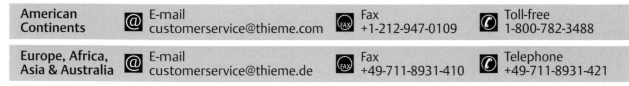